Control and Automation in Anaesthesia

Springer
Berlin
Heidelberg
New York
Barcelona
Budapest
Hong Kong
London
Milan
Paris
Tokyo

H. Schwilden   H. Stoeckel (Eds.)

Control and Automation
in Anaesthesia

With 106 Figures and 24 Tables

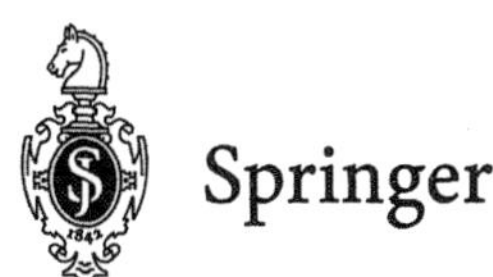

Springer

Professor Dr.Dr.med. H. Schwilden
Professor Dr.med. Dr.med. h.c. Stoeckel
Universität Bonn
Klinik und Poliklinik
für Anästhesiologie
und spezielle Intensivmedizin
Sigmund-Freud-Str. 25
53105 Bonn, Germany

ISBN-13:978-3-642-79575-6   e-ISBN-13:978-3-642-79573-2
DOI: 10.1007/978-3-642-79573-2

Library of Congress Cataloging-in-Publication Data. Control and automation in anesthesia/[edited
by] H. Schwilden, H. Stoeckel. p. cm. Includes bibliographical references and index.
ISBN-13:978-3-642-79575-6   1. Anesthesia – Data processing – Congresses.
2. Anesthetics – Administration – Automatic control – Congresses. 3. Patient monitoring – Data
processing – Congresses. I. Schwilden, Helmut. II. Stoeckel, Horst, 1930– .
[DNLM: 1. Anesthesia – congresses. 2. Monitoring, Physiologic methods – congresses.
3. Signal Processing, Computer-Assisted – congresses. 4. Drug Delivery Systems –
congresses. 5. Automatic Data Processing – congresses. WO 200 C764 1995] RD80.95.C66
1995 617.9′6′0285 – dc20 DNLM/DLC for Library of Congress 95-1211

Typesetting: Best-set Typesetter Ltd., Hong Kong

SPIN: 10492356   19/3130/SPS – 5 4 3 2 1 0 – Printed on acid-free paper

Preface

This book records the presentations given at a workshop held in Bonn in May 1994. The aim of the meeting was to bring together scientists from various disciplines and clinicians to discuss within a group of experts the theoretical, medical, engineering, and regulatory aspects of automated control of therapeutic interventions in anaesthesiology.

The meeting was considered a continuation of a preceding workshop on "Quantitation, Modelling and Control in Anaesthesia" [1], which was held also in Bonn 10 years ago in May 1984. That workshop dealt with problems of how to quantitate concepts like anaesthetic depth, how to model anaesthetic drug disposition, how to link pharmacokinetics and pharmacodynamics, and how to use such concepts for the control of anaesthetic drug delivery. With respect to these topics the current proceedings have simultaneously both a broadened and a narrowed perspective. It is broadened in so far as the topics of the workshop did not focus exclusively on anaesthetic drugs and the control of their delivery, but did also discuss anaesthesia machine monitoring and patients therapeutic monitoring as well as control of blood pressure and artificial ventilation. The proceedings have narrowed the perspective insofar as they do not intensively discuss the processes of quantitation and modelling but presuppose them and give more room to control, especially automated control.

During the past 10 years informatics has tremendously expanded its knowledge and methods applicable to control problems. Of special interest to medicine and anaesthesiology are the developments of fuzzy logic and neuronal networks. Fuzzy logic may represent the right formalism to "calculate" with fuzzy variables as are common in a clinical setting and to support decision making under uncertainty. Neuronal networks represent an intensively investigated type of synthetic objects which have the ability to learn. They have been successfully applied to quite a number of control problems. With respect to the management of anaesthesia, this methodology seems to be espe-

---

1. Stoeckel H (ed) (1985) Quantitation, modelling and control in anaesthesia. Thieme, Stuttgart

cially suited for the automated control of multiple input-multiple output systems, such as the simultaneous infusions of different agents controlling, for instance, simultaneously antinociception, vigilance, haemodynamic quantities and muscle relaxation. The organizers of the meeting had the impression that these two topics in conjunction with artificial intelligence and expert systems will be the very methodology in designing future automated control systems. It was, therefore, decided to review these methodologies at the beginning of the meeting.

By definition, control requires the measurement or estimation of at least one quantity or variable which should be controlled. Such quantity is in general only a surrogate variable of the underlying process to be controlled. Instead of the EEG, the anaesthesiologists actually would like to control anaesthetic depth; instead of endtidal CO_2, he would like to control adequate artificial ventilation; and instead of monitoring the EMG for the abductor pollicis longus, he would like to control the muscle relaxation of the patient. Hence the evaluation and the assessment of the measured signal with respect to the actual process one would like to control is of special importance and provokes the essential question as to what can and what should be monitored for the control of what process. This question is discussed with respect to the anaesthesia machine as well as with respect to a patient's anaesthetic therapy.

The various modes and approaches to the control and automation of artificial ventilation and the control and automation of i.v. and inhalational anaesthetic drug delivery are presented and discussed in detail in Parts III–IV. As automatically controlled systems are entering clinical practice, the non-medical and non-engineering aspects of automated control, namely the liability and the requirements with respect to technical, regulatory, manufacturer's and even ethical points of view, are becoming important. This is discussed in the final part of the book. The recent development of guidelines, laws and other statements of regulatory character give particular emphasis to this part.

We hope that the proceedings will contribute to the discussion on control and automation in medicine and, in particular, in anaesthesiology and may thus eventually contribute to an advancement in anaesthetic therapy.

Our sincere thanks go to the distinguished group of speakers, chairmen and discussants who made the excellent contributions and shared freely their deep knowledge, expertise and experience.

Bonn, September 1994   HELMUT SCHWILDEN
                                                            HORST STOECKEL

Contents

Contributors

Bender, H.J.

Institut für Anästhesiologie
und spezielle Intensivmedizin
Klinikum der Stadt Mannheim
68135 Mannheim, Germany

Billard, V.

Anesthesiology Service (112A)
Stanford University
School of Medicine
3801 Miranda Avenue
Palo Alto, CA 94304, USA

Booij, L.H.D.J.

Department of Anaesthesia
Critical, Intensive and Emergency Care
Academisch Ziekenhuis Nijmegen
Geert Grooteplein 10
6500 HB Nijmegen, The Netherlands

Bovenkamp, U.

TÜV-Rheinland
Sicherheit und Umweltschutz GmbH
Abt. Medizintechnik
51101 Köln, Germany

Eckmiller, R.

Institut für Informatik VI
Universität Bonn
Römerstr. 164
53117 Bonn, Germany

Frankenberger, H.

Labor für Biomedizinische Technik
Fachhochschule Lübeck
Stephensonstr. 3
23562 Lübeck, Germany

Gaba, D.M.

Anesthesiology Service, 112A
Palo Alto VAMC
3801 Miranda Avenue
Palo Alto, CA 94304, USA

Glass, P.S.A.

Department of Anesthesiology
Duke University Medical Center
Durham, NC 27710, USA

Gravenstein, J.S.

Department of Anesthesiology
College of Medicine
University of Florida
1600 SW Archer Road
Gainsville, FL 32610-0254, USA

Hermanrud, B.

Siemens
16 Electronics Avenue
Danvers, MA 01923, USA

Kenny, G.N.C.

Department of Anaesthesia
Royal Infirmary
8–16 Alexandra Parade
Glasgow G31 2ER, UK

Kochs, E.

Institut für Anästhesiologie
Klinikum Rechts der Isar
Technische Universität München
Ismaninger Str. 22
81675 Munich, Germany

König, P.

Hôpital Cantonal Universitaire de Genève
Department d'Anesthésiologie
24, rue Michelin-du-Crest
1211 Geneva 4, Switzerland

Olkkola, K.T.

Department of Anaesthesia
Helsinki University Central Hospital
Haartmaninkatu 4
00290 Helsinki, Finland

Scharmer, E.-G.

Drägerwerk Aktiengesellschaft
Produktbereich Anästhesie
Moislinger Allee 53/55
23542 Lübeck, Germany

Schüttler, J.

Klinik für Anästhesiologie
und spezielle Intensivmedizin
Universität Bonn
Sigmund-Freud-Str. 25
53105 Bonn, Germany

Schwender, D.

Institut für Anästhesiologie
Klinikum Großhadern
Ludwig-Maximilians-Universität
Marchioninistr. 15
81377 Munich, Germany

Schwilden, H.

Klinik für Anästhesiologie
und spezielle Intensivmedizin
Universität Bonn
Sigmund-Freud-Str. 25
53105 Bonn, Germany

Sear, J.W.

Nuffield Department of Anaesthetics
Level I
The John Radcliffe Hospital
Hadington
Oxford OX3 9DU, UK

Tschöpe, E.

Institut für Arzneimittel
des Bundesgesundheitsamtes
Seestr. 10
13353 Berlin, Germany

Ty Smith, N.

Department of Anesthesia
University of California
3350 La Jolla Village Drive
San Diego, CA 92161, USA

Viby-Mogensen, J.

Department of Anaesthesia
University Hospital
Rikhshospitalet
9 Blegdamsvej
2100 Copenhagen, Denmark

Westenskow, D.R.

Department of Anesthesiology
University of Utah
50 North Medical Drive
Salt Lake City, UH 84132, USA

Zbinden, A.M.

Institut für Anästhesiologie
und Intensivbehandlung
Inselspital
3010 Bern, Switzerland

Zimmermann, H.-J.   Institut für Wirtschaftswissenschaften
Rheinisch-Westfälische
Technische Hochschule
Templergraben 64
52056 Aachen, Germany

I General Methods of Control and Automation

Decision Support via Fuzzy Technology

H.-J. Zimmermann

Introduction

The first article on fuzzy set theory appeared in 1965 [8]. Since then, the number of publications in this area has grown to over 15 000. Many of these contributions are in mathematical areas (topology, analysis, graph theory, logic). To an increasing degree, however, this theory has been applied to various areas and has resulted in methods, tools, and approaches which could be called "fuzzy technology". In particular, since the end of the 1980s, when Japanese successes triggered the "fuzzy boom" in Europe and somewhat later in the USA, fuzzy set theory has been applied to decision-support systems, to diagnostic problems, to control problems, to pattern recognition, and to other problems, and medicine is one of the areas into which fuzzy sets entered first. One of the major reasons for this might be the fact that a majority of the problem structures found in medicine are not of the crisp black-or-white type but rather of the more complicated more-or-less type. This contribution will introduce the basic paradigms, principles, and methods of fuzzy set theory and then sketch some of the better-known applications to decision support in the medical area.

What is Fuzzy Technology?

Major Goals of Fuzzy Technology

From an application point of view, the major goals of fuzzy technology can be summarized as follows.

Modeling of Uncertainty

The best known "uncertainty theory", i.e., Kolmogorow's probability theory, focuses on uncertainty due to randomness. Fuzzy set theory does not compete with this theory but focuses on uncertainty caused by other reasons, and it tries to complement probability theory wherever it is appropriate. Only two types of uncertainty will be discussed here. *"The probability of hitting the target is 0.7"*. This is obviously a probabilistic statement. Two conditions are implied: The event about which a probabilistic statement is made (hitting the target) has to be crisp, two-valued; i.e., there must be no doubt about whether it has happened or not. No probabilistic statements can be made about other phenomena, e.g., "satisfactory profits", "dangerous illnesses", "nice summer days".

Second, the probability has to be known as a real number between 0 and 1 (on an absolute scale level); i.e., 0.7 is read as 0.7000! In some cases this information might be available. In many cases, particularly in knowledge-based systems with human experts' knowledge, it will not be available in this form and probability theory cannot be properly applied. In a probabilistic statement such as "The probability of becoming very sick is low" the conditions for applying probability theory are obviously not satisfied.

Quite another type of uncertainty is the so-called *linguistic, lexical uncertainty*, which refers to the contents or the semantic meaning of terms like "large stones", "high fever", "old men", etc. The meanings of these words obviously depend very much on the context (situation, person, time). If the context is not clear, the words have no well-defined meaning. Human beings normally circumvent this problem by deriving the appropriate context from the situation. If linguistically formulated "expert knowledge" is to be used in and by a computer such an interpretation is not possible, leaving the word meaningless. As will be shown in the next paragraph, fuzzy sets can be used to define the contents of such words formally and meaningfully.

Relaxation

Many of the very powerful classical mathematical tools for modeling and optimization have a crisp, two-valued character, distinguishing, e.g., between optimal and suboptimal, feasible and unfeasible, true and false. These conditions are very often not given in real situations. Fuzzy set theory is used to adapt such crisp methods to real situations while maintaining the power of the mathematical method.

Reduction of Complexity

Often problem situations are characterized by amounts of data which exceed the human ability to recognize the informational structures hidden in these data. Fuzzy set theory in the framework of fuzzy data analysis or datamining tries to reduce the complexity of data (e.g., in diagnosis) by using either fuzzy cluster algorithms or linguistic variables, which will be described below.

Meaning-Preserving Reasoning

In expert system technology, in which either nonexisting mathematical models of problems or unavailable algorithms are substituted by human expertise, which is stored in knowledge bases and processed by inference engines, usually symbol processing is used; i.e., if-then statements are stored in the computer and their relevance is evaluated solely on the basis of their truth values – true or false – which again have to be entered by human users and cannot be obtained directly by the computer.

Fuzzy set theory – via linguistic variables and special inference methods – attaches the meaning to the words and statements and ensures that this meaning is preserved in the inference process.

Basic Fuzzy Set Theory (FS)

The core of FS is naturally the fuzzy set, originally defined as follows. If X is a collection of objects denoted generically by x, then a fuzzy set $\tilde{A}$ in X is a set of ordered pairs:

$$\tilde{A} = \{(x, \mu_{\tilde{A}}(x))|\ x \in X\}$$

$\mu_{\tilde{A}}(x)$ is called the membership function (generalized characteristic function) which maps X to the membership spaced M. Its range is the subset of non-negative real numbers whose supremum is finite. For sup $\mu(x) = 1$ the set is called "normalized". Of the many existing special types of fuzzy sets only one will be mentioned here: the linguistic variable. A linguistic variable (strictly defined as a quintuple) is a variable, the possible values of which are not numbers but words or statements. These words are called "terms". The meaning of these terms is defined via fuzzy sets on a "base variable". See Fig. 1 for an example.

Operations with fuzzy sets or fuzzy statements are defined via their membership functions, $\mu(x)$. The set theory operations intersection, union and comple-

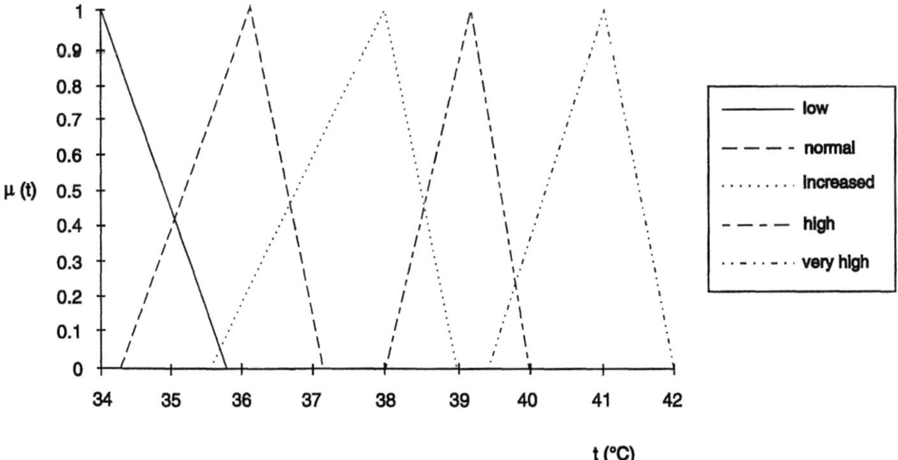

Fig. 1. The linguistic variable "temperature"

ment (of fuzzy sets) correspond to the logic connectives "and", "incl. or", and "negation" of statements.

Intersection: (logical and). The membership function of the intersection of two fuzzy sets $\tilde{A}$ and $\tilde{B}$ is defined as:

$$\mu_{\tilde{A} \cap \tilde{B}}(x) = \text{Min}(\mu_{\tilde{A}}(x), \mu_{\tilde{B}}(x)) \forall x \in X$$

Union (inclusive or). The membership function of the union is defined as:

$$\mu_{\tilde{A} \cup \tilde{B}}(x) = \text{Max}(\mu_{\tilde{A}}(x), \mu_{\tilde{B}}(x)) \forall x \in X$$

Complement: (negation). The membership function of the complement is defined as:

$$\mu_{\tilde{A}}(x) = 1 - \mu_{\tilde{A}}(x) \forall x \in X$$

In the meantime, a large number of context dependent operators have been suggested and partly tested as alternative operators for those mentioned above. The operators can be structured into t-Norm (for the intersection/log. and), t-Conorms (for the union/log. or), and compensatory operators (to model the linguistic "and") [11].

Applications in Decision Support

Areas of Application

From a methods point of view, applications of fuzzy technology can be summarized as follows:

Model based (relaxation)
- Fuzzy optimization (Fuzzy LP)
- Fuzzy clustering
- Fuzzy Petri nets
- Fuzzy multi-criteria analysis
- Fuzzy CPM methods

Information processing (complexity reduction)
- Fuzzy data banks
- Fuzzy programming languages
- Fuzzy library systems

Knowledge based (meaning-preserving reasoning)
- Fuzzy expert systems
- Fuzzy control

Hybrid applications
- (Fuzzy) data analysis (complexity reduction)
- Concurrent engineering
- Creditworthiness evaluation

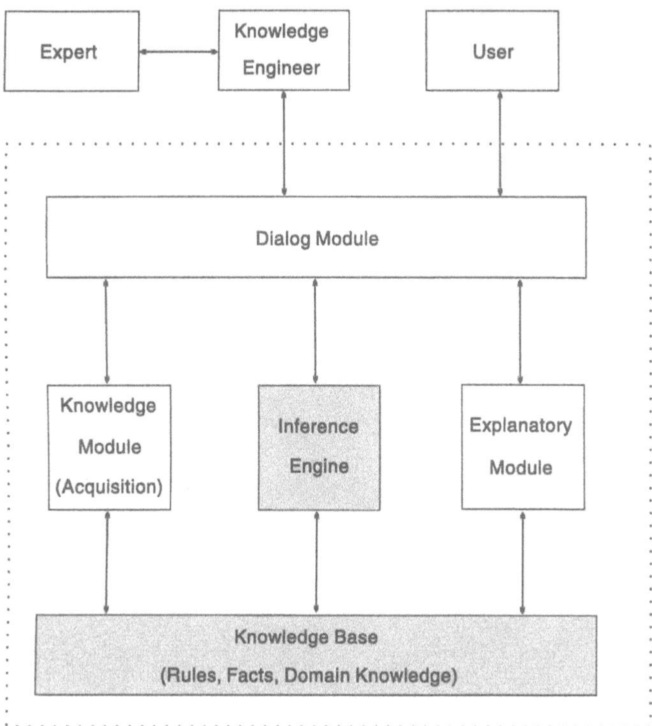

Fig. 2. Structure of an expert system

Here we shall elaborate only on the knowledge-based applications, because they seem to be the most relevant in medicine. Figure 2 shows the structure of an expert system. As already mentioned, knowledge enters the system in linguistic form. It is stored in a knowledge base and processed in the inference engine in the form of fuzzy sets. The interface with the users should also be (quasi) linguistic or graphical.

If expert system technology is to be used to control something automatically, the input information, e.g., temperatures, pressures, etc., is not in a linguistic form; neither is the output, e.g., settings of values, switches, burners, etc. The first solution to this type of problem was suggested and tested in the mid 1970s and has become known as Mamdani's "Fuzzy Controller" [5]. In contrast to the expert system, real numbers which were received from and transmitted to the process to be controlled were transformed into linguistic form (fuzzy sets) to compute the appropriate control action and retransformed into real numbers for control signals (Fig. 3).

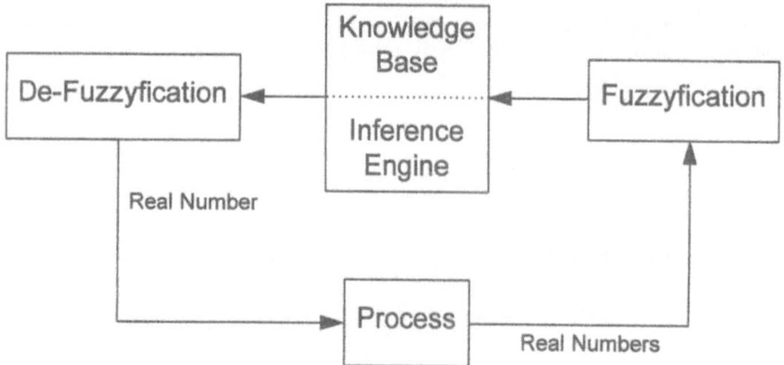

Fig. 3. Structure of a Fuzzy Controller

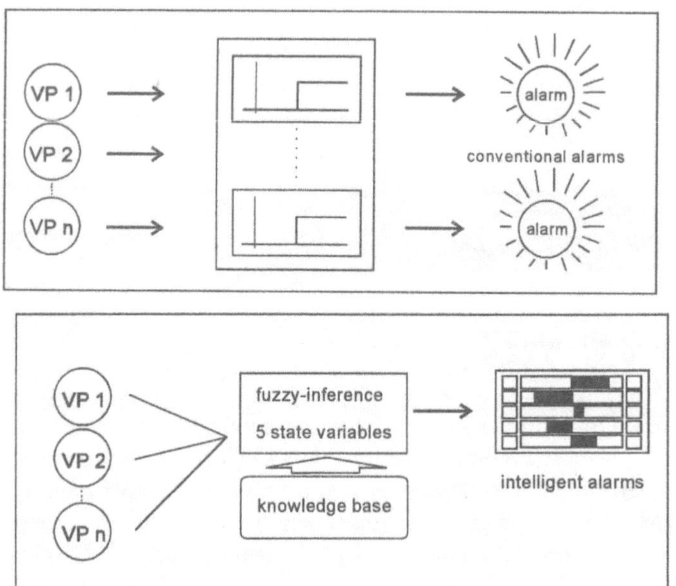

Fig. 4. Alarm function of monitoring devices – conventional versus intelligent alarms. (From [4])

Medical Applications

Medical applications are of the fuzzy control type as well as of the expert system type. Ongoing research on the control of a totally artificial heart, for instance, and blood pressure control use the fuzzy control approach successfully [6, 7]. One of the best-known expert systems for diagnostic problems which used fuzzy technology is CADIAC-2 [1, 2]. It contains disease profiles and diagnostic rules for 267 diseases which are various diagnostic groups and allow differential diagnoses.

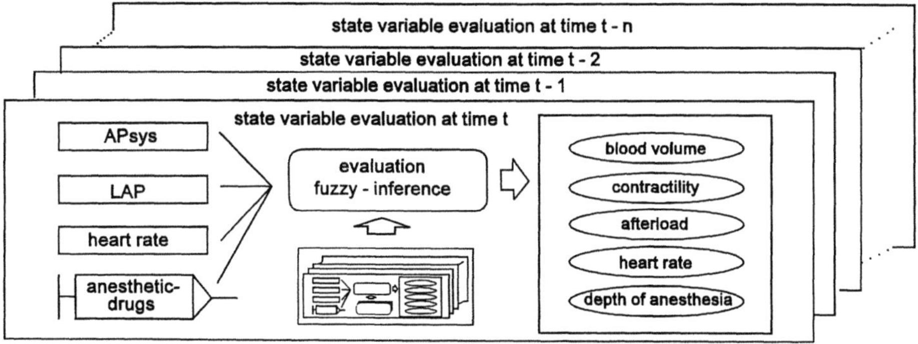

Fig. 5. State variable evaluation by the cardioanesthetist. (From [4])

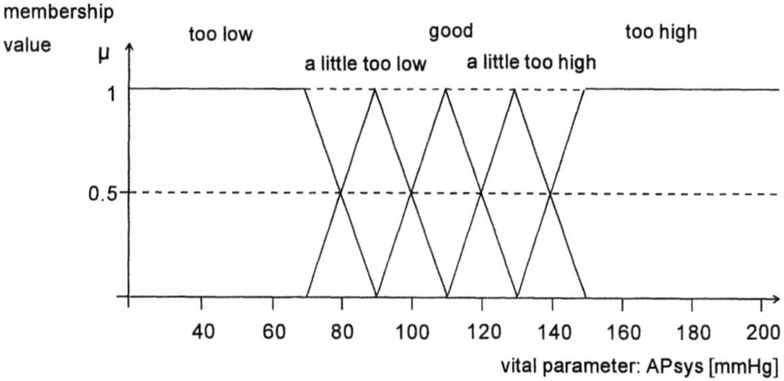

Fig. 6. Membership functions for the linguistic variable "arterial systolic pressure" (*AP sys*)

Another decision-support system based on fuzzy technology that supports cardioanesthetists while they perform anesthesia during complicated surgical operations is IAC (Intelligent Alarm in Cardioanesthesia). It focuses on supporting the anesthetist while evaluating the patient's hemodynamic state. While classical monitoring devices which present vital parameters like blood pressure, temperatures, and blood volume trigger optical or acoustical alarms whenever any parameter exceeds a predetermined threshold, IAC models the anesthetist by evaluating the most important vital parameter constellations via fuzzy inference and visualizing five hemodynamic state variables. Figure 4 illustrates the differences between classical systems and IAC. The state variables evaluated are shown in Fig. 5.

Linguistic variables used for fuzzy inference are shown for "arterial systolic pressure" in Fig. 6. Since the input into IAC are data provided by measuring devices and the output is visualized graphically, IAC has the structure of fuzzy control even though it does not control any process automatically (Fig. 7).

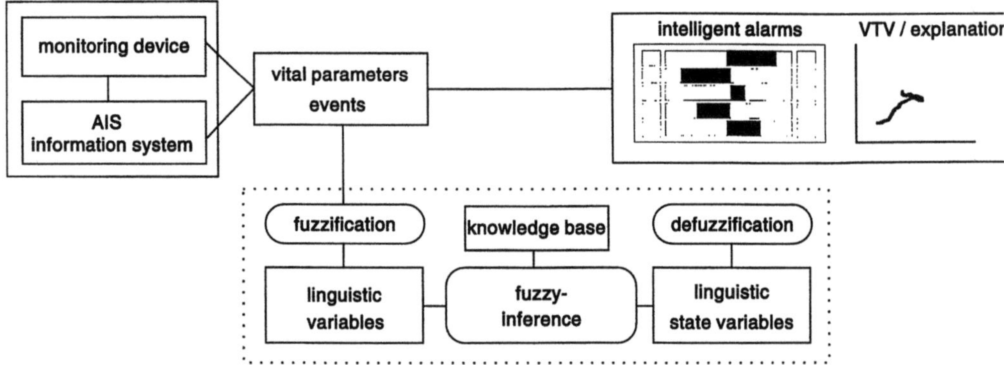

Fig. 7. Structure of the intelligent alarm system

Particular care was taken to offer additional informative pictures to the anesthetist from which the development of the vital parameters of a patient can be judged statically and dynamically. Success with existing medical decision-support systems has been encouraging, and it is anticipated that more of these tools will be available in various areas in the not too distant future.

References

1. Adlassnig K-P (1986) Fuzzy set theory in medical diagnosis. IEEE Transactions on Systems, Man and Cybernetics SMC-16: 260–265
2. Adlassnig K-P, Leitich H, Kolarz G (1993) On the applicability of diagnostic criteria for the diagnostic of rheumatoid arthritis in an expert system. In: Expert systems with applications, vol 6. pp 441–448
3. Becker K, Käsmacher H, Juffernbruck K, Rau G, Kalff G, Zimmermann H-J (1993) An intelligent alarm system using fuzzy inference. In: Proc. 2nd European Congr Eng Med, Amsterdam, pp 57–58
4. Becker K, Käsmacher H, Rau G, Kalff G, Zimmermann H-J (1994) A fuzzy logic approach to intelligent alarms in cardioanaesthesia. IEEE Proceedings, WCCI
5. Mamdani EH (1977) Applications of fuzzy set theory to control systems. In: Gupta, Saridis, Gaines (eds) Fuzzy automation and decision process. Amsterdam, New York, pp 71–88
6. Meier R, Nieuwland J, Zbinden AM, Hacisalihzade SS (1992) Fuzzy logic control of blood pressure during anesthesia. IEEE Control Systems: 12–17
7. Rau G, Becker K, Kaufmann R, Zimmermann H-J (1994) Fuzzy logic and control: principal approach and potential applications in medicine. Artif Organs (submitted for publication)
8. Zadeh LA (1965) Fuzzy sets, information and control. 8:338–353
9. Zadeh LA (1973) Outline of a new approach to the analysis of complex systems and decision processes. IEEE Trans Syst, Man, Cybern SMC-3, pp 28–44
10. Zimmermann H-J (1987) Fuzzy sets, decision making and expert systems. Boston
11. Zimmermann H-J (1991) Fuzzy set theory – and its applications, 2nd edn. Boston
12. Zimmermann H-J, Zysno P (1980) Latent connectives in human decision making. Fuzzy Sets Systems 4:37–54

Principles of Adaptive Neural Networks for Control

R. Eckmiller

History

The young research field called "neural networks for computing", or "neuroinformatics", or "connectionism" has the goal of transferring concepts of the structure and function of biological neural systems (brains) to the design of novel, adaptive computers, which are not driven by software, but rather by learning.

The development of software-driven computers began around 1940. Any mathematical problem to be solved by such a computer has to be represented algebraic-analytically in order to be entered as software. This basic fact has the dramatic and generally overlooked consequence that the use of software-driven computers typically limits the user to algebraic-analytical representations of a given problem. Around 1960, research efforts were initiated to generate so-called intelligent functions (a special domain of biological neural networks), such as pattern recognition, associative memory, and movement control of redundant robots or autonomous vehicles. Given the two alternative approaches of special software (e.g., new symbolic languages) for conventional computers or special hardware (e.g., perceptron-like neural net hardware), most researchers concentrated on novel software for intelligent functions, thus starting the new field of "artificial intelligence" (AI).

About 25 years later (around 1985), it became more and more evident among AI experts that the special software approach would find its limits at the level of "expert systems". One of the most plausible reasons for the limits of conventional (software-based) AI research was the notion that algebraic-analytical representations require mathematical theories of the underlying "intelligent" functions. However, such theories for pattern recognition or redundant robot control in real time in a natural environment are presently not available.

This sobering evaluation in the early 1980s was the decisive reason for a strong revival of the special hardware approach in AI research under various headings such as neural networks (NN) for computing, connectionism, or neuroinformatics. The most important merit of this approach is the fact that numerous examples of biological existence proof exist. Any fly (presumably born with a hard-wired net of well under 1 million neurons which does not change too much during its lifetime) is capable of mapping visual trajectories in real time onto obstacle-avoiding flight trajectories (before gracefully landing on the ceiling).

Many frogs (with considerably larger neural nets and the ability to change their net topology by means of self-organization during learning) can motionlessly monitor a fly's flight trajectory and with reasonable success generate a prey-catching movement.

Such biological neural networks (NNs) are information-processing systems, which presumably (a) do not represent the numerous sensorimotor mapping operations (or behavior) algebraic-analytically as in a software-driven computer, but rather (b) embed the mapping operations in the highly parallel dynamic neural net topology, and (c) acquire these geometric-topological representations partly during evolution and partly during their lifetime by means of self-organization and learning in interaction with the physical environment. It is postulated here that software-driven conventional computers and self-organization-driven neural networks (neural computers) correspond to two separate mathematical theory spaces with only limited overlap [10, 11].

Current State

At present, most research in neuroinformatics, which can be considered a novel approach in AI, is still based on software simulations of artificial NNs (with the same synchronicity and real-time problems as in simulations of highly parallel electronic circuits) with certain algebraically derived learning rules. The radical change from algebraic-analytical to geometric-topological representations is just beginning. This development will be boosted by the commercial availability of fully parallel and asynchronously operating NN hardware with user-specifiable initial net topology and dynamics, as well as learning rules being embedded in the net topology (rather than separate from the net, as in most current software simulations). Several companies and research institutes are currently designing NN hardware, which will operate as a new kind of co-processor in conventional work stations or as stand alone systems. The available NN software simulators and the emerging hardware simulators offer information processing far beyond cur-rent mathematical theories. In other words, neuroinformatics is at present largely an experimental research field like experimental physics or engineering. Intuition and concepts borrowed from other areas (especially neuroscience) spur this field; one never knows in advance whether the combination of a certain initial net topology, a certain learning rule, and a certain set of learning opportunities will yield a satisfying self-organization with convergence toward a final net topology and – most importantly – mapping functions with the desired precision and generalization.

Most of the mathematical theories and methods presently being used for simulation of artificial NNs belong to the algebraic-analytical theory space. They include:

1. Linear systems theory
2. Adaptive filter theory

3. Dynamic systems theory
4. Variation calculus
5. Fuzzy set theory

Future Developments

The biological existence proof guarantees that NNs are (in principle) capable of generating various mapping operations, which were acquired by self-organization of the dynamic net topology during a learning phase. Accordingly, biological and artificial NNs can be described as geometrical mapping machines. However, no mathematical theory is available which could predict the relation between dynamic neural net topology, learning rule, set of learning opportunities, and the desired mapping operation. Given the fact that more than half of our present knowledge in mathematics was discovered only in the past 50 years, there is hope that future research efforts can be successfully directed towards novel mathematics of information processing in neural networks. The expected emphasis on geometry and dynamic net topology will certainly also be valuable for theories of other parallel information-processing systems (e.g., optical computers and molecular computers).

A number of mathematical theories and methods with origins in the geometric-topological theory space could form a base for the new theory to be developed. They include:

1. Various geometry theories
2. Various topology theories
3. Graph theory
4. Cellular automata theory
5. Theory of fractal geometry
6. Knot theory

As in most other previous technological developments (e.g., feedback-control systems, mechanical clocks and automata, conventional computers), the experimental, engineering design of self-organizing NN hardware (neural computers) for various special purposes (sensory, associative learning, or motor) precedes the development of the corresponding theory of geometrical mapping machines. Geometry and topology play a more crucial role in NN design than in any other information technology. This demands a new breed of experts ("network architects"), who will be as important as software engineers were for conventional computers.

In summary, neuroinformatics is heading toward computer technologies which are capable of geometric-topological representations of specific mapping functions. Progress is under way to merge the technologies of neural computers with those of conventional computers, thus creating a genuinely novel hybrid computer generation.

Neural Computers for Robot Control

The standard task of robot control is to map a desired workspace trajectory $q^*(t)$ onto n torque time functions $\tau_i(t)$ for the corresponding n joints of a manipulator, such that its tool center point (tcp) moving along $q(t)$ remains as close as possible to $q^*(t)$ (Fig. 1). During the past 50 years research has focused on various aspects of this task, such as: path planning [e.g., finding an appropriate obstacle-avoiding desired trajectory $q^*(t)$], inverse kinematics (finding the corresponding n joint angle increments for a step along the desired trajectory), and inverse dynamics (finding the corresponding n torques to move tcp along the desired trajectory, even in the presence of unexpected load changes).

At present, most industrial robotic applications are restricted to simple point-to-point movements with unspecified trajectories, without compliance control, with negligible dynamic coupling, and without kinematic redundancy. These severe functional restrictions, as compared with typically elastic, redundant, nonlinear biological motor systems, are due to a combination of the excessive computing power required for processing the various matrix operations and sets of coupled linear differential equations in real time and theoretical limitations in dealing with elastic, redundant, nonlinear manipulators.

Conventional approaches to the design of robot controllers (with the aim of combining stability and parameter adjustment in real time with position and force control) led from the principles of self-optimizing controllers by Kalman [25], model reference adaptive controllers by Whitaker [29], and self-tuning regulators by Åström [5, 21] to decoupling of nonlinear controllers by Freund [19], learning controllers by Arimoto [4, 8], index of performance in optimal controllers [21], and nonlinear adaptive model-based controllers by Craig [6]. Relevant research on the design of adaptive systems for control, which has connections to prediction, has also been published in the fields of digital filters [30], adaptive lattice filters [21], and time series analysis [35].

In the light of current limitations of conventional robot control regarding lack of sufficient algebraic-analytical representations of the required mapping operations (Fig. 1) and/or computing power to meet the real-time requirements, several novel approaches using artificial neural networks are being presented here [15]. Although the field of neural computing will take many more years to mature, this research is guided not only by the manifold biological evidence of complex motor systems under neural network control, but also by an increasing number of very promising results in industrial application areas in which the conventional approach has reached its limits. This fact has been acknowledged already by a number of prominent robotics scientists (see, for example [10, 11, 27, 39]).

Path Planning and Obstacle Avoidance

The potential of neural networks with intrinsic features such as adaptability, fine-grained parallelism, combinations of local and global information processing, and graceful degradation for generation of desired trajectories with obstacle avoidance

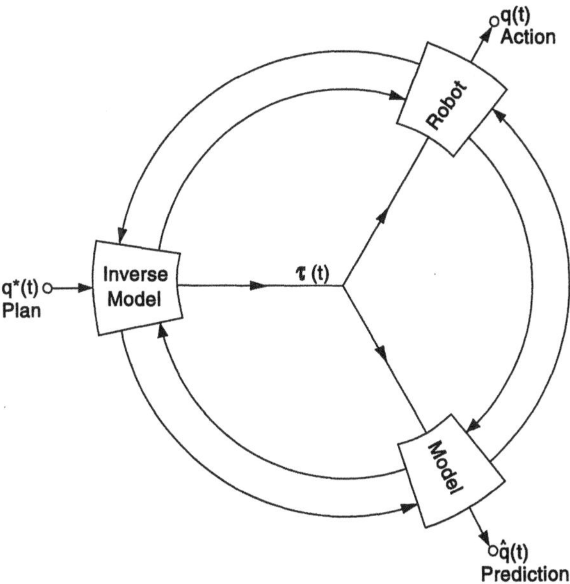

Fig. 1. Robot control paradigm. Desired trajectory $q^*(t)$ is mapped by the inverse model (inverse kinematics plus dynamics control) onto a torque vector $\tau(t)$ for the n joints of the robot, which in turn moves its tcp along the actual trajectory $q(t)$. The model serves for system identification of the robot dynamics and generates a predicted trajectory $\hat{q}(t)$

in real time – a very difficult task for present robot control systems – is currently being explored by several groups. Their approaches include heuristic dynamic programming [38] and temporal difference learning [34].

In our laboratory we develop various networks for internal representation of the workspace in order to store desired trajectories and representations of obstacles and generate corresponding obstacle-avoiding trajectories. A neural triangular lattice (NTL) with a traveling activity peak was developed for storage and generation of desired 2-D trajectories [9]. Alternatively, another net topology consisting of a temporal pattern generator (TPG) connected with two activity memory neurons (AM) with adaptive synapses was designed to store 2-D trajectories during a brief learning phase [20]. Currently, these approaches are being expanded to represent the 3-D workspace, including visually detected obstacles for generation of obstacle-avoiding 3-D trajectories. In a third approach to path planning, we used a higher-order neural net implementation of a sequential dynamic programming algorithm [18].

Inverse Kinematics

Several groups have recently proposed neural networks for the mapping of the desired trajectory coordinates onto the corresponding set of joint angles even in cases of redundant planar manipulators [1, 26, 32]. In our laboratory, we developed a neural kinematics net (NKN) for real-time processing of the inverse kinematics of a redundant planar manipulator [9, 22]. The NKN processes the inverse kinematics for each trajectory element at a time by means of various geometric measurement and mapping operations in modules with predefined (rather than acquired during a learning phase) net topologies. The NKN model has been further improved recently. A locally operating adaptive network, based on connection assignment and topographical encoding (CATE), was developed [23] to keep the number of neurons optimally small, while maintaining a given mapping accuracy.

System Identification and Control

Probably the biggest challenge for neural computing with regard to robotics is the development of adaptive neural networks with real-time capabilities to replace and significantly surpass conventional controllers as well as corresponding models for system identification (Fig. 1). The controller receives a desired time course for the joint rotation angles at the input and generates appropriate control signals at the output. In general, the controller can be treated as a filter, usually an adaptive nonlinear filter, the dynamics of which may be difficult, if not impossible, to describe analytically. Adaptation of the controller dynamics may be necessary not only during a learning phase, but also in real-time during operation, due to unexpected load changes, etc. Accordingly, any improvements by means of neural net controllers have to be evaluated relative to the various conventional adaptive controllers, systems, or filters. It is noteworthy that, on the one hand, various methods of parameter estimation, self-adjusting performance, error minimization, and gradient descent have already been developed in control theory and related fields, while, on the other hand, several adaptive neural networks, such as Adaline [40] and CMAC [2] have been known in the robotics and control community for a number of years. More recent, very promising designs of adaptive neural networks for control include gradient methods [27], a combination of nets for system identification and control [28], and reinforcement maximation over time [38].

Example: 4-Joint Machine

Based on various neurobiological studies, we began a project on controlling a redundant 4-joint machine by means of neural networks, which includes the design of pulse-coded neural net hardware. Figure 2 shows the two required neural net modules, the neural space net (NSN) and the neural kinematics net (NKN), as well as the 4-joint machine on the right side. In short, the NSN on the left is supposed to store desired trajectories, such as the trajectory for the hand-written letter b. When b is being called, an activity peak AP travels along the path of b on a neural lattice [9]. The NSN output provides time functions for the two-dimen-

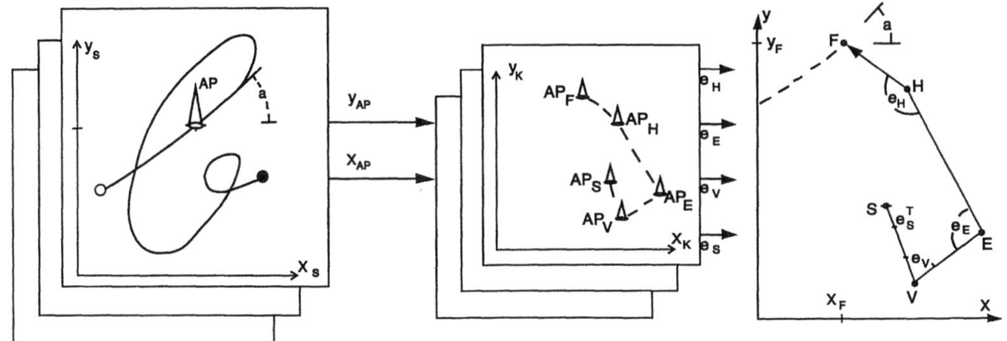

Fig. 2. Neural net control of a 4-joint machine (*right*). *Left*: Neural net space for storage of various trajectories by means of a travelling activity peak (*AP*) on a neural lattice. *Middle*: Neural kinematics net for mapping of the desired trajectory $(x_{AP}(t), y_{AP}(t))$ onto four simultaneous time functions (e_H, e_E, e_V, and e_S) for the rotary control signals of the four actuators

sional coordinates of the activity peak while AP travels. These time functions y_{AP} and x_{AP} form the input for the neural kinematics net NKN. NKN is assumed to consist of several neural net components in order to perform the required mapping operation, thus generating time functions for the four actuators indicated here as angle signals e_H, e_E, e_V, and e_S for hand, elbow, virtual joint, and shoulder.

In principle, NKN operates locally, in that it receives the current direction angle a from NSN for the next trajectory element and finds the corresponding combination of actuator control signals on the basis of its internal position model (POM) of the 4-joint machine. The POM can be thought of as a continuously updated bookkeeping system for all geometric parameters of the 4-joint machine.

Neurotechnology

The emerging field of "neurotechnology" deals with *compensation of functional deficits of the human nervous system by means of novel computer and microsystems technologies*. Accordingly, neurotechnology requires the development of adaptive biology-inspired pulse-processing neural networks (BPN) [12, 16], as well as novel multicontact neural interfaces (MNI) to allow for functional substitution of and bidirectional communication with specific parts of the nervous system in real time [13]. Thus, it is essential for technical neural systems (BPN) to be adjustable in response to signals from the implant-carrying patient, as well as to encode and decode neural signals.

The aim of neurotechnology is the development of a new generation of prosthetic devices, such as novel functional electrical stimulation (FES) systems, or retina implants as indicated by the two schemas of Fig. 3. The top schema depicts a BPN as an adaptive neural encoder to map signals from a technical sensor array

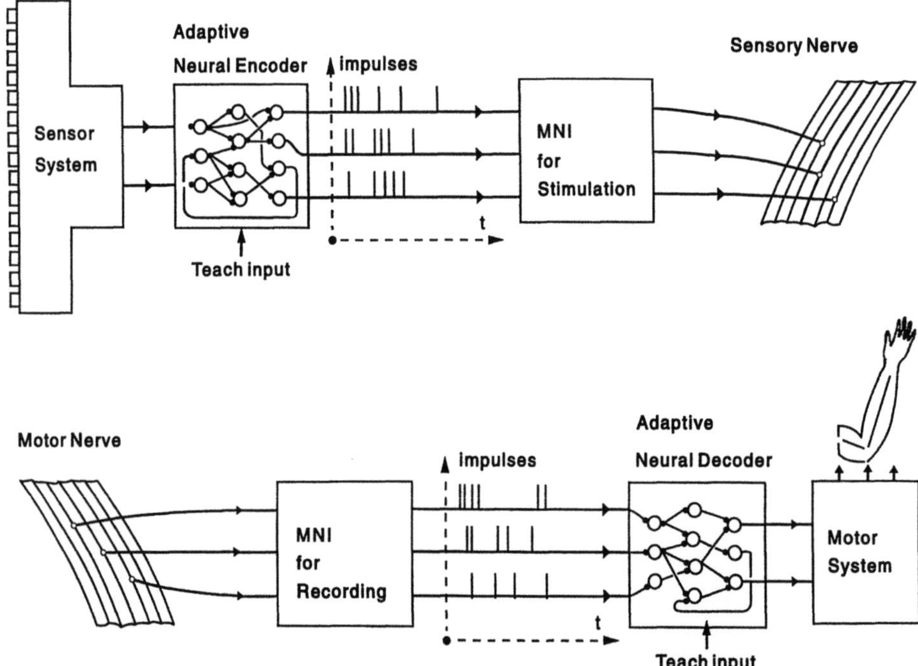

Fig. 3. Two typical neuroprosthetic applications of neuro-technology. *Top*: Technical sensor system (prosthesis) supplies an adaptive neural computer as a biology-inspired pulse-processing neural network (BPN, which serves here as neural encoder) with sensory signals. The BPN generates corresponding encoded impulse trains as input (stimulation) for a sensory nerve via a multicontact neural interface (*MNI*). *Bottom*: Motor control signals, which are recorded as impulse trains from a motor nerve via a multicontact neural interface (*MNI*), are decoded by a BPN and fed into a technical motor system (prosthesis)

onto (several hundred) separate neural impulse trains, which are being connected with single nerve fibers by means of an MNI. In contrast, the bottom schema in Fig. 3 indicates the reverse situation of another MNI for recording of (several hundred) separate neural impulse trains from human nervous tissue, and a subsequent BPN as an adaptive neural decoder to map the spike trains onto appropriate control signals for technical devices (e.g., prostheses or monitors).

Concept of a Retina Implant

A significant number of visually impaired human subjects suffer from retinal defects, especially retinitis pigmentosa (RP) or macula degeneration (MD); the former typically begins in RP with night blindness (loss of rod photoreceptors), deteriorates into tunnel vision, and finally leads to total blindness (additional loss of all cone photoreceptors). However, significant portions of retinal ganglion cells and subsequent parts of the visual system remain intact [33]. In a recent pioneering study [24], it was demonstrated that local electrical stimulation of the retinal ganglion cell layer in blind RP patients yields localized visual sensations.

We are currently developing components for a retina implant for RP patients in cooperation with several partners from microelectronics, microsystems, and retina surgery research centers. The conceived retina implant (Fig. 4) consists of a retina stimulator for ganglion cell stimulation and a retina encoder designed as a neural net with flexible antagonistic receptive field properties (RF-BPN). The currently developed RF-BPN module, handling both slow potentials and impulse events, allows for modification of ten spatial and/or temporal parameters in order

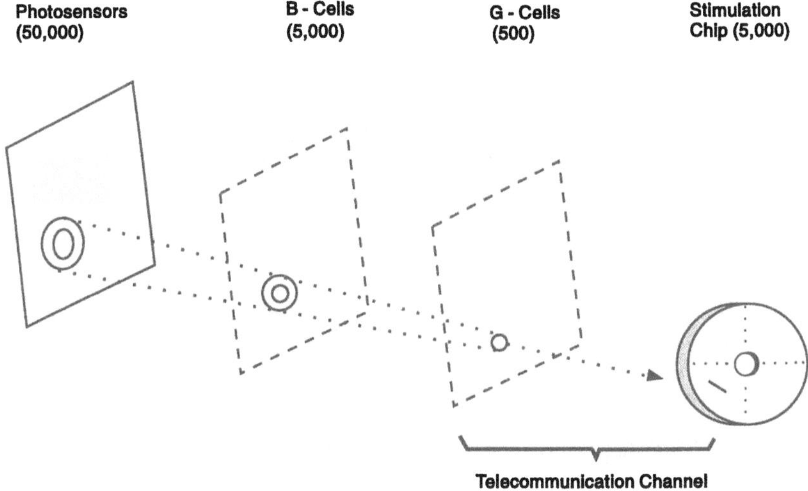

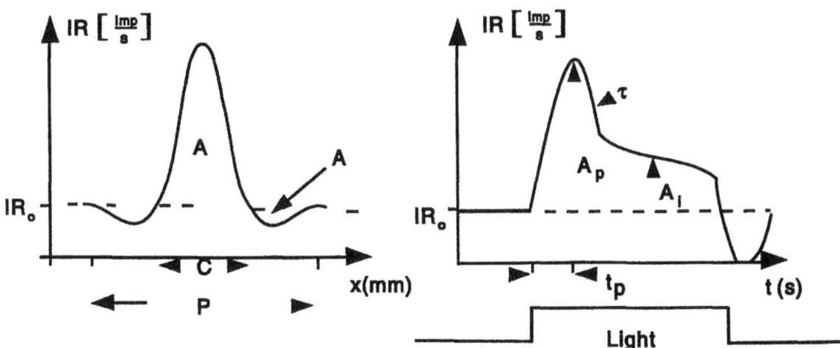

Fig. 4. Plan for a retina implant. *Top*: RF-BPNs consisting of photo sensors, bipolar cells, and about 500 ganglion cells, as well as an implanted ganglion cell stimulator with about 5000 microcontacts. *Bottom*: Modifiable parameters of the receptive field properties of RF-BPNs

to adjust the RF-BPN to the desired receptive field properties of a given ganglion cell [7, 37]. Specifically, each RF-BPN module can be tuned in a learning process to the receptive field properties of a retinal X-cell type (about 60% of the total ganglion cell population in the primate retina) or a Y-cell type (about 25%) with regard to parameters such as RF center, or time constants [14].

References

1. Ahmand Z, Guez A (1990) On the solution to the inverse kinematic problem. In: Proc IEEE Int Joint Conf. Robotics and Automation, IEEE, Cincinnati, 13–18 May 1990, pp 1692–1697
2. Albus JS (1975) A new approach to manipulator control: the cerebellar model articulation controller (CMAC). J Dyn Syst Measurement Control 97:220–227
3. Aleksander I (ed) (1989) Neural computing architectures. North Oxford Academic, London
4. Arimoto S, Kawamura S, Miyazaki F (1984) Bettering operation of robots by learning. J Robotics Systems 1:123–140
5. Åström KJ, Wittenmark B (1989) Adaptive control. Addison-Wesley, Reading, M
6. Craig JJ, Hsu P, Sastry SS (1987) Adaptive control of mechanical manipulators. Int J Robotics Res 6:16–28
7. Dacey DM, Petersen MR (1992) Dendritic field size and morphology of midget and parasol ganglion cells of the human retina. Proc Natl Acad Sci USA 89:9666–9670
8. Dillmann R (1988) Lernende Roboter. Springer, Berein Heidelberg New York
9. Eckmiller R (1989) Neural nets for sensorimotor trajectories. IEEE Control Systems Magazine 9:53–59
10. Eckmiller R (ed) (1990) Advanced neural computers. Elsevier, Amsterdam
11. Eckmiller R (1990) Concerning the emerging role of geometry in neuroinformatics. In: Eckmiller R, Hartmann G, Hauske G (eds) Parallel processing in neural systems and computers. Elsevier, Amsterdam, pp 5–8
12. Eckmiller R (1991) Pulse processing neural systems for motor control. In: Kohonen T, Mäkisara K, Simula O, Kangas J (eds) Artificial neural networks, vol 1. Elsevier, Amsterdam, pp 345–350
13. Eckmiller R (1993) Concerning the challenge of neurotechnology. In: Bothe M-W Samii M, Eckmiller R (eds) Neurobionics. Elsevier, Amsterdam, pp 21–28
14. Eckmiller R (ed) (1994) Final report of the feasibility study for a neurotechnology program. Bundesministerium für Forsching und Technologie, Bonn
15. Eckmiller R, Kreimeier B (1991) Improvement of robot control by neural computers. In: Proc IEEE Int Joint Conf. Neural Networks, Singapore, November 1991, vol II. pp 1837–1843
16. Eckmiller R, Napp-Zinn H (1993) Information processing in biology-inspired pulse-coded neural networks. In: Proc Int Joint Conf on Neural Networks, Nagoya, vol 1. pp 643–648
17. Eckmiller R, Hartmann G, Hauske G (eds) (1990) Parallel processing in neural systems and computers. Elsevier, Amsterdam
18. Fahner G, Eckmiller R (1994) Implementation of an AI-approach for path planning by a neural net-based hybrid system. J Artif Neural Networks 1:115–125
19. Freund E (1982) Fast nonlinear control with arbitrary pole-placement for industrial robots and manipulators. Int J Robotics Res 1:65–78
20. Goerke N, Schöne M, Kreimeier B, Eckmiller R (1990) A network with pulse-processing neurons for generation of arbitrary temporal sequences. In: Proc IEEE Int Joint Conf. Neural Networks, San Diego, pp 315–320

21. Goodwin GC, Sin KS (1984) Adaptive filtering, prediction and control. Prentice Hall, Englewood Cliffs
22. Hakala J, Steiner R, Eckmiller R (1990) Quasi-local solution for inverse kinematics of a redundant robot arm. In: Proc IEEE Int Joint Conf. Neural Networks, San Diego, pp 321–326
23. Hakala J, Fahner G, Eckmiller R (1991) Rapid learning of inverse robot kinematics based on connection assignment and topographical encoding (CATE). In: Proc IEEE Int Joint Conf. Neural Networks, Singapore, vol II. pp 1536–1541
24. Humayun MS, Propst RH, Hickingbotham D, de Juan E, Dagnelie G (1993) Visual sensations produced by electrical stimulation of the retinal surface in patients with end-stage retinitis pigmentosa (RP). Invest Ophthalmol Vis Sci 34[Suppl]:835
25. Kalman RE (1958) Design of a self-optimizing control system. Trans Am Soc Mech Eng 80:468–478
26. Kuperstein M (1988) Neural model of adaptive hand-eye coordination for single postures. Science 239:1308–1311
27. Narendra NS, Parthasarathy K (1991) Gradient methods for the optimization of dynamical systems containing neural networks. IEEE Trans Neural Networks 2:252–262
28. Nguyen DH, Widrow B (1990) Neural networks for self-learning control systems. IEEE Control Systems Mag 10:18–23
29. Osburn PV, Whitaker HP, Kezer A (1961) New development in the design of model reference adaptive control systems. In: Proc Inst Aerospace Sci, IAS paper no 61-39, pp 1–26, New York
30. Pitas I, Venetsanopoulos AN (eds) (1990) Nonlinear digital filters. Kluwer, Boston
31. Richert P, Hosticka BJ, Kesper M, Scholles M, Schwarz M (1993) An emulator for biologically inspired neural networks. In: Proc Int Joint Conf on Neural Networks, Nagoya, vol. 1. pp 841–844
32. Ritter HJ, Martinez TM, Schulten KJ (1989) Topology-conserving maps for learning visuo-motor coordination. Neural Networks 2:159–168
33. Stone JL, Barlow WE, Humayun MS, de Juan E, Milam AH (1992) Morphometric analysis of macular photoreceptors and ganglion cells in retinas with retinitis pigmentosa. Arch Ophthalmol 110:1634–1639
34. Sutton RS (1990) First results with Dyna, an integrated architecture for learning, planning and reaching. In: Miller TK III, Sutton RS, Werbos PJ (eds) Neural networks for control. MIT Press, Cambridge, pp 179–189
35. Tong H, (1990) Non-linear time series. Oxford University Press, Oxford
36. van den Bout DE, Miller TK III (1990) Graph partitioning using annealed neural networks. IEEE Trans Neural Networks 1:192 203
37. Wässle H Boycott BB (1991) Functional architecture of the mammalian retina. Physiol Rev 71:447–480
38. Werbos PJ (1990) A menu of designs for reinforcement learning over time. In: Miller TK III, Sutton RS, Werbos PJ (eds) Neural networks for control. MIT Press, Cambridge, pp 67–95
39. White DA, Sofge DA (1992) Handbook of intelligent control. Van Nostrand Reinhold, New York
40. Widrow B, Gupta NK, Maitra S (1973) Punish/reward: learning with a critic in adaptive threshold systems. IEEE Trans Syst Man Cybern 3:455–465

Artificial Intelligence and Expert Systems

D.M. Gaba

Introduction

Control and automation in anesthesia imply the intelligent manipulation of anesthetics or adjuvant drugs to provide satisfactory medical conditions for the dynamically changing patient undergoing surgery and anesthesia. Traditionally, the intelligence is supplied totally by the human anesthetist. The focus of this workshop is on new methods in which the manipulation of drugs or other interventions is handled by computers. When the computer makes these changes in response to specific measurements made on the patient, this is termed "closed-loop control". Other forms of automation (that is, machines conducting activities formerly conducted by a person) are also possible. These range from the relatively mundane – such as the mechanical ventilator or the standard electromechanical infusion pump – to truly autonomous computer agents which could conduct diagnosis and therapy on the patient in the operating room or the intensive care unit (ICU).

Closed-loop control has been known for many years and is present in a wide variety of applications in the industrial world. Whole branches of mathematics and engineering are devoted to "control theory" – the techniques of translating measurements of the system into control inputs to the system. In this paper I will review a different set of techniques for dealing with information about a system. These techniques can be summarized under the name "artificial intelligence", commonly abbreviated as AI. What they have in common is that, for the most part (there are exceptions), they represent ways to deal with information *symbolically* rather than strictly mathematically. In practice, there is no definite division between AI and other mathematical, logical, or symbolic systems, and some aspects of traditional control theory are incorporated into what are typically viewed as AI applications.

The literature on AI is now enormous. It is far beyond the scope of this paper to review the field in general. Rather, my intention is to provide an introduction to the nature of several different techniques and approaches, outlining some of their positive and negative features. I will briefly allude to some of their applications to anesthesia and intensive care, and I will discuss potential applications, both to the application of closed-loop control in anesthesia and to the broader issues of automation in anesthesia and intensive care. In the final section of this paper I will address another problem – the question of the interaction between human beings and automated systems. These interactions are the source of many potential problems in the application of automation to real work environments.

Techniques of Artificial Intelligence

There are literally hundreds or thousands of alternative AI techniques which have been promulgated over the past 40 years. I have chosen to address five broad classes of these techniques (not an exhaustive sampling by any means) which differ in their representation of clinical knowledge and the means of relating such knowledge to changing information about the patient in the real world. The techniques are:

1. Rule-based production systems ("expert systems")
2. Neural network systems
3. Bayesian belief network systems
4. Physiologic modeling systems
5. General-purpose monitoring architectures

Rule-Based Production Systems

The earliest AI systems were largely rule based. Their knowledge base consists of a (possibly very large) set of *rules*, each of which is an IF/THEN statement connecting one or more premises to one or more conclusions. Given a set of input data which may satisfy some of the rules' premises, conclusions will be drawn. These, together with the original input data, may then satisfy yet other rules, generating new conclusions, and so on. Rules which are activated successfully (are "fired") are called "productions," hence another name for such systems is "production systems." The assumption is that a sufficient set of rules can capture sufficient knowledge to translate incoming clinical information into diagnoses and appropriate actions. Table 1 shows an admittedly simplistic illustrative example.

Of course, there are many issues not easily resolved by such simple application of rules. Rule-based systems require additional rules about what to do when

Table 1. Simple example of rule-based productions

Rule 1:	If the systolic blood pressure is less than 92 then hypotension is present.
Rule 2:	If the heart rate is greater than 105 then tachycardia is present.
Rule 3:	If hypotension is present and tachycardia is present then hypovolemia is present.
Rule 4:	If hypovolemia is present then administer colloid at a rate of 100 ml per min up to a maximum of 1000 ml.
Input data:	Heart rate = 130 Systolic blood pressure = 8 mmHg
Conclusions:	Hypotension is present; tachycardia is present; hypovolemia is present.
Actions:	Administer colloid at 100 ml per min up to a maximum of 1000 ml.

multiple competing rules have fired. Such rules about rules are called "meta-rules" and they embody strategic information about the most useful approaches to different goals. Another extra feature that has to be added is a means for handling uncertainty. The value of each measured variable has some uncertainty. Uncertainty is also a feature of the inferences represented in the rules. For example, hypotension and tachycardia do *not* always imply hypovolemia, although hypovolemia is a common cause of these two signs occurring together. When multiple chained inferences are made, each of them possessing a certain amount of uncertainty, the uncertainty of the final conclusion is likely to be higher than that associated with each of the intermediate states. Rule-based systems have utilized a variety of ad hoc empirical heuristics to deal with uncertainty. These have gone by names such as "certainty factor", "causal strength", and "evoking strength/ frequency-weight". However, these ad hoc solutions have not been highly effective. In the words of one of the developers of the "certainty factor" approach, these "ad hoc models were imprecise meldings of probabilistic and utility notions" [1].

Systems have been generated with hundreds, or thousands of rules. Nonetheless, only a few prototype systems for anesthesia or intensive care have been described [2–4].

Advantages and Disadvantages of Rule-Based Systems

The main advantage of rule-based systems is their simplicity. Rules can be readily expressed, either in standard programming languages or in generic shell programs designed for this purpose. Furthermore, domain experts have a relatively easy time generating some sorts of rules. Whether the experts can express the richness of their knowledge in the form of rules and meta-rules is another matter, however. Rule-based systems support explanation, since the sequence of rules leading to a conclusion can be retrieved and can be used to generate a readable plain-text explanation. A final advantage is that rule-based systems can be very successful. When the system to be dealt with can be described well in the form of a moderate number of straightforward rules, the performance is quite good. Rule-based expert systems are in use for a variety of purposes in the military and in industry (American Express is rumored to use an expert system to determine whether to approve or disapprove a charge). However, few if any rule-based expert systems are in routine use in either the OR or the ICU.

The main disadvantages of rule-base systems have been partially alluded to already. One is the difficulty in handling uncertainty when propagating chains of rules. Another is the fact that rule sets may be contradictory or inconsistent. Rules which are reasonable by themselves may chain together to produce contradictory conclusions. Weeding out the inappropriate conclusions may be difficult. In many cases the rules fail to identify the limitations on their scope of application. The expert knows these limitations but has a difficult time articulating them. Some types of knowledge are particularly difficult to encode as rules. Examples might include physiologic relationships and topographical or topological relationships between components or body systems. These relationships might be more easily encoded and utilized using another AI technique. Note also that fuzzy logic techniques (as described in this volume by Professor Zimmerman) may be added to rule-based systems so that they are not so dependent on the exact classification breakpoints and categories of "crisp logic".

Advantages and Disadvantages of Neural Networks

Neural networks are the topic of the paper by Professor Eckmiller in this volume, so I will not discuss them in detail, but I would like to comment on their advantages and disadvantages. To review, however, a typical neural network contains three layers of "neurons": the input layer, the middle layer, and the output layer. By means of training the network on a set of "training cases", for which the set of inputs and the set of outputs are known in advance, and using special training algorithms, the most common of which "back-propagates" changes in the weighting of the inputs and outputs of each neuron, the network will become trained or "tuned" to generate reasonably correct outputs from a given input.

Neural networks have many advantages. Using an appropriate neural network shell, they are, by definition, easy to program, since there is no program. The network itself instantiates its "knowledge" by the connectionist whole of its topology and the learned input/output weights. Neural networks are extremely fast in operation. Once trained, the neural network can nearly instantaneously translate inputs into outputs. Furthermore, because of the connectionist style of such a technique, the network may be sensitive to features that are not readily apparent to the domain experts. Given a rich training set, subtle combinations of inputs that reliably indicate a given output will be recognized.

Neural networks also have disadvantages, many of them related to training of the network. As James A. Reggia has written, in a review of neural computation in medicine: "Training can be slow and computationally expensive. These models require a large, representative database of training cases which can be difficult and costly to obtain" [5]. In any case, providing training cases can be most tractable if the number of inputs and outputs is small, and if cases can be unequivocally categorized to a specific output. These criteria may be met when a small number of inputs or sensors classifies a restricted set of diagnoses, and when the input data can be reliably generated by electronic or physical simulation with known fault conditions. The experiments of Westenskow's laboratory [6–8] are examples of successful application of neural networks to the analysis of faults in the anesthesia breathing circuit. However, extrapolating these techniques to more complex clinical conditions will be difficult. The number of inputs and the number of possible outputs will be much larger. Also, it will be impossible to generate reliable training data strictly through simulation (as did Westenskow's group), since there exists no fully reliable simulator of the wide spectrum of patient states that need to be recognized. If actual clinical data must be used to train the network there will be difficulty in unequivocally assigning a specific output (diagnosis) to a given set of input data. There will almost always be uncertainty as to the true underlying diagnosis and as to whether additional (hidden) co-existing faults or conditions may be confounding the network. As Reggia states: "Connectionist models based on methods such as error back-propagation have not been demonstrated to perform well for multiple disorder problems . . . and in fact there is evidence that they perform rather poorly" [5].

These difficulties are compounded by another property of neural networks; the same features that allow the network to recognize subtle combinations of features also mean that the network cannot readily provide an explanation for its outputs. The middle-layer neurons have no semantic meaning. One could list the strengths of activation for each node, but this would tell the user nothing. Therefore, when tuning the network it is impossible to determine whether unexpected confounding is occurring. The network can be *tested*, but it cannot be *inspected*. Finally, neural networks do not explicitly handle uncertainty, although active research in this area is going on.

Therefore, it is not surprising that neural network techniques can be extremely successful in restricted domains. Their high speed makes them particularly suitable for incorporation into real-time engineered systems, in which they will be relied on to conduct fault diagnosis or state recognition and classification with restricted sets of inputs and outputs. New techniques for designing and training neural networks may improve their applicability to more complex clinical decision paradigms, but this remains to be seen.

Bayesian Belief Networks

In the search for better ways to deal with probabilistic aspects of medical reasoning and the representation of uncertainty, a new technique was first described by Pearl in 1982 [9]. This technique, called Bayesian belief network (BBN) is "a directed acyclic graph in which the *nodes* represent stochastic variables and arcs between the nodes represent probabilistic relationships" [10, 11]. A prototypical example is shown in Fig. 1. In medicine, such a network can be established in advance from an analysis of known physiology or by expert assessments of which of these elements influence each other (BBNs are also known as "probabilistic influence diagrams"). The state of each higher node will affect the probability of occurrence of each state of the nodes connected to it below. The a priori probabilities of these influences can be adjusted in advance, based on what is known about the system.

The lowest nodes in these networks are typically *observables*, whose value can be measured in the real world by clinical examination, history, electronic monitoring, or laboratory testing. Using algorithms based on Bayes' theorem (which relates the a posteriori probability of an item to its a priori probability and the known values below it) the probability of each state of each node in the network can be recalculated as observed evidence arrives at the lowest-level (observable) nodes. Typically, the diagnoses or alarm states are the highest-level nodes, whose probabilities are of interest to the clinician. Thus, the typical output of such a

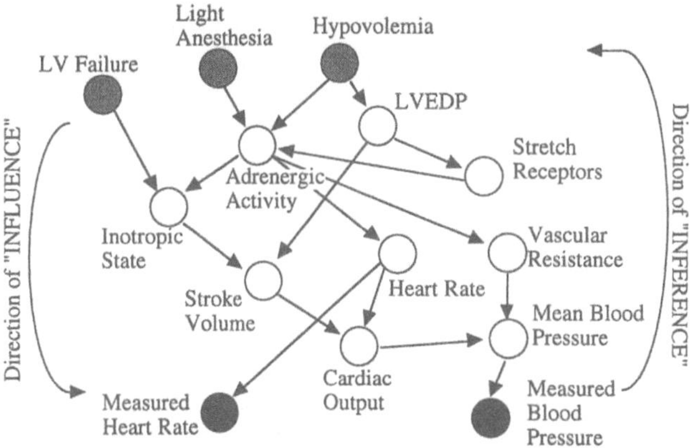

Fig. 1. A portion of a prototypical Bayesian belief network for anesthesia alarms. Each node has a set of possible values or states. The state of a node may affect the probability of the occurrence of states connected to it below. The network thus links states by probabilistic influence. Special algorithms update the probability of occurrence for each state of each node, using Bayes' theorem applied to actual data arriving at the lowest level nodes. (Based in part on the ALARM system [12])

network will be a list of probabilities of occurrence for each state of each node of interest. Further processing from this list can display an alarm or message whenever an important state (or combination of states) reaches a high enough probability.

Many such belief networks have been constructed for medical applications. This approach has become one of the dominant techniques used by the Medical Information Sciences Department at Stanford University School of Medicine, directed by the inventor of the first medical rule-based production system, Edward Shortliffe. This laboratory has adopted the belief network approach because it gives a precise definition of uncertainty. Ingo Beinlich, an anesthesiologist from Professor Stoeckel's program at the University of Bonn, performed graduate work at Stanford in which he developed belief networks for anesthesiologists. One early prototype called ALARM underwent bench testing in 1989 [12], and was also used as a vehicle to test another program which generated explanations from belief networks [10]. However, no fully capable belief network system of this type has been tested in real or simulated OR or ICU conditions.

There are advantages to the belief network approach. Each of the nodes is included in the network because medical knowledge has already established (even if imprecisely) a relationship between it and another node. Thus, a belief network can be built without the need to learn from a large set of training cases. However, it has been shown that a belief network can be trained from a database of inputs and outputs [11, 13]. Furthermore, the intermediate nodes of a belief network represent real conceptual entities that will be meaningful to domain experts. Because of this fact, it is possible to generate explanations from belief networks, and to guide the thinking of domain experts in this way. Therefore, the belief networks combine some of the advantages of neural networks while avoiding the disadvantages of hidden layers and abstract connection weights.

One of the major disadvantages of belief networks is that instantiating the initial probabilities between each state of each of the nodes is very tedious and labor intensive for expert(s), in spite of the availability of graphical tools to simplify the process of establishing nodes and linking them together. Furthermore, existing medical knowledge may not easily yield the kinds of probabilities between states that are required. Some preliminary work has been done on developing a translation between the kinds of terms that clinicians typically use and the probabilities (or probability distributions) needed by the network [14]. As yet, there appears to be no simple solution to this problem. Another limitation is that the updating algorithms for the belief networks, while markedly improved over the last few years, are still relatively slow. For large and complex networks it may not be possible to conduct the updating process in real time. While it is possible that some applications may not require quick updates, this is certainly the goal in very dynamic domains like anesthesia. Faster algorithms may be developed, and computational speed for a given cost is constantly improving. Still, it is not clear whether sufficient improvements will be made in the foreseeable future to make belief networks a feasible approach for complex automation in the OR and the ICU.

Physiologic Modeling

Another set of techniques of artificial intelligence deals with physiologic modeling. If one has a good model of physiologic processes, it should be relatively easy to adapt the model to a given patient, so as to explain and predict the patient's behavior. The mathematical techniques of quantitative modeling are well known to members of this workshop and will be dealt with in more detail in other presentations. Thus, with one exception, I will not address standard mathematical modeling techniques. The exception has to do with the complexity of the mathematical models. Dealing with mathematical models of ventilation, Rutledge et al. [15, 16] have shown that the most complete mathematical models have no analytic solutions and thus require very time-consuming numerical integration, making them inappropriate for most real-time applications. But only a few clinical situations require a very complex model. Most clinical questions can be answered with simpler models. Rutledge and colleagues have demonstrated how to define a hierarchy of models with differing levels of complexity and then choose the appropriate model based on the questions to be answered, the time available, and the speed of the computing resources at hand.

Another approach to physiologic modeling is to perform it in a qualitative rather than a quantitative fashion. Most clinical questions do not demand an exact quantitative solution. There has been considerable work on producing qualitative models in medicine. In anesthesia and ICU, Dawant and Uckun at Vanderbilt University have put together the YAQ qualitative modeling process ontology, which is then used in the SIMON monitoring architecture [17, 18]. YAQ is an extension of qualitative process theory, in which "the model equations are defined as qualitative *proportionalities* and *influences*" [17]. An example would be that blood pressure is qualitatively proportional to cardiac output, and that cardiac output is influenced by afterload. These qualitative relationships can be linked together much as differential equations are combined in mathematical models.

Advantages of qualitative modeling are that it requires less computing time than does quantitative modeling, and it may be easier to define an appropriate qualitative model compared with a fully quantitative model. However, qualitative modeling is still a rather new technique, and it is unclear how well the qualitative predictions can be used for patient management.

General-Purpose Monitoring Architectures

Finally, some artificial intelligence researchers are taking a more ambitious approach by attempting to define very complex general-purpose monitoring architectures which can use multiple techniques to provide diagnostic support and even closed-loop control. One example, with which I am associated, is the Guardian system developed at the Knowledge Systems Laboratory at Stanford University. Guardian's overall architecture is shown in Fig. 2. The heart of Guardian is a blackboard architecture – a knowledge and memory management scheme to which each component of the system can write information, and from which each component can read information [19]. Having a common blackboard allows the system, in principle, to use multiple reasoning systems at one time. A key feature of Guardian is that, like human beings, it adjusts its own monitoring of data streams based on the situation at hand. It can, for example, focus attention on certain items while ignoring others. Guardian is able to recognize patterns of signs and symptoms and classify them into relevant disease entities. At the present time the system has three diagnostic systems, although not all of them are fully functional. One, termed ReAct [20], recognizes critical conditions and recommends stereotypical but appropriate therapies. Another is based on parsimonious covering theory and yields probabilities of the existence of different disease states. This component can be thought of as a belief network which directly connects observables to diagnoses, based on the probability of occurrence of the observable, given the disease. Still another component, based on multilevel flow models (a type of qualitative modeling) can determine which physiologic goals are not being met and what would be necessary to meet them [21]. A new program, called the Skeletal Plan Instantiator (SPIN) is designed to control the selection and implementation of actions from the list of those relevant to the current diagnoses.

The main advantages of a general-purpose system like this are its flexibility and adaptability. In principle, it can have all manner of cognitive resources to deal with different levels of temporal need (like ReAct, which is optimized for rapid responses) or different levels of diagnostic complexity. It is also able to modify its

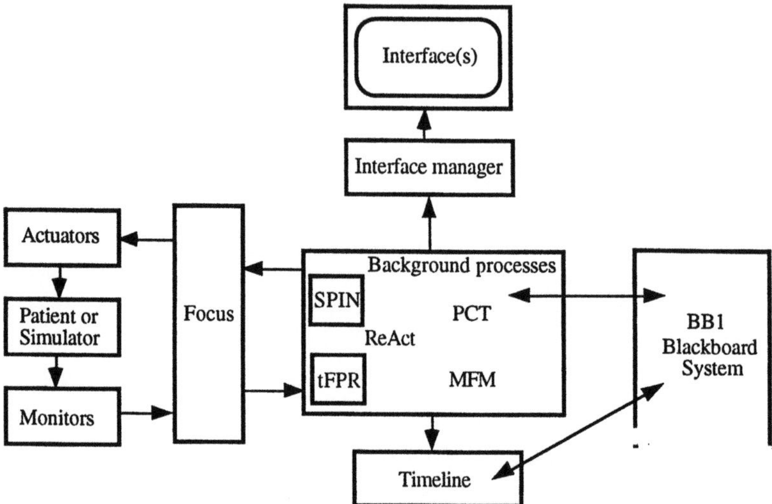

Fig. 2. Overall structure of the Guardian general-purpose monitoring system. Data from the patient (or a test simulator) enter on the left and are filtered and abstracted by a program called *Focus*. Static and temporal patterns are recognized by a program called the Temporal Fuzzy Pattern Recognizer (*tFPR*), which presents the patterns to other knowledge resources. These include *ReAct*, a system designed to react rapidly to high criticality conditions, and the diagnostic components *PCT* and *MFM* (described in the text). Actions are generated by ReAct and may be recommended by PCT and MFM. The implementation of actions is controlled through the Skeletal Plan Instantiator (*SPIN*), which can make recommendations to the clinician or (in principle) signal actuators (pumps, ventilators, etc.) directly. The *BB1 blackboard* is a shared memory and control structure for the diverse reasoning systems. (Adapted from a diagram drawn by Serdar Uckun, Knowledge Systems Laboratory, Stanford University)

own behavior in real time, adjusting the amount of information coming into the main part of the program. These features are essential when and if intelligent agents are to work semiautonomously or in closed-loop control of complex situations. Without such flexibility and adaptability an AI system is almost certain to be incapable of handling dynamically changing, complex situations with multiple problems, multiple manifestations, and multiple constraints.

The disadvantages of a general-purpose system are its complexity and the difficulty of coordinating and controlling all of the (potentially disparate) components. Furthermore, in the current implementation the system is rather slow, and as more cognitive features are added it is likely to become even slower.

AI Components as Adjuncts
to Traditional Closed-Loop Control

Artificial intelligence techniques are not only of use for the more complex tasks of diagnosis. They may also be useful as adjuncts to traditional types of closed-loop

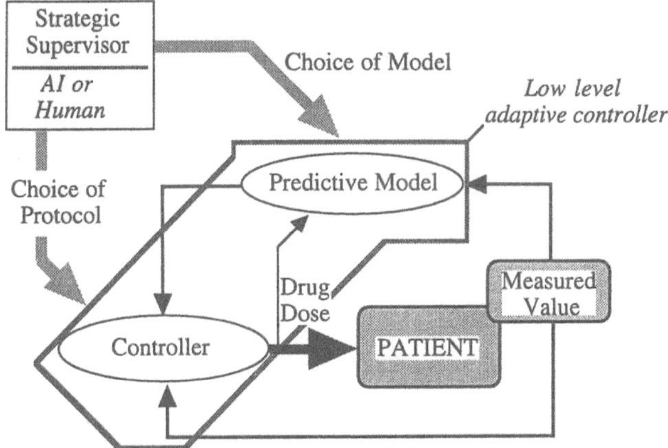

Fig. 3. An artificial intelligence (*AI*) or human clinician "supervisor" that alters the behavior of a standard "low-level" adaptive closed-loop controller. The supervisor can control changes both in the predictive model of future behavior, as well as in the choice of response protocols. The supervisor may increase safety by making the system responsive to context and other clinically relevant features of the patient

control. Standard (PID) closed-loop controllers base their control signals on one or more of the following: differences between the current and desired values of the variable being controlled (proportional control), the derivative of the difference, or the integral of the differences. However, these mathematical techniques may not suffice to allow control of all patients during rapidly changing clinical circumstances. Martin et al. (including N.T. Smith) have described a supervisory "shell" which modifies the control actions of a standard controller of a vasodilator (controlling blood pressure) in order to safeguard the patient from excessively aggressive control [22, 23]. In the case of Martin et al., the safety shell uses primarily if-then rules, but any other kind of AI technique could be imagined for this purpose. Similar supervisory shells have been described by others [24]. It is even possible for the supervisor to modify both the mathematical model of the process *and* the model of the effects or choices of control actions. This is shown diagramatically in Fig. 3.

Human-Device Interactions with Automated Systems and Closed-Loop Controllers

Automated systems under consideration for anesthesia and intensive care will not operate autonomously – they will be operated and monitored by human beings. Experience in industries like commercial aviation should make us wary of some of the pitfalls of introducing automated systems into the human work environment in anesthesia. Over the past 20 years psychologists, human factors engineers, and cognitive engineers have described a number of problems in the interaction of human operators and automated systems [25–30]. Some of these have already resulted in lethal accidents, while others have demonstrated the potential for adverse outcomes. In our own research and analysis of anesthesia safety we have begun to see the same phenomena occurring with existing rudimentary automation (automated blood pressure cuffs, infusion pumps), and it is highly likely that such problems will intensify if and when more complex and more powerful automated systems are introduced [31–34]. Thus, it is important to review these problem areas and to consider ways to avoid the pitfalls.

Automation May (Paradoxically) Increase Workload for Certain Tasks

Although one of the main reasons for introducing automation is to reduce the physical and mental workload on the operator, for some automated systems (especially those whose design makes them "clumsy" automation [27]) using and monitoring them to ensure correct operation imposes more workload than does performing the task manually. This is even more likely to be true for tasks that (when performed manually) rely on highly perceptual-motor skills. Thus, one cannot *assume* that automation will necessarily reduce workload. That is an empirical question which must be determined by experiment.

Automation May Reduce Some Errors But Induce Others

Automation is advocated for control of a process or a variable more precisely and with less constant attention by the anesthetist. In this regard, automation is usually thought of as reducing errors by providing constant, uniform control. However, the experience in aviation is that while automated systems often do prevent many kinds of errors, new types of errors have occurred. For example, it is widely believed that the KAL flight 007 event, in which a Korean airliner was shot down after straying into Soviet airspace, occurred because of a keyboard entry error by one of the pilots, and their subsequent failure to monitor their position by other means [27]. The use of key entry systems in anesthesia is increasing (especially with infusion pumps) and will be even greater for closed-loop controllers. Means for recognizing and trapping keyboard entry errors, and for making the results of key entries highly visible to the anesthetist will be important features of automated systems.

Mode Errors

Complex devices nearly always have multiple "modes" of operation. This increases their flexibility and usefulness in a larger variety of situations, or to support different styles of practice. Thus, an infusion pump could have modes for "ml/min", "μg/min", or "μg/kg per min." A more complex computer-controlled pump could also have modes for achieving a specified blood or effect compartment target level ("ng/ml"). A closed-loop controller could add other modes, for example, a "target median EEG frequency" mode. Because the same display screen and keyboard will be used for each of these modes, it will be very important to identify in which mode the device is operating and what the displayed and entered values mean. Errors made by human operators because they are confused as to which mode is active are called "mode errors" [26], and they have been found to be particularly problematic with aviation automation.

One aviation example of a mode error has to do with the autopilot/autoland system of a certain type of commercial airliner. The system can be used in a "glide slope" mode, in which the angle of descent (glide slope) is entered (3°, for example). Another mode is "descent rate", in which the descent rate is entered in feet per minute (or meters per minute). A numerical display such as "3.0" in glide slope mode would be quite normal, but if the device is in the descent rate mode, the same display would mean 3000 feet per minute, an excessively steep rate of descent (4–5 times steeper than that of a 3° glide slope). Such an error was probably the cause of an airliner crash in Europe several years ago.

Similar mode errors have been observed in anesthesiology and intensive care. One example involved a computer-controlled infusion pump. A nurse on the night shift in an ICU which used the pump to provide target concentration control of sedative drugs put the pump into a different mode of operation, for which the entered values caused a rapid infusion of sedative into the patient. Fortunately, this was noticed and the pump was stopped before a catastrophe ensued.

Complex devices often make it hard to determine what mode is active, how that mode was selected, and what the settings mean for that mode. There are many ways to prevent and mitigate mode errors, most of which depend on making such things *very* clear to the operator. Another strategy is to reduce the number of possible modes, eliminating those that are not absolutely necessary for patient care.

Automation-Induced Complacency

To the extent that successful automation *is* achieved, there are other, broader concerns. If the operator becomes used to reliable automated systems, will he or she still have the skill and experience to take over if the automation fails, or if the situation evolves outside the envelope of the automated system? Will the operator continue to monitor the automated system satisfactorily so as to recognize a failure or an unforeseen problem? Will automation reduce the overall level of vigilance of the operator?

These questions have not been systematically addressed for automated systems in anesthesiology. There is a case report [33] of anesthesiologists failing to recognize that an automated blood pressure cuff had not cycled for over 30 min, leading them to aggressively treat apparent hypertension, which in fact had changed to profound hypotension. There is also a report that many anesthesiologists cannot calculate the correct infusion rate for vasoactive drugs during a crisis [35]. An automated infusion pump capable of being set in micrograms per kilogram per minute might assist such individuals, but what would happen if this mode failed and the doses had to be calculated by hand?

Training Requirements for Safe Use of Automated Systems

For the reasons mentioned above and many others, practitioners must be thoroughly trained in the use of each automated system. Previous experience in anesthesiology does not bode well for the willingness or ability of many practitioners to acquire this training. The theoretical advantages of automated systems may accrue only to those who are fully familiar with them. When they are put into the hands of the average anesthesiologist or intensivist, there are enhanced risks of errors, especially when the equipment must be used in highly time pressured and dynamic situations. Thus, the net cost-effectiveness of automated equipment must consider the costs of errors made with it in the real world, in addition to device costs.

Careful Human Factors in Design and Thorough Realistic Testing Are Musts for Automated Systems in Anesthesia

The only way to avoid these pitfalls and reap the potential benefits of automation in the real world is to carefully design automated equipment and then to test it under a wide variety of stringent and realistic conditions in which failure is likely. Cognitive engineers now have better ways of preventing mode errors, by providing clear feedback about a device's operation to the user. The number of operating modes should be kept to a minimum. Appropriate cognitive analyses of the task to be supported and the device's operation will help to generate optimum designs. Average users should be tested with devices in (simulated) high-pressure crisis situations in which errors are likely to be more frequent. The errors and pitfalls made by individuals who have *not* received substantial training with the device should be documented, and designs revised to minimize or eliminate these error pathways. Without such safeguards it is likely that a number of catastrophes will occur with the introduction of automated systems. The backlash generated by such catastrophes could wipe away any hope of reaping benefits from them.

Conclusion

The application of standard mathematical control techniques to automation in anesthesia still has much to offer. However, it is likely that they will need to be supplemented by other techniques typically described as artificial intelligence. Simple rules or rule-based expert systems may suffice to supplement traditional mathematical techniques for many specific applications. Neural networks may be most effective for the rapid analysis of restricted sets of input data, while more complex analyses of large input sets will probably require a combination of techniques working in a cooperative, distributed architecture. Great care will need to be taken to ensure that fielded systems can be used effectively by human anesthesia and intensive care unit staff. This need will affect the design and testing of the devices, as well as the way they are sold and supported by manufacturers.

References

1. Shortliffe EH (1992) AI meets decision science: emerging synergies for decision support. In: Evans DA, Patel VL (eds) Advanced models of cognition for medical training and practice. Springer, Berlin Heidelberg New York, pp 71–89
2. van Oostrom JH, van der Aa JJ, Nederstigt JA, Beneken JEW, Gravenstein JS (1989) Intelligent alarms in the anesthesia circle breathing system (abstract). Anesthesiology 71:A336
3. Watt RC, Navabi MJ, Mylrea KC, Hammeroff SR (1989) Integrated monitoring "smart alarms" can detect critical events and reduce false alarms (abstract). Anesthesiology 71:A338
4. Loeb RG, Brunner JX, Westenskow DR, Feldman B, Pace NL (1989) The Utah anesthesia workstation. Anesthesiology 70:999–1007
5. Reggia JA (1993) Neural computation in medicine. Artif Intell Med 5:143–157
6. Westenskow DR, Orr JA, Simon FH, Bender HJ, Frankenberger H (1992) Intelligent alarms reduce anesthesiologist's response time to critical faults. Anesthesiology 77:1074–1079
7. Farrell RM, Orr JA, Kuck K, Westenskow DR (1992) Differential features for a neural network-based anesthesia alarm system. Biomed Sci Instrum 28:99–104
8. Orr JA, Westenskow DR (1994) A breathing circuit alarm system based on neural networks. J Clin Monit 10:101–109
9. Pearl J (1982) Reverend Bayes on inference engines: a distributed hierarchical approach, Proc AAAI-82 National Conference on Artificial Intelligence, Pittsburgh, PA. MIT Press, Cambridge, MA, pp 133–136
10. Suermondt HJ (1992) Explanation in Bayesian belief networks. PhD thesis, Stanford University
11. Pearl J (1988) Probabilistic reasoning in intelligent systems: networks of plausible inference. Morgan Kaufmann, San Mateo, CA
12. Beinlich IA, Gaba DM (1989) The ALARM monitoring system – intelligent decision making under uncertainty (abstract). Anesthesiology 71:A337
13. Herskovitz E, Cooper GF (1991) Kutato: an entropy-driven system for construction of probabilistic expert systems from databases. In: Bonissone PO, Henrion M, Kanal LN, Lemmer JF (eds) Uncertainty in Artificial Intelligence. North-Holland, Amsterdam
14. Beinlich IA (1990) Prototypical structures for probabilistic networks. Masters thesis, Stanford University
15. Rutledge GW (1993) Dynamic selection of models for a ventilator-management advisor. Proc Annu Symp Comput Appl Med Care (SCAMC): 344–350
16. Rutledge GW, Thomsen GE, Farr BR, Tovar MA, Polaschek JX, Beinlich IA, Sheiner LB, Fagan LM (1993) The design and implementation of a ventilator-management advisor. Artif Intell Med 5:67–82
17. Uckun S, Dawant BM (1992) Qualitative modeling as a paradigm for diagnosis and prediction in critical care environments. Art Intell Med 4:127–144
18. Uckun S, Dawant BM, Lindstrom DP (1993) Model-based diagnosis in intensive care monitoring: the YAQ approach. Art Intell Med 5:31–48

19. Hayes-Roth B (1985) A blackboard architecture for control. Art Intell 26:251–321
20. Ash D (1993) Diagnosis using action-based hierarchies for real-time performance. PhD thesis, Stanford University
21. Larsson JE (1992) Knowledge-based methods for control systems. Department of Automatic Control, Lund Institute of Technology, Lund, Sweden
22. Martin JF, Schneider AM, Quinn ML, Smith NT (1992) Improved safety and efficacy in adaptive control of arterial blood pressure through the use of a supervisor. IEEE Trans Biomed Eng 39: 381–388
23. Martin JF, Smith NT, Quinn ML, Schneider AM (1992) Supervisory adaptive control of arterial pressure during cardiac surgery. IEEE Trans Biomed Eng 39:389–393
24. Isaka S, Sebald AV (1993) Control strategies for arterial blood pressure regulation. IEEE Trans Biomed Eng 40:353–363
25. Woods DD (1990) Modeling and predicting human error. In: Elkind JI, Card SK, Hochberg J, Huey BM (eds) Human performance models for computer-aided engineering. Academic, Boston, pp 248–274
26. Sarter NB, Woods DD (1995) "How in the world did I ever get into that mode?" Mode error and awareness in supervisory control. Hum Factors (in press)
27. Wiener EL (1988) Cockpit automation. In: Wiener EL, Nagel DC (eds) Human factors in aviation. Academic, San Diego, pp 433–461
28 Norman DA (1988) The psychology of everyday things. Basic Books, New York
29. Norman DA (1992) Turn signals are the facial expressions of automobiles. Addison-Wesley, Reading, MA
30. Norman DA (1993) Things that make us smart. Addison-Wesley, Reading, MA
31. Cook RI, Potter SS, Woods DD, McDonald JS (1991) Evaluating the human engineering of microprocessor-controlled operating room devices. J Clin Monit 7:217-226
32. Cook RI, Woods DD, Howie MB, Harrow JC, Gaba DM (1992) Unintentional delivery of vasoactive drugs with an electromechanical infusion device. J Cardiothoracic Anesth 6:238–9244
33. Howard SK (1993) Failure of an automated noninvasive blood pressure device: the contribution of human error and software design flaw (abstract). J Clin Monit 9:232–233
34. Botney RI, Gaba DM (1995) Human factors issues in monitoring. In: Blitt C (ed) Monitoring in anesthesia and intensive care. Churchill Livingstone, New York, pp 23–54
35. Schwid HA, O'Donnell D (1992) Anesthesiologists' management of simulated critical incidents. Anesthesiology 76:495–501

II Assessment and Evaluation of Signals and Measurements

a) Anesthesia Machine Monitoring

Which Monitoring Qualities Ensure
Proper Machine Function?

H. Frankenberger

Introduction

Anaesthetists are in the relatively unusual position of administering potent lethal drugs to patients via medical devices. Their main objective is the safety of the patient and the production of conditions that are appropriate to the surgery being performed [1]. In general anaesthesia, anaesthetists have to affect, in a reversible controlled process, the patient's central nervous system in order to cause, for the period of surgery:

- Analgesia
- Unconsciousness
- Muscle relaxation
- Sedation and tranquilization

with minimal effects on the respiratory and cardiovascular systems. In any case, ventilation has to be assured for delivering oxygen to the lungs.

In many countries of the western world the current state of the art for reaching these goals is to administer different specific drugs, each drug to be controlled separately. The administration of drugs can be achieved via inhalation or via intravenous administration.

Anaesthetic Incidents and Consequences

The overwhelming majority of anaesthetics proceed uneventfully, but a routine anaesthetic may give rise to a dangerous or life-threatening situation; some of these situations can be avoided with appropriate monitoring. Cooper et al. [2], analysing "preventable anaesthesia mishaps", examined 359 incidents. Equipment failure was involved in 40% and, of these, 12% were associated with functional failure of anaesthetic machines [3]. Not included in these figures were, e.g., accidental disconnections of breathing circuits. In their report on anaesthetic mortality, Lunn and Mushin [4] analysed 6060 deaths and identified a group of 58 "for which the assessors believed anaesthesia was totally responsible." Thompson [3] states that "inadequate provision of essential monitoring instruments is a factor which cannot be ignored." He requires that the "safe design of anaesthetic equipment cannot be considered without referring to monitoring" [3]. Calkins [5] suggests that "some improvement and reduction of human error and equipment hazards is possible by monitoring the performance of the anaesthetic delivery system, consisting of the machine, ventilator and patient-breathing system". This kind of monitoring can assist in the prevention of anaesthetic incidents by providing information about the performance of medical devices.

DIN *13252*: "Inhalational anaesthetic apparatus: requirements for safety and testing"

In many countries the anaesthesia equipment used in the late 1970s was mainly inhalational anaesthetic equipment and consisted of the following basic components:

- Gas supply system (oxygen, nitrous oxide, air)
- Gas delivery system (oxygen–nitrous oxide, oxygen–air)
- Anaesthetic delivery system (halothane, enflurane, isoflurane)
- Breathing system (rebreathing system, nonrebreathing system)
- Ventilator
- Scavenging system

Various discrete instruments and devices of different manufacturers for parameters such as tidal volume, airway pressure, inspired oxygen concentration, ECG, and blood pressure were attached to the anaesthesia machine. No requirements for safety of anaesthesia equipment were formulated at that time.

From a technical point of view, this kind of anaesthesia machine can be considered as three actuators, operating in an open-control appliance via the breathing system on the patient. As long as the technical components are functioning properly, the anaesthesia machine ventilates the patient, delivers oxygen and delivers the anaesthetic drug according to the set values. The patient receives adequate concentrations if there are no leakages or obstructions in the system. The concept of open-control appliance does not allow for recognition of deviations from the set values if these values are not monitored. Without adequate machine monitoring the anaesthetist as the operator of the patient–machine system will recognise deviations from the set values only if there are observed undesirable reactions from the patient.

In 1979 the German Association for Anaesthesia and Intensive Care [6] published recommendations for the safety of anaesthesia machines. These recommendations included 15 points to be respected for the design and use of anaesthesia machines. Mandatory for each anaesthesia machine were the following monitors:

- O_2 monitor with low-oxygen alarm
- Airway pressure monitor with disconnect and stenosis alarm
- Ventilation volume monitor

These recommendations were the basis for the German standard DIN 13252: "Inhalational anaesthetic apparatus: requirements for safety and testing" published in 1984 [7]. The safety features required the above-mentioned monitors; the CO_2 monitor was included as an option for alternative ventilation monitoring. Further requirements were the following protection features against hazardous output:

- Noninterchangeable gas connections
- Gas-specific color coding
- Calibrated vaporizers
- Single vaporizer use
- Maximum concentration limitation for vaporizers
- Vaporizer back pressure-related concentration accuracy $\pm20\%$
- Agent-specific key filler
- Zero adjust for vaporizers
- O_2-supply failure alarm
- N_2O cut-off
- Haptic differentiation for O_2 and other flowmeter control knobs
- Maximum pressure limitation for ventilators
- Manual ventilation bag
- ISO 5356 conical connectors for breathing systems
- Checklist – at the beginning of an operating session
- Instructions for use, including methods for cleaning, disinfection, and sterilisation and recommended intervals for inspection.

Anaesthetic agent monitoring was not included; no reliable measuring equipment was available at that time.

The DIN 13252 safety standard was the result of a risk analysis. The following consequences were studied with the aim of avoiding or recognising at a very early stage:

- Hypoxia
- Hyperoxia
- Alveolar collapse
- Barotrauma
- Anaesthetic drug application too high
- Anaesthetic drug application too low
- Hypocapnia
- Hypercapnia

Anaesthesia machine-related causes of hypoxia can be:

- Lack of oxygen
- Inadequate oxygen flow
- Wrong gas (only N_2O) flowing to the patient

The following components for monitoring and avoiding hypoxia are required for each anaesthesia machine in the German DIN standard:

- Oxygen monitor with low alarm setting
- Oxygen-supply failure alarm
- N_2O cut-off

- Ventilation volume monitor
- Disconnect alarm
- Stenosis alarm
- Noninterchangeable gas connections
- Gas-specific color coding
- Haptic differentiation for O_2 and other flowmeter control knobs
- Manual ventilation bag
- ISO 5356 conical connectors for breathing systems

The cause of barotrauma can be excessive pressure in the lungs of the patient. The following components for monitoring and avoiding barotrauma are required in the German DIN standard:

- Airway pressure monitor with stenosis alarm
- Maximum pressure limitation for ventilators
- Adjustable pressure limitation (APL)

The cause of inhalation anaesthesia being too deep can be:

- Excessive anaesthetic drug administration
- Administration of the wrong anaesthetic drug

The following components for keeping inhalation anaesthesia from being too deep are given in the German DIN standard:
- Calibrated vaporizers
- Single vaporizer use
- Maximum concentration limitation for vaporizers
- Agent-specific key filler
- Zero adjust for vaporizers

No anaesthetic agent monitor was required at that time.

CEN TC *215* Standardisation Activities: Anaesthetic Work Stations and Their Modules – Essential Requirements

In 1987, the European Community agreed to develop the internal European market in which the free movement of goods is ensured. For the safety and health protection of patients and users of medical devices, these devices must meet the "essential requirements" set out in the annexes to the European Medical Device Directive [8] as a prerequisite for free trade. The "essential requirements" are best transposed into harmonised European standards which can be used for conformity assessment. The European standard organisation CEN initiated the European standard committee CEN TC 215 in February 1990 to develop an anaesthesia work-station standard with cross-reference to the "essential requirements" of the European Medical Device Directive.

The anaesthesia work-station concept for inhalation anaesthesia administration is a spin-off of Cooper's analysis and his concept of an "electronic anaesthesia machine with integrated monitoring" for increasing patient safety through reduction of the risk of human error and machine hazards. This concept no longer tolerates the "add-on" of medical devices and monitors to the anaesthesia work station. The monitoring of inhalation agents is mandatory in the proposed standard prEN 740: "Medical electrical equipment; anaesthetic work stations and their modules; particular requirements" [9]. The anaesthetic work station is defined in [9] as a "system for administration of inhalation anaesthesia which includes one or more actuator modules, its essential monitoring and alarm modules and essential hazard-protection modules." An actuator module performs the task of delivery of energy or substances in controlled quantities. The work station consists of the following actuator modules (Table 1):

- Driving power module (electrical, pneumatic)
- Anaesthetic gas delivery module
- Anaesthetic vapour delivery module
- Anaesthetic ventilator module
- Anaesthetic breathing system

The following monitor and alarm modules have to be integrated in the anaesthesia work station:

- The driving power actuator module has to include a power failure alarm module for the gas and electrical power. The power failure alarm module has to activate an audible alarm signal for at least 7s duration if the driving power falls below the minimum level specified.
- The anaesthetic gas delivery actuator module – if there is one on the anaesthetic work station – has to include:

Table 1. Anaesthetic workstation (pr EN 740-1994)

Actuator module	Monitoring + alarm module	Protection module
Driving power	Power failure alarm	
Anaesthetic gas delivery	O_2-supply failure alarm FiO_2 monitor + alarm	N_2O cut-off AGS
Anaesthetic vapour delivery	Anaesthetic agent monitor + alarm	AGS
Anaesthetic ventilator	Airway pressure monitor + alarm Expired volume monitor Breathing circuit integrity	Max. pressure limitation APL
Anaesthetic breathing system	CO_2 monitor + alarm Breathing system integrity Expired volume monitor Airway pressure monitor	Max. pressure limitation APL

APL, Adjustable pressure limitation; *AGS*, Anaesthetic gas scavenging system.

- - The oxygen supply failure alarm module. The anaesthetic gas delivery module shall be operated with an oxygen supply failure alarm module which generates an auditory alarm signal to indicate failure of the oxygen supply. The alarm signal shall be derived from the oxygen supply pressure.
  - The oxygen monitor and alarm module. The anaesthetic gas delivery module shall be operated with an oxygen monitor for the measurement of the inspiratory oxygen concentration. The monitor shall be provided with an operator-adjustable lower alarm limit.
- The anaesthetic vapour delivery actuator module – if there is one on the anaesthetic work station – has to include:
  - The anaesthetic gas monitor and alarm module. If the anaesthetic vapour delivery module can cause a safety hazard under single fault condition it shall be operated with an anaesthetic gas monitor and alarm module for monitoring the concentration of anaesthetic agent vapour in the inspiratory gas.
- The anaesthetic ventilator actuator module – if there is one on the anaesthetic work station – has to include:
  - The airway pressure monitoring and alarm module. If the anaesthetic work station is in use with an anaesthetic ventilator module it shall be operated with a means of monitoring the pressure in the anaesthetic breathing system during the complete breathing cycle. The monitoring module has to activate a high-priority alarm signal when the pressure exceeds the limit for high pressure. In case of disconnection of the patient from the anaesthetic ventilator or anaesthetic breathing system an alarm has to be activated.
  - The expired volume monitor and alarm module. If the anaesthetic work station is in use with an anaesthetic ventilator module it shall be operated with a means of monitoring the patient's expiratory tidal or minute volume. The low expired volume alarm shall not be delayed for more than 120 s.
  - The anaesthetic breathing system integrity (disconnect) alarm module. In case of disconnection of the patient from the anaesthetic ventilator or anaesthetic breathing system an alarm has to be activated.
- The anaesthetic breathing system module – if there is one on the anaesthetic work station – has to include:
  - The carbon dioxide monitor and alarm module. The breathing system shall be operated with a means of monitoring the patient's respired CO_2. A low expiratory carbon dioxide concentration alarm shall be provided.
  - The anaesthetic breathing system integrity alarm module. In case of disconnection of the patient from the anaesthetic ventilator or anaesthetic breathing system an alarm has to be activated.

Each anaesthesia work station has to be equipped with protection modules which, without intervention of the operator, perform the task of protecting the patient against hazardous output due to incorrect delivery of energy and substances. Included is also the protection of the operator and the atmosphere in the operating room from expired and/or excess anaesthetic gases. The following protection modules have to be integrated into the anaesthesia work station:

– Protection module for cut-off gases other than oxygen

If the anaesthetic work station is in use with an anaesthetic gas delivery module for gases other than oxygen, air or premixed gases as, e.g. Entonox, it shall be operated with a gas cut-off device. This gas cut-off device shall be activated when the oxygen supply pressure falls below a specified value. It shall either cut off the supply of all gases other than oxygen, air and premixed gases with an oxygen content above 21%, or progressively reduce the flow of all other gases (except air or the above-mentioned premixed gases) while maintaining the proportion of oxygen until the supply of oxygen finally fails, at which point the supply of all other gases (except air or the above mentioned premixed gases) shall be cut off. The gas cut-off device shall not be activated before the oxygen supply failure alarm.

– Maximum airway pressure protection module

If the anaesthetic work station is in use with an anaesthetic ventilator module and/ or an anaesthetic breathing system it shall be operated with a maximum pressure protection module which ensures that a pressure of 125 cm H_2O not be exceeded at the patient connection port.

– Adjustable airway pressure limitation protection module

If the anaesthetic work station is in use with an anaesthetic ventilator module and a maximum airway pressure protection module set at a maximum pressure it shall be provided with an adjustable airway pressure limitation protection system to prevent a pressure build-up in excess of 80 cm H_2O.

– Anaesthetic gas pollution protection module

If the anaesthetic work station is in use with an anaesthetic gas delivery module for gases other than oxygen and air, or with an anaesthetic vapour delivery module, it shall be used with an (AGS) anaesthetic gas scavenging system.

Conclusion

The question: "Which monitoring quantities ensure proper anaesthesia machine function?" has been discussed for inhalational anaesthesia machines and work stations under the aspect of different standardisation activities. Bases for deciding about the adequate monitoring quantities are risk analysis and methods for investigating in a systematic manner what kind of safety measures have to be integrated in a technical system – such as an anaesthesia work station – to avoid undesired mishaps. The actuator functions of the inhalational anaesthesia work station such as anaesthetic gas delivery, anaesthetic vapour delivery, anaesthetic ventilation have to be safeguarded by adequate monitoring and alarm modules. If the anaesthetist decides about the necessary actuator functions of the anaesthesia work station he also decides about the necessary monitoring quantities, as laid down in the proposed European standard prEN 740.

If in future anaesthesia workstations are going to be on the market based on liquid administration of anaesthetic agents via infusion pumps, risk analyses will have to be applied to evaluate the parameters to be monitored. If the safety of the patient is to have the same predominant role as for inhalational anaesthesia work stations, monitoring devices will be necessary to indicate if the preset values on the infusion pumps are administered to the patient. This means that some kind of liquid flow monitoring is necessary to ensure proper infusion pump function. Following the essential requirements of the European Medical Device Directive, this is absolutely mandatory.

References

1. Crankshaw DP, Beemer GH (1991) How should we administer intravenous anaesthetic drugs? Baillieres Clin Anaesthesiol 5:327
2. Cooper JB, Newbower RS, Long CD, McPeek B (1978) Preventable anesthesia mishaps. Anesthesiology 49: 399
3. Thompson PW (1987) Safer design of anaesthetic equipment. Br J Anaesth 59:913
4. Lunn JN, Mushin WW (1982) Mortality associated with anaesthesia. Nuffield Provincial Hospitals Trust, London
5. Calkins JM (1985) Monitoring the anesthetic delivery system. In: Blitt CD (ed) Monitoring in anaesthesia and critical care medicine. Churchill Livingstone, New York
6. Ahnefeld FW (1979) Die Sicherheit medizinisch-technischer Geräte und Anlagen. Anasthesiol Intensivmed 11:279
7. DIN 13252 (1984) Inhalationsnarkosegeräte: sicherheitstechnische Anforderungen und Prüfung. Beuth, Berlin
8. Council Directive 93/42/EEC of June 14, 1993 concerning medical devices. Official J. of the Europ. Communities No. L 169. vol 36, July 12
9. DIN EN 740 (1992) Medizinische elektrische Geräte; Anästhesie-Arbeitsplätze und deren Module; Besondere Anforderungen; Deutsche Fassung prEN 740. Beuth, Berlin

Reliability, Testability, Alarms, and the Fail-Safe Concept

J.S. Gravenstein

Introduction

Reliability and testability of equipment used in anesthesia, alarm technology, and the fail-safe concept can be discussed from the perspective of the investigator or as experienced by the clinician in 1994. In this presentation I will present the view of the North American clinician working with modern and well-established equipment rather than with experimental or advanced research systems. Therefore, I shall focus on current systems in terms of their reliability; I shall mention testing practices, delineate alarms, and examine how far we have come to realize fail-safety. Finally, I shall address conceptual issues surrounding the question of reliability, testability, alarm technology, and the fail-safe system.

Reliability

It is well established that the majority of mishaps in anesthesia are attributable to mistakes and errors committed by the user, that is, to human failures rather than to malfunction of equipment [1, 2]. One might expect that such observations would lead to the adoption of strict standards that describe the level of skill expected of the operator of anesthesia equipment. The airline industry, where human failure is also far more common than equipment malfunction, operates with well-defined performance standards that pilots must meet before they are permitted to fly commercial aircraft. At least in the United States, such human performance standards do not exist for anesthesia personnel. Even though the problems lie primarily with human performance and not with malfunction of equipment, we have many standards describing how equipment is to be manufactured and what features the equipment must have in order to make it as safe as possible within reasonable economic restraints. A multitude of agencies have formulated standards that describe how the equipment is to be built and what features the equipment should have. An abbreviated list of national and international, governmental and voluntary agencies that have issued recommendations, regulations, and standards appears in Table 1. These agencies deal with relatively readily definable problems, such as the diameters of connectors, the colors of cylinders containing a medical gas, or the need for monitors and alarms; yet the work of the regulating committees and agencies progresses exceedingly slowly and

Table 1. Selected standard-setting organizations

International Standards Organization (ISO)
Deutsche Industrienorm (DIN)
International Electrotechnical Committee (IEC)
European Standards Organization (CEN)
Food and Drug Administration (FDA)
Medizinische Geräteverordnung (MedGv)
American Society for Testing & Materials (ASTM)
American National Standards Institution (ANSI)

---

often with disparate results. Consequently, in some instances the well-intended efforts of these agencies have led to confusion and incompatibilities, particularly across national borders. Indeed, the pace of progress is sometimes so slow that standards, when they finally appear, fail to keep up with developments and practices.

Testability

Interesting cross-currents mark the questions of testing of equipment. On the one hand, manufacturers attempt more and more to incorporate in their devices the automatic protocols for testing and calibration of the equipment; on the other hand, clinical personnel are being urged to adopt routine testing conventions. A study by the Food and Drug Administration of the United States (FDA) had demonstrated that clinicians do not understand the operation of their equipment well enough to discover malfunctions [3]. In response to this troublesome observation, the FDA, in close cooperation with clinical and engineering experts, published in 1986 its version of an adequate "pre-check list" of an anesthesia machine containing 24 steps (Table 2) that were to be completed daily before such a machine was to be used [4]. However, experience soon demonstrated that the requirements were too laborious. Execution of a proper FDA-recommended pre-test took

Table 2. Anesthesia apparatus checkout recommendations of 1986 (From [4])

This checkout, or a reasonable equivalent, should be conducted before administering anesthesia. This is a guideline that users are encouraged to modify to accommodate differences in equipment design and variations in local clinical practice. Such local modifications should have appropriate peer review. Users should refer to the operator's manual for special procedures or precautions.

1. Inspect anesthesia machine for:
    a. Machine identification number
    b. Valid inspection sticker
    c. Undamaged flowmeters, vaporizers, gauges, supply hoses; complete, undamaged breathing system with adequate CO_2 absorbent
    d. Correct mounting of cylinders in yokes
    e. Presence of cylinder wrench

Table 2 (*Contd.*)

---

*2. *Inspect and turn on:*
Electrical equipment requiring warm-up (ECG/pressure monitor, etc.)

*3. *Connect waste-gas scavenging system:*
Adjust vacuum as required

*4. *Check that:*
   a. Flow-control valves are off
   b. Vaporizers are off
   c. Vaporizers are filled (not overfilled)
   d. Filler caps are sealed tightly
   e. CO_2 absorber by-pass (if any) is off

*5. *Check oxygen (O_2) cylinder supplies:*
   a. Disconnect pipeline supply (if connected) and return cylinder and pipeline
      pressure gauges to zero with O_2 flush valve.
   b. Open O_2 cylinder; check pressure; close cylinder and observe gauge for evidence
      of high-pressure leak.
   c. With the O_2 flush valve, flush to empty piping.
   d. Repeat as in *b* and *c* above for second O_2 cylinder, if present.
   e. Replace any cylinder less than about 600 psig.
   f. Open less full cylinder.

*6. *Turn on master switch (if present)*

*7. *Check nitrous oxide (N_2O) and other gas cylinder supplies:*
Use same procedure as described in *5a* & *b* above, but open and *CLOSE*
flow-control valve to empty piping. Note: N_2O pressure below 745 psig indicates that
the cylinder is less than 1/4 full.

*8. *Test flowmeters:*
   a. Check that float is at bottom of tube with flow-control valves closed (or at min.
      O_2 flow if so equipped).
   b. Adjust flow of all gases through their full range and check for erratic movements
      of floats.

*9. *Test ratio protection/warning system (if present):*
Attempt to create hypoxic O_2/N_2O mixture, and verify correct change in gas flows
and/or alarm.

*10. *Test O_2 pressure failure system:*
   a. Set O_2 and other gas flows to mid-range.
   b. Close O_2 cylinder and flush to release O_2 pressure.
   c. Verify that all flows fall to zero. Open O_2 cylinder.
   d. Close all other cylinders and bleed piping pressures.
   e. Close O_2 cylinder and bleed piping pressure.
   f. CLOSE FLOW CONTROL VALVES.

*11. *Test central pipeline gas supplies:*
   a. Inspect supply hoses (should not be cracked or worn).
   b. Connect supply hoses, verifying correct color coding.
   c. Adjust all flows to at least mid-range.
   d. Verify that supply pressures hold (45–55 psig).

*12. *Add any accessory equipment to the breathing system:*
Add PEEP valve, humidifier, etc., if they might be used (if necessary, remove after
step 18 until needed).

Table 2 (*Contd.*)

---

13. *Calibrate O_2 monitor:*
    *a. Calibrate O_2 monitor to read 21% in room air.
    *b. Test low alarm.
    c. Occlude breathing system at patient end; fill and empty system several times with 100% O_2.
    d. Check that monitor reading is nearly 100%.

14. *Sniff inspiratory gas:*
    There should be no odor.

*15. *Check unidirectional valves:*
    a. Inhale and exhale through a surgical mask into the breathing system (each limb individually, if possible).
    b. Verify unidirectional flow in each limb.
    c. Reconnect tubing firmly.

##16. *Test for leaks in machine and breathing system:*
    a. Close APL (pop-off) valve and occlude system at patient end.
    b. Fill system via O_2 flush until bag just full, but negligible pressure in system. Set O_2 flow to 5 l/min.
    c. Slowly decrease O_2 flow until pressure *no longer rises* above about $20\,cm\,H_2O$. This approximates total leak rate, which should be not greater than a few hundred ml/min (less for closed-circuit techniques).
    CAUTION: Check valves in some machines make it imperative to measure flow in step *c* above when pressure *just stops rising.*
    d. Squeeze bag to pressure of about $50\,cm\,H_2O$ and verify that system is tight.

17. *Exhaust valve and scavenger system:*
    a. Open APL valve and observe release of pressure.
    b. Occlude breathing system at patient end and verify that negligible positive or negative pressure appears with either zero or 5 l/min flow and exhaust relief valve (if present) opens with flush flow.

18. *Test ventilator:*
    a. If switching valve is present, test function in both bag and ventilator mode.
    b. Close APL valve if necessary and occlude system at patient end.
    c. Test for leaks and pressure relief by appropriate cycling (exact procedure will vary with type of ventilator).
    d. Attach reservoir bag at mask fitting, fill system and cycle ventilator. Ensure filling/emptying of bag.

19. *Check for appropriate level of patient suction.*

20. *Check, connect, and calibrate other electronic monitors.*

21. *Check final position of all controls.*

22. *Turn on and set other appropriate alarms* for equipment to be used.
    (Perform next two steps as soon as is practical.)

23. *Set O_2 monitor alarm limits.*

24. *Set airway pressure and/or volume monitor alarm limits* (if adjustable).

---

* If an anesthetist uses the same machine in successive cases, the steps marked with an asterisk need not be repeated or may be abbreviated after the initial checkout.
A vaporizer leak can be detected only if the vaporizer is turned on during this test. Even then, a relatively small but clinically significant leak may still be obscured.

almost 20 min, too long to be acceptable in clinical practice. A revised, abbreviated pre-check list was therefore published in 1993 [5]. It had been reduced to 14 steps (Table 3) and was assumed to require only about 5 min for completion. It was also understood that the complete check had to be executed only once a day. Then, before subsequent anesthetics were used with the same machine and on the same day, only an abbreviated check of steps was considered necessary. How the profession will accept this list and whether clinicians will adhere to it remains to be seen.

Now a word about testing of personnel. In the United States, committees of the American Society of Anesthesiologists and of the Anesthesia Patient Safety Foundation have raised the question of whether anesthesia personnel should be "credentialed" in the use of complex equipment in order to ensure competency of the user. Some have suggested that an anesthetist would need to invest about 2 days of learning in order to become thoroughly familiar with a new, modern anesthesia machine. However, the production pressure experienced by clinicians working in the United States makes it unlikely that such thorough preparations will be adopted. Indeed, in many instances, new equipment is brought to a hospital and an "in-service" exercise is offered by the person representing the manufacturer. Typical in-service exercises are scheduled for less than an hour, are not attended by all clinicians, some of whom cannot free themselves from clinical responsibilities, and are not repeated. Even colleagues who manage to attend an in-service demonstration may forget what they were told and, half a year later, may find themselves confronted with a machine or device they have never used and have not thought about for many months. Of course, there are operating manuals that should help. Many of them are written by engineers who tend to stress aspects of engineering design rather than clinical utility. Manufacturers' attorneys add legal language that makes the document even harder to scan for clinical guidance. Finally, anesthesia equipment is commonly operated by many different users, not every one of whom has seen or can find the operating manual.

Manufacturers need to realize that clinicians often do not know as much about the equipment as the designers of the equipment assume [6]. To alleviate that deficiency, in-service exercises should be enhanced, instruction of clinical personnel intensified, and the design of the equipment improved. Manufacturers need to realize that anesthetists are as unlikely to read instruction manuals as travelers are unlikely to read the manuals that come with rental cars. Perhaps manuals will be read more often if they are better written. In the United States the FDA has now published a manual giving useful suggestions on how to write a good manual [7].

A good test of a well-designed piece of equipment is to let it be used (perhaps in a simulator) by a clinician who has never seen the device before. It will quickly become apparent whether the device meets the "intuitively obvious" test. As a minimum, new equipment should come with built-in instructions that enable the newcomer to operate the equipment at a basic, safe level.

Table 3. Anesthesia apparatus checkout recommendations, 1993

This checkout, or a reasonable equivalent, should be conducted before administration of anesthesia. These recommendations are vaild only for an anesthesia system that conforms to current and relevant standards and includes an ascending bellows ventilator and at least the following monitors: capnograph, pulse oximeter, oxygen analyzer, respiratory volume monitor (spirometer) and breathing system pressure monitor with high- and low-pressure alarms. This is a guideline that users are encouraged to modify to accommodate differences in equipment design and variations in local clinical practice. Such local modification should have appropriate peer review. Users should refer to the operator manual for specific procedures and precautions.

Emergency ventilation equipment
*1. Verify backup ventilation equipment is available and functioning.

High-pressure system
*2. Check O_2 cylinder supply
    a. Open O_2 cylinder and verify at least half full (about 1000 psi).
    b. Close cylinder.

*3. Check central pipeline supplies
    a. Check that hoses are connected and pipeline gauges read about 50 psi.

Low-pressure system
*4. Check initial status of low-pressure system
    a. Close flow control valves and turn vaporizers off.
    b. Check fill level and tighten vaporizers' filler caps.

*5. Perform leak check of machine low-pressure system
    a. Verify that the machine master switch and flow control valves are OFF.
    b. Attach "Suction Bulb" to common (fresh-) gas outlet.
    c. Squeeze bulb repeatedly until fully collapsed.
    d. Verify bulb stays *fully* collapsed for at least 10 s.
    e. Open one vaporizer at a time and repeat *c* and *d* as above.
    f. Remove suction bulb, and reconnect fresh-gas hose.

*6. Turn on machine master switch and all other necessary electrical equipment.

*7. Test flowmeters
    a. Adjust flow of all gases through their full range, checking for smooth operation of floats and undamaged flowtubes.
    b. Attempt to create a hypoxic O_2/N_2O mixture and verify correct changes in flow and/or alarm.

Scavenging system
*8. Adjust and check scavenging system
    a. Ensure proper connections between the scavenging system and both APL (pop-off) valve and ventilator relief valve.
    b. Adjust waste gas vacuum (if possible).
    c. Fully open APL valve and occlude Y-piece.
    d. With minimum O_2 flow, allow scavenger reservoir bag to collapse completely and verify that absorber pressure gauge reads about zero.
    e. With the O_2 flush activated, allow the scavenger reservoir bag to distend fully, and then verify that absorber pressure gauge reads $<10\,cm\,H_2O$.

Table 3 (*Contd.*)

Breathing system

*9. Calibrate O$_2$ monitor
   a. Ensure monitor reads 21% in room air.
   b. Verify low O$_2$ alarm is enabled and functioning.
   c. Reinstall sensor in circuit and flush breathing system with O$_2$.
   d. Verify that monitor now reads greater than 90%.

10. Check initial status of breathing system
   a. Set selector switch to "Bag" mode.
   b. Check that breathing circuit is complete, undamaged and unobstructed.
   c. Verify that CO$_2$ absorbent is adequate.
   d. Install breathing circuit accessory equipment (e.g., humidifier, PEEP valve) to be used during the case.

11. Perform leak check of the breathing system
   a. Set all gas flows to zero (or minimum).
   b. Close APL (pop-off) valve and occlude Y-piece.
   c. Pressurize breathing system to about 30 cm H$_2$O with O$_2$ flush.
   d. Ensure that pressure remains fixed for at least 10 s.
   e. Open APL (pop-off) valve and ensure that pressure decreases.

Manual and automatic ventilation systems

12. Test ventilation systems and unidirectional valves
   a. Place a second breathing bag on Y-piece.
   b. Set appropriate ventilator parameters for next patient.
   c. Switch to automatic ventilation (Ventilator) mode.
   d. Turn ventilator ON and fill bellows and breathing bag with O$_2$ flush.
   e. Set O$_2$ flow to minimum, other gas flows to zero.
   f. Verify that during inspiration bellows delivers appropriate tidal volume and that during expiration bellows fills completely.
   g. Set fresh gas flow to about 5 l/min.
   h. Verify that the ventilator bellows and simulated lungs fill and empty appropriately without sustained pressure at end expiration.
   i. *Check for proper action of unidirectional valves.*
   j. Exercise breathing circuit accessories to ensure proper function.
   k. Turn ventilator OFF and switch to manual ventilation (Bag/APL) mode.
   l. Ventilate manually and ensure inflation and deflation of artificial lungs and appropriate feel of system resistance and compliance.
   m. Remove second breathing bag from Y-piece.

Monitors

13. Check, calibrate and/or set alarm limits of all monitors
   Capnograph   Pulse oximeter   O$_2$ analyzer
               Respiratory volume monitor (spirometer)
            Pressure monitor with high and low airway pressure alarms

Final position

14. Check final status of machine
   a. Vaporizers off   d. All flowmeters to zero (or minimum)
   b. APL valve open   e. Patient suction level adequate
   c. Selector switch to "Bag"   f. Breathing system ready to use

---

* *If an anesthesia provider uses the same machine in successive cases, these steps need not be repeated or may be abbreviated after the initial checkout.*

Alarms

The institution of alarms was the natural consequence of the introduction of automated monitors that sense and measure biologic signals. It was a relatively easy task to designate thresholds, the crossing of which was deemed to signal an unacceptable deviation from normal. Alarm thresholds were built in by the manufacturer – so-called default alarms – based on estimates made by consulting clinicians. Most thresholds were made adjustable to enable clinicians to use them with patients with pathologic vital signs. Every transgression triggered an alarm. These alarms were initially a beep; later designs included a written message, and most recently the auditory signal was modulated to enable the clinician to identify the source of the alarm by the nature of the sound. Today monitors of numerous variables come equipped with alarms that sound at the crossing of upper and lower levels. With some 20 or more potential alarms in an operating room, it is small wonder that we now talk of "alarm pollution", where clinicians report hearing so many alarms that they no longer know which threshold has been crossed or whether a beeper or telephone has sounded.

Alarm pollution is not the only issue. Difficult to answer are questions of where to set the threshold for every single variable, where to set thresholds for multiple variables forming a pattern (for example, hypotension and tachycardia as contrasted to hypotension and bradycardia), and whether alarms should be sounded for short-lasting as well as for protracted deviations. Finally, we must ask whether an alarm should be sounded when developing conditions suggest an adjustment of the clinical management, or whether alarms should be reserved for true emergencies that are judged to be life threatening [8]. Problems also occur because false alarms are common [9]. The difficulties engulfing the alarm technology have not yet been resolved to the satisfaction of most clinicians. Because of artifacts causing false alarms and the problems surrounding current alarm technology and philosophy, it is still common for clinicians to disable alarms, sometimes with disastrous consequences for the patient.

The Fail-Safe System

The evolution of anesthesia machines has been powerfully influenced by mishaps reported to the manufacturers. For every item listed in Table 4 there are examples of mishaps and disasters that the manufacturer hoped to avert by modifying the machine or adding features. The majority of these features were designed to protect the patient from the hazards of receiving not enough oxygen, the wrong gas, excessive pressure in the breathing circuit, or no ventilation because of a disconnection or misconnection. One system designed to protect the personnel in the operating room was the gas-scavenging system. It may not have contributed anything to the safety of the anesthetist, but it may have caused some fatalities of patients when the system was used improperly [10]. In general, the growing complexity of equipment introduces new potential hazards because complex equip-

Table 4. Safety features of modern anesthesia machines

 1. 25% Oxygen
 2. Standing bellows
 3. Integrated vaporizer
 4. Ventilator low-pressure alarm
 5. Latching and bayonet-type connections
 6. Size-dissimilar fittings
 7. Special vaporizer manifold
 8. Integrated bag/ventilator selector switch
 9. CO_2 absorber with internal gas circuits
10. Low-pressure oxygen shut-off
11. Oxygen analyzer

ment contains more possibilities of malfunction and misuse. Thus, complexity may bring advantages but often only at a price. Overall, I submit that the advantages of more sophisticated and complicated design outweigh the problems introduced by added complexity.

Conceptual Issues

As a challenge, let me state three tenets:

1. Many measurements in anesthesia are contaminated by uncontrolled and often unknown variables.
2. Many alarms do not reflect physiologically meaningful events.
3. The fail-safe concept is a chimera.

Ad 1:
Analogies have been drawn between anesthetists and pilots (both operate complex systems and must make rapid decisions) and between anesthesia machines and automobiles (experienced users should be able to operate different models without additional training). Such analogies can be useful, but they fail when we consider that pilots do not fly sick planes and drivers of automobiles are not expected to pinpoint problems with the equipment when the car breaks down. Yet, the anesthetist takes care of patients with unpredictable physiologic responses that may affect the signals monitored during anesthesia, and the anesthetist is expected to pinpoint malfunction of the equipment even while using it. Three examples can illustrate these points.

a) We must ensure that the anesthesia machine delivers oxygen in volumes and concentrations chosen by the anesthetist. Ideally, we should identify the gas that flows from the central piped gas supply and measure its rate of flow before it enters the breathing circuit. This we do not do. Instead, we only measure the concentration of oxygen in the breathing circuit – often using instruments with slow response times that do not enable us to distinguish inspired from expired concentrations of oxygen. Many clinicians can recall cases where oxygen and nitrous oxide pipelines had been crossed during repairs and where the anesthesia machine delivered nitrous oxide from the oxygen flow meter. The problem could not be discovered as long as both gases were used at approximately equal flow rates. A lower than normal average oxygen concentration in the breathing circuit could have many explanations, including a leak in the machine itself or the breathing circuit, through which some of the fresh gas escaped.

b) We wish to ensure that the patient's arterial carbon dioxide tension remains in a range desired by the clinicians. We therefore measure inspired and expired concentrations of the gas with the help of a capnograph. If, during general anesthesia of a paralyzed patient whose lungs are ventilated mechanically, the end-tidal carbon dioxide tension is observed to decrease, we cannot tell whether a leak in the collecting capillary, hyperventilation, or increased alveolar dead space is responsible for the finding. An elevated end-tidal PCO_2 may be the consequence of malfunction of a one-way valve, exhausted carbon dioxide absorber, hypoventilation, or malignant hyperthermia [11].

c) We wish to present the patient with a concentration of inhalation anesthetic designed to achieve a desired effect. We adjust the vaporizer accordingly, but we do not know what it delivers because the gas analyzer sampling inspired and expired gas will show values that are quite different from the one we have selected. The time constant of the system, the fresh-gas flow chosen, the patient's uptake of anesthetic, and the anesthetic concentration of the expired gas – all will affect the inspired anesthetic concentration. We cannot tell whether the vaporizer is accurate.

Ad 2:

Unphysiologic values may be well tolerated if they last only a short time; nearly physiologic values may not be tolerated if they last a long time: The relationship between duration and threshold is not linear.

Alarm conditions are context sensitive. For example, a reduction of systolic pressure from 120 to 90 mmHg signals no trouble at all if it occurs in response to deepening anesthesia, but it signals severe trouble if it occurs in response to tracheal intubation under light anesthesia.

Large differences exist among patients and their ability to tolerate abnormal physiologic values. In a patient with a space-occupying lesion in the brain the reduction of mean arterial pressure from 120 to 100 mmHg may be accompanied by loss of consciousness, while such a change in the majority of patients is tolerated without consequence. We cannot predict threshold values for different patients.

Ad 3:

The manufacturers of anesthesia machines have responded to uncounted anecdotal experiences of hypoxia reported to have occurred during anesthesia. Hypoxic gas mixtures were attributed to crossed pipelines, inadequate oxygen supply pressure, improperly attached cylinders, leaks, inappropriate setting of flowmeters, and disconnections. Each one of these mechanisms was rendered less likely by the introduction of safeguards that have become standards for anesthesia machines and anesthesia ventilators. Several years ago, the president of a major manufacturer of anesthesia machines told me that significantly fewer lawsuits based on anesthestic mishaps had been brought against his company in recent years as compared with the past. He attributed this to the introduction of safety features on his machines, because there appeared to be a chronologic relationship between more safety features and fewer lawsuits. His competitor had similar experiences. This anecdote exemplifies the process that has been observed throughout the anesthesia machine industry. It is a natural process. It is the process we expect of ethical manufacturers. A feature is recognized that – without a malfunction – can lead to a mishap. For example, older machines had two separate oxygen flowmeters; one for flow rates below 1000 ml/min, the other for liters per min. When the anesthetist misread the correctly labeled flowmeters and administered 200 ml/min instead of 2000 ml/min of oxygen with 2 l/min nitrous oxide, the patient suffered hypoxic brain damage. In response to this potential misuse, the oxygen flowmeters were redesigned. We would expect a reduction or elimination of this type of mishap with the introduction of the new flowmeter. However, were we challenged to show with scientific rigor that the more expensive machine with new safety features was safer, we would fail. We could not document that the high purchase price of an anesthesia machine with many safety features is justified by ensuring a better outcome for our patients than could be achieved with the continued use of an older machine without safety features. Accidents have not disappeared, and it is still possible to harm patients with modern anesthesia equipment.

A Perspective

We believe that we have made progress. Today we use equipment that has many safety features; we use monitors that present physiologic data of many variables known to signal trouble when they change all too much during anesthesia and when nothing is done about correcting them. Yet we have failed on two counts:

1. Anesthesia is not yet fail-safe. Anesthetic mishaps still exact a toll. Most of the mishaps are probably linked to human failure. Even though we cannot document it scientifically, most anesthesiologists are convinced that the design of modern anesthesia equipment has helped to reduce the incidence of preventable mishaps. Many examples come to mind. Here are but three: First, although an alert clinician would not attach a nitrous oxide cylinder to an oxygen yoke, the pin-index system makes it almost impossible to do so. Second, although an alert clinician would detect a disconnected breathing hose anyway, a disconnect alarm would make it almost impossible not to recognize it. Third, although an alert clinician would discover excessive pressure in the breathing system, a pressure alarm would make it almost impossible to miss such a development with potentially fatal consequences.

Despite these safety features, disasters continue to happen, if infrequently. Hypoxic gas mixtures can still be given, for example, when an inadequate fresh gas flow may have been selected. The causes of many disasters are complex and multifactorial. Sometimes, the very complexity of modern equipment may contribute to human errors. We can predict that new safety features will be incorporated in the next generation of equipment. Perhaps they will further decrease the already low frequency of disasters. But even they are not likely to make anesthesia 100% safe because there is no such thing as a completely fail-safe system.

2. We have failed to document the benefit of the new safety features of anesthesia machines and monitors. Thrifty administrators, therefore, might argue that there is no point in spending money on expensive anesthesia equipment as there is no evidence that it will improve the patients' fate or reduce cost.

Why have we failed to document the effects of advances in our specialty? Runciman, in an excellent editorial [12], reminds us that the well-established, prospective, randomized, double-blind quantitative methods suffer from several weaknesses. Political, ethical, and financial constraints may make them difficult to execute. A priori hypotheses are required, which may preclude the identification of interesting outliers. Values must often be reduced to numbers that describe only one facet (perhaps not the most interesting) of a multifaceted phenomenon. Runciman believes that we should examine the applicability of qualitative research to our field.

In future studies of anesthesia morbidity I would like to suggest that we look beyond mortality and focus on morbidity. We should not limit ourselves to an examination of the all too obvious morbidity that includes broken teeth and nerve palsies. Instead, we should listen to what the patients tell us about their experiences. How did they feel after anesthesia? Did they notice cognitive deficits after the anesthetic and operation? Such deficits may affect 10% or more of our patients and may last for weeks to months. We do not know yet whether they are related to anesthesia (the most likely candidate) or to other perioperative events. Nor do we know what causes them. If they are linked to anesthesia, this important outcome variable would require intensive study.

Perhaps the incidence of such cognitive deficits was higher in years gone by when older anesthetics and equipment were used. We need to measure these variables and determine if they are linked to what we do. Then we can initiate an informed discussion of the desirable safety features and procedures that may affect outcome of anesthesia.

References

1. Cooper JB, Newbower RS, McPeek B (1978) Preventable anesthesia mishaps: a study of human factors. Anesthesiology 49:399–406
2. Weinger MB, Englund CE (1990) Ergonomic and human factors affecting anesthetic vigilance and monitoring performance in the operating room environment. Anesthesiology 73:995–1021

3. Lee DE (1991) Pre-operative check-list revisited. ASA Newslett 55:9
4. Carstensen P (1986) FDA issues pre-use checkout. Anesthesia Patient Safety Foundation Newslett 1:13–15
5. Morrison JL (1994) FDA Anesthesia apparatus checkout recommendations, 1993. ASA Newslett 58:25
6. Gravenstein JS, Larkin CR jr (1994) Equipment competency – we might have a problem. J Clin Monit 10:1–3
7. Food and Drug Administration (1994) Write it right. J Clin Monit (in press)
8. van Oostrom JH, Gravenstein C, Gravenstein JS (1993) Acceptable ranges for vital signs during general anesthesia. J Clin Monit 9:321–325
9. McIntyre JWR (1985) Ergonomics: anaesthetists' use of auditory alarms in the operating room. Int J Clin Monit Comput 2:47–55
10. Keats AS (1990) Anesthesia mortality in perspective. Anesth Analg 71:113–119
11. Gravenstein JS, Paulus DA, Hayes T (1994) Gas monitoring in clinical practice. Butterworth, London (in press)
12. Runciman WB (1993) Qualitative versus quantitative research – balancing cost, yield and feasibility. Anaesth Intensive Care 21:502–505

The Differences Between Closed-Circuit, Low-Flow, and High-Flow Breathing Systems: Controllability, Monitoring, and Engineering Aspects

L.H.D.J. Booij and J.G.C. Lerou

Introduction

During inhalation anaesthesia the breathing system serves to control the composition of the alveolar gas mixture. As shown in Fig. 1, the breathing system has a crucially important place in a very complex system composed of many subsystems. The breathing system is the interface between the patient and the anaesthesia system, and therefore it should be properly designed and adequately monitored.

Fundamental requirements for the administration of anaesthesia are accuracy, reproducibility, reliability, controllability, ease of administration, cost-effectiveness and safety. Anaesthetic equipment has to fulfil the same requirements. It must allow us to control physiological and other variables in an accurate, reproducible, reliable, controllable, easy, cost-effective and safe way. Only 10% of anaesthesia mishaps are the direct result of equipment failure, whereas 90% are due to human error [1]. However, one third of human errors are involved in an interaction with the anaesthesia machine or the breathing system. Thus many human-machine interfaces between the components of the anaesthesia system (Fig. 1) and the practitioner are areas of possible improvement, regardless of the fresh-gas flow used. Well-designed anaesthesia systems may prevent or at least reduce the incidence of human error.

The essence of low-flow and closed-circuit anaesthesia is to control the alveolar gas mixture without delivering a high flow of fresh gas into the breathing system. Closed-circuit anaesthesia must be considered a safe technique, because it has been shown that a difference in outcome between "open" and closed-circuit anaesthesia does not exist (Table 1) [2]. However, this does not mean that every breathing system and every anaesthesia machine is suitable for closed-circuit anaesthesia. Although there are many common aspects in the design and the use of breathing systems, there are also clinically important differences. We will deal with some engineering, monitoring, and controllability aspects of the differences between closed-circuit, low-flow, and high-flow breathing systems.

Definitions

Anaesthesiologists have used a variety of criteria to classify anaesthesia breathing systems. A functional classification was proposed by Hamilton [3], who used the

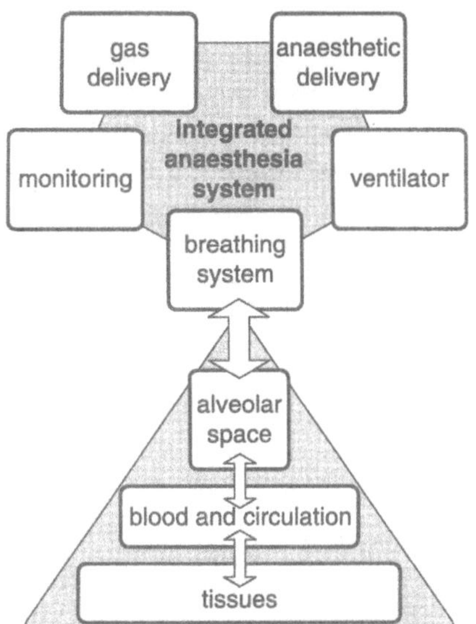

Fig. 1. Complex system composed of patient and anaesthesia system. Note the unique place of the breathing system

Table 1. Comparison of outcome of open- versus closed-circuit anaesthesia (300 patients). (From [29])

	Open mean (SE)	Closed mean (SE)	p-Value for difference
Emergence (min)	11.25 (1.43)	8.24 (1.46)	0.07
PARS on arrival	8.31 (0.11)	8.57 (0.12)	0.05
RR-time (min)	114.15 (6.87)	120.46 (7.06)	0.44
Δ Temp (°C)	−1.74 (0.11)	−1.73 (0.10)	0.95
Complications	3	5	0.24
Patient's rating (0–10)	9.58 (0.10)	9.77 (0.10)	0.09
Undesirable cardiovascular effects (%)	14.85 (3.32)	14.80 (4.44)	0.98

PARS, Post anaesthesia recovery score; *RR-time*, time in recovery room.

total delivery flow rate to define the type of system. Because of the complexity and the semantics of the material we will limit ourselves to the circle system. A well-designed circle system, including a carbon dioxide absorber and one-way valves, allows the anaesthesiologist to use fairly different rates of fresh-gas flow. This leads to the terms "closed-circuit", "low-flow" and "high-flow", as defined below. In addition, we introduce the term "low-flow techniques".

Closed-circuit

In a closed circuit the fresh-gas flow equals the patient's uptake; thus, closed-circuit anaesthesia requires a *unique* flow rate. In an average "normal" adult patient total gas uptake is less than 500 ml/min, e.g., 250 ml/min oxygen, 150 ml/min nitrous oxide, and 10 ml/min isoflurane. A carbon dioxide absorber is absolutely necessary because all exhaled gases are recycled. Thus the efficiency of the system is optimal. This is an important feature because anaesthetic agents, including nitrous oxide, are expensive. The *efficiency* of a breathing system is defined as the amount of gas taken up by the patient divided by the amount of gas delivered. For example, the efficiency of a closed system for oxygen is 250/250 = 1. In contrast, the efficiency of a system using 3 l/min oxygen is 250/3000 = 0.083. Since the efficiency of a closed system equals 1 for all gases and vapours, it cannot be improved.

Low-flow

With low flow, the fresh-gas flow is much smaller than the respiratory minute volume, say 0.5–1.5 l/min. There is partial rebreathing; thus a carbon dioxide absorber is mandatory. Low-flow systems have been defined on a rather arbitrary basis. Three authors have introduced three different definitions. Aldrete uses Brody's number, i.e. $10\,BW^{0.75}$, multiplies it by an arbitrary factor 6, and thus obtains $60\,BW^{0.75}$ as the upper limit for the fresh-gas flow during low-flow anaesthesia (note: BW = body weight) [4]. According to this definition, the fresh-gas flow must be smaller than 1.45 l/min for a 70-kg patient. Foldes et al. have proposed a total of 1 l/min (500 ml/min of oxygen and 500 ml/min nitrous oxide) [5]. Virtue has introduced the term "minimal-flow" for his technique with a total of 0.5 l/min (300 ml/min of oxygen and 200 ml/min of nitrous oxide, i.e., 60% oxygen in the fresh gas) [6]. We advocate the definition of Aldrete because it has an objective basis. We preserve the term "minimal flow" for the unique combination proposed by Virtue, since it helps to remember the rule of thumb: "The longer the anaesthetic procedure, and the lower the fresh-gas flow, the higher the oxygen concentration in the fresh gas."

The efficiency of a low-flow breathing system is intermediate. For example, suppose 15 ml/min isoflurane is administered to the circle system, while the patient's uptake is 10 ml/min. Thus the efficiency for isoflurane is 10/15 = 0.67.

High-flow

With high flow, the fresh gas flow equals or exceeds the ventilatory minute volume. There is little or no rebreathing, and a carbon dioxide absorber is not really necessary. Therefore, an alternative nonrebreathing system other than the classical, rather complex, circle system may be used. The efficiency of such a system is extremely low. For example, suppose a fresh-gas flow of 6000 ml/min nitrous oxide, while 100 ml/min is taken up. The efficiency is 100/6000 = 0.02. In other words, 98% of the nitrous oxide is vented to the atmosphere. This represents a large portion of anaesthetic pollution and cost.

Low-flow Techniques

Below, we will use the single term "low-flow techniques" to designate all techniques using less than 1.45 l/min for a 70-kg patient. Thus, the term includes low-flow and closed-circuit anaesthesia as defined above.

The Relationship Between Engineering, Monitoring, and Controllability

Concentrating on traditional questions about low-flow and closed-circuit breathing systems, we will deal with a – necessarily incomplete – list of their specific features. The following list of real or supposed characteristics of low-flow techniques will be discussed:

1. *Engineering aspects*: Low-flow techniques require special leak-proof equipment, including calibrated flow meters, accurate vaporizers, and a standing bellows ventilator, all in excellent condition.
2 *Monitoring aspects*: Low-flow techniques place severe demands on the quality and quantity of monitoring equipment because the gas concentrations are unpredictable in breathing systems using low rates of fresh-gas flow.
3 *Controllability aspects*: Low-flow techniques prevent the rapid increase or decrease of the concentration of volatile anaesthetic.

These three aspects are strongly interrelated. Engineers, using modern technology, have already solved some putative controllability problems associated with low-flow techniques. There are well-known solutions for others, but manufacturers hesitate to introduce them, fearing that their innovations will not find widespread acceptance. To illustrate the relationship between engineering, monitoring, and controllability we give an example: the control of the alveolar isoflurane concentration. Figure 2 shows a specific example of the general theoretical scheme of a control loop. A control loop consists of a controlled variable, a sensor, a comparator, and an effector. Our example shows the controlled variable, i.e., the alveolar isoflurane concentration, and a sensor that measures the value of the controlled variable, e.g., a mass spectrometer. The measured value is compared with a target value or set point. If a difference is present, proper intervening action has to be selected and effectuated to restore the controlled variable to within the desired range. The effectors in the example are the anaesthetic delivery and absorption systems. The target value is part of a model of the system to which the controlled variable belongs.

The sensor is an essential part of the control loop. Hence, no sensor, no control. Adequate sensors are the products of good engineering and should be part of our monitoring equipment. Thus, controllability depends on engineering and well-devised monitoring equipment.

Using traditional technology for the delivery of a volatile anaesthetic, the anaesthesiologist – acting as comparator and selector – selects and manipulates a

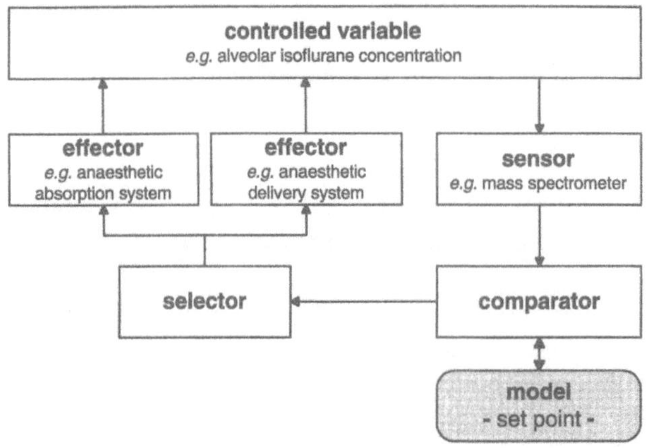

Fig. 2. Control loop for the alveolar isoflurane concentration

vaporizer to keep the alveolar isoflurane concentration within narrow limits (Fig. 2). The vaporizer output is the product of concentration and gas flow. With a traditional vaporizer outside the circle, anaesthetic mass flow is therefore limited during closed-circuit operation. This suggests that the low-flow technique prevents the rapid increase of the concentration of volatile anaesthetic. However, this is an engineering problem. The peculiar problem can be solved by injecting liquid isoflurane directly into the gas stream in very small boluses. Inserting a charcoal filter into the closed circuit absorbing all isoflurane rapidly decreases the alveolar isoflurane concentration without disturbing closed-circuit conditions (Fig. 2). This points out again that controllability is a subject of engineering.

Furthermore, adequate control is possible only if a valid model exists of the system that is to be controlled. Adequate knowledge of a model of the behaviour of isoflurane in the entity "patient-circle system", for instance after its injection as a liquid in a closed circuit, is a prerequisite for safe and accurate control. Real control of the isoflurane concentration is therefore possible only if we have at least: (a) an adequate sensor, (b) a clinically validated model, and (c) adequate and effective effectors. This again demonstrates the relationship between controllability, engineering, and monitoring.

Differences Between the Breathing Systems

We will review the real or supposed characteristics of low-flow techniques listed above.

1. *Low-flow techniques require well-maintained leakproof specialized equipment, and accurate gas and anaesthetic delivery systems.*

Well-maintained Leak-proof Equipment

All anaesthesia equipment should be maintained in excellent condition and thoroughly tested before use, whatever the required fresh-gas flow. The effects of leakage on the breathing system – and thus on the control of the patient's alveolar gas – may be more marked under low-flow conditions than in high-flow systems. However, this depends only on the size of the leakage in proportion to the fresh-gas flow. Even small leaks prevent the successful use of low-flow techniques. Obviously, the low-flow advocate will pay utmost attention to the integrity of the breathing system [7]. However, a leak check should be part of the pre-use checkout and inspection procedure of the components of the anaesthesia machine (Fig. 1), regardless of the fresh-gas flow [8].

Specialized Equipment: Standing Bellows Ventilator

During closed-circuit anaesthesia the volume of the breathing system is maintained constant. A constant circuit volume can be ascertained through a standing (rising) bellows ventilator. This respirometer type of ventilator exhausts gas only when the bellows expands to the top of its housing. If fresh gas is added to the breathing system so that the bellows height is maintained below the top of the housing, no gas is vented to the atmosphere. The flowmeters then reflect the uptake of oxygen and nitrous oxide. An accurate gas delivery unit in the range of 0–500 ml/min is therefore required (see further).

The standing bellows is not merely a part of the ventilator; it has added value as a noninvasive monitoring device. Because of its considerable size, it can be satisfactorily observed from a distance too great for deciphering the information on an electronic display. Under low-flow conditions, the bellows rises to its end-tidal position only if the tidal volume has successfully entered and left the patient. Thus the bellows measures and monitors the movement of gas to and from the patient's alveolar space (Fig. 1). Consequently, the rate of rising of the bellows mirrors the rate of the passive exhalation. Exhalation is completely patient dependent, and a too-slow rising of the bellows reveals bronchospasm or kinking of the expiratory limb of the circle system. Furthermore, the bellows reflects gas uptake and thus the factors governing uptake. A sudden drop in gas uptake, e.g., owing to a drop in cardiac output, causes a sudden higher end-tidal position of the bellows. In addition, slight diaphragmatic motion, indicating recovery from a muscle relaxant, or changes in intrathoracic volume (cardiogenic oscillations) show up as tiny movements of the bellows at its end-tidal position. These benefits are lost under high-flow conditions because the excessive fresh-gas flow – and not the exhaled gas – forces the bellows to expand.

A standing bellows ventilator is usually combined with the continuous delivery of fresh gases into the circuit. Consequently, the amount of fresh gas entering the system during inspiration is passed to the patient in addition to the tidal volume the ventilator delivers. Thus the fresh-gas flow rate [9] and the inspiratory-expiratory ratio (I:E ratio) affect the tidal volume [10]. With I:E = 1:2, one third of the fresh-gas flow contributes to the volume delivered to the patient. For example, suppose 6000 ml/min of fresh gas is used, the breath rate is 10 per min, and I:E = 1:2. With these settings, 200 ml is added to the tidal volume set on the ventilator. If the fresh-gas flow is 600 ml/min, the added volume is only 20 ml. This means that by simply reducing the fresh-gas flow from 6000 to 600 ml/min, the tidal volume delivered to the patient will be cut down by 180 ml (200 minus 20).

The unwanted effects on the tidal volume can be prevented by a reservoir. The fresh gases are delivered to this reservoir and do not enter the breathing system during the inspiratory phase. Consequently, the monitoring function of the standing bellows is lost, and the administration of closed-circuit anaesthesia is virtually impossible since there is no means of monitoring the constant volume of the breathing system. The practitioner has to balance the pros and cons of the standing bellows principle. We think the pros outweigh the cons.

The complete picture may be puzzling for the clinician because a part of the delivered tidal volume is lost to the breathing system compliance. This compliance is due to (a) the compressibility of the gases within the system, and (b) the distensibility of the breathing system components. The breathing system compliance therefore depends on the dimensions and the distensibility of the system components. An example will clarify the impact of system compliance. System compliance can be measured, but let us assume that it is 100 ml/kPa (or 10 ml/cm H_2O). In addition, suppose an atmospheric pressure of 100 kPa and a peak inspiratory pressure of 2 kPa (or 20 cm H_2O). Owing to the compressibility of a gas, the gas volume is compressed by 2% (ratio of the absolute pressures is 102/ 100). This loss is relatively small. The total loss will be 100 ml/kPa times 2 kPa, or 200 ml. This means that the tidal volume delivered to the patient will be reduced by 200 ml.

We summarize the effects of the fresh gas flow and the breathing system compliance on the tidal volume as follows:

predicted, effective tidal volume = tidal volume set on ventilator + G−L

where G is the volume added by the fresh-gas flow, and L is the volume lost by compliance. Specifying the two factors G and L, we obtain:

$$V_{pe} = V_s + \frac{\dot{V}R}{fR + f} - CP$$

where V_{pe} is the predicted effective tidal volume, V_s is the tidal volume set on the ventilator, $\dot{V}$ is the fresh gas flow, f is the ventilatory rate, R is the I:E ratio, C is the breathing system compliance, and P is the peak inspiratory pressure.

As an example, we calculate V_{pe} for $V_s = 1000$ ml, $\dot{V} = 6000$ ml/min, $R = 0.5$ (I:E is 1:2), $f = 10$/min, $C = 100$ ml/kPa, and $P = 2.5$ kPa. V_{pe} then equals 950 ml. Under the same conditions but with $\dot{V} = 300$ ml/min and a decline of P to 2 kPa, V_{pe} equals 810 ml.

The equation presented above is nothing more than a rule of thumb. The alveolar ventilation should be controlled by means of adequate sensors, i.e., the combination of volume measurement in the expiratory limb of the breathing system, capnometry at the lips of the patient, pulse oximetry, and blood-gas analysis. However, this is mandatory for any anaesthetic procedure, whatever the fresh-gas flow rate is.

Patient Breathing System

As for the impact of different fresh-gas flows, relevant properties of the patient breathing circuit are: the unidirectional valves, the fresh-gas utilization, and the CO_2 removal. In a circle system three valves exist: two unidirectional breathing valves and the adjustable pressure-limiting valve (APL). The first two valves force the circulation of gas into one direction. The movable part in the valve, i.e., a flat disc, should be specifically constructed to prevent the build-up of water, because considerable condensation occurs within the valve during prolonged use of low-flow techniques. The presence of water droplets may cause a reversed flow of the gases or even sticking of the valve. In some designs of the circle system, the unidirectional valves are replaced by a fan causing unidirectional gas flow.

The concentration of both respiratory gases and anaesthetic agents in a circle system depends on the particular design chosen by the engineer. For example, the differences in design have an impact on (a) the elimination of alveolar gas [11], and (b) the fresh-gas utilization (FGU). Zbinden and co-workers defined the FGU of a circle system as the ratio of the amount of gas reaching the patient's lungs to the total amount of fresh gas [12]. They have shown that some circle systems use the fresh gas more efficiently than others. An ideal breathing system has an FGU of 100%, no matter what is the rate of fresh-gas flow. Under low-flow conditions the FGU was higher than 90% for all circle systems studied. However, the FGU decreased rapidly in all systems when fresh-gas flows greater than 3 l/min were used. With a fresh gas flow equal to the respiratory minute volume (8 l/min) the FGU ranged from 40 to 85%. This points out the greater economy of low-flow breathing systems, the relationship between engineering and controllability, and the value of gas analysis even in high-flow systems.

A rebreathing system relies on the efficiency of the carbon dioxide absorption. The nonrebreathing system has a definite advantage in this respect, because its very nature precludes all possible problems associated with the removal of carbon dioxide from rebreathed gas.

Whatever the fresh gas flow, the pressure in the breathing circuit must be monitored accurately to detect excessive alveolar pressure. As to the detection of disconnections, we believe that capnometry at the Y-piece is superior to a pressure-sensitive monitor, because many circumstances may fool the latter.

Gas Delivery System

The usual gas delivery unit consists of a rotameter and a needle valve; one delivery unit is used with each gas. Clinical practice requires that flows with a range of two magnitudes, say 0.1–10 l/min, can be delivered. To overcome the engineering problems associated with this great range of flows, low and high flowmeters are used in series. Thus two flowmeters arranged in series are used for each gas, i.e., oxygen, nitrous oxide and air, This arrangement may add to the physical dimensions of the anaesthesia system, especially if long flow tubes are used to maximize readability, adjustability and ease of use. In addition, safety devices are incorporated to guarantee at least 20% oxygen in the fresh gas. Although this conventional set-up allows us to safely administer high-flow and closed-circuit anaesthesia, it prevents easy and optimal control of the circle gas during low-flow techniques.

To illustrate, we focus on the implications of the conventional gas delivery system for the practice of closed-circuit anaesthesia: (a) Frequent manual adjustments of the fresh-gas flows are necessary to compensate for changes in gas uptake; (b) although the buffering effect of a closed breathing system prevents rapid changes in gas concentrations, the interdependence of oxygen and nitrous oxide delivery further impedes optimal control.

These problems can be solved by a feedback-control system to control the circuit volume and the oxygen concentration in a closed breathing system. It has been shown that existent technology can control the circuit volume through the nitrous oxide flow and the inspired oxygen concentration via the oxygen flow [13, 14]. This again illustrates the utmost importance of appropriate sensors and effectors in a control loop [15], as well as the relationship between engineering, monitoring and controllability.

Anaesthetic Delivery System

Volatile anaesthetic agents have narrow therapeutic ranges. Thus, gas delivery systems should be accurate and reliable, not only under low-flow but also under high-flow conditions. With the arrival of reliable inhalation agent monitors it has become, in our opinion, less important which technique is used to introduce the agent into the circuit (e.g., vaporizer, manual injection, infusion pump, electronically controlled vaporizer). The attention should be focused on the ability to rapidly change the amount of agent delivered. The output of most vaporizers is not only limited, but also nonlinear at gas flows below 1 l/min and depends on the ratio of oxygen/nitrous oxide in the fresh-gas flow [16].

The methods using injection of a liquid anaesthetic agent have some definite advantages when compared with the plenum vaporizers currently in use. From an engineering standpoint, it is advantageous that injectors do not require mixed technology to make them computer controlled. In contrast, with the use of a vaporizer outside the circle, the manual injection of liquid anaesthetic achieves total independence of the fresh-flow rate and the composition of the fresh gas. Unfortunately, the frequent interventions necessary while injecting the liquid boluses add to the array of tasks of the anaesthesiologist. Liquid injection, however, lends itself to computer control, and a feedback-controlled infusion system is the direction for the future. Stable alveolar concentrations can be rapidly achieved and maintained with an automated anaesthetic delivery system [17, 18]. Designing such a system benefits from the use of clinically validated models.

Injection of anaesthetic liquid in combination with closed-circuit anaesthesia allows us to quantitate the patient's uptake. Anaesthesiologists have been used to administering a certain percent of an inhalation anaesthetic into a high-flow system. They have been totally unaware of the actual amount of anaesthetic taken up by the patient through the lungs. In contrast, they know the exact dosages of the anaesthetics administered via the intravenous route and enter them meticulously on the anaesthetic record. The exact dose of the potent inhalation anaesthetic with its narrow therapeutic range should not remain unknown. This is feasible through the use of injectors of liquid anaesthetic while providing closed-circuit anaesthesia.

2. *Gas concentrations are unpredictable; low-flow techniques therefore have severe demands on the quality and quantity of monitoring equipment.*

We have developed a model to predict the behaviour of volatile agents in closed circuits [19]. Clinical studies yielded the predictive performance of this model for isoflurane [20] and enflurane [21]. Figure 3 suggests that an extended version of our system model might be capable of predicting the enflurane concentrations under low-flow conditions. There is close agreement between the predicted concentrations and those we measured by respiratory mass spectrometry (200 MGA, Centronics, England). Other models exist for other gases. Thus, it is safe to conclude that it is feasible to predict the composition of alveolar gas concentrations, even if there is increasing difficulty as fresh-gas flow is reduced.

However, the anaesthesiologist should never rely solely on model predictions. The interpatient variability in uptake prevents the blind use of calculated drug regimens [22]. These should be accompanied by the measurement of the gases and vapours present in the breathing system. Adequate monitoring is thus mandatory. Some recent developments invalidate the argument that low-flow techniques require too much and too expensive monitoring in comparison with high-flow

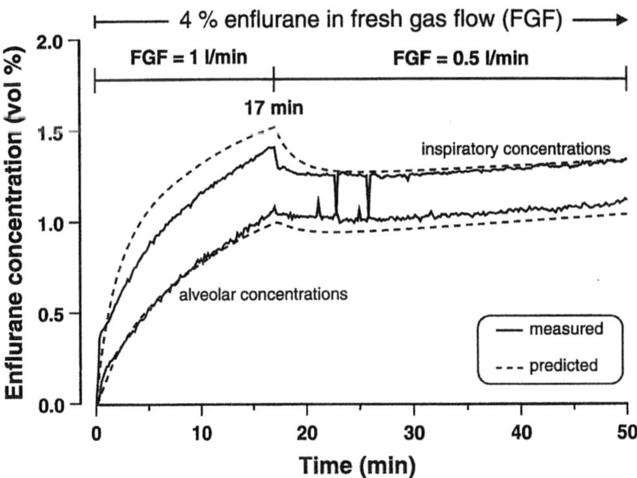

Fig. 3. Low-flow anaesthesia in a 56-year-old male patient (weight 63 kg; height 1.72 m). There is good agreement between the measured concentrations and those predicted by our model

techniques. The anaesthetic community is now convinced that fairly extensive monitoring, including the measurement of gases, is essential during any anaesthetic procedure, whatever the fresh-gas flow is. Accordingly, the standards of care – published in many countries – for monitoring equipment do not differentiate between the different breathing systems.

Whatever the type of system in use, monitoring of the breathing system includes measuring and recording the concentrations of oxygen, carbon dioxide and inhaled agents, as well as respiratory frequency, minute volume and airway pressures. The new user-friendly multigas analysers are capable of analysing not only oxygen and carbon dioxide, but also nitrous oxide, inhaled anaesthetics and even nitrogen. These gas analysers are appearing more and more often in daily routine practice, either as stand-alone units or as modules in integrated anaesthesia systems (Fig. 1).

Each device has its own specific problems and errors. Side-stream monitors sample a particular amount of gas from the circle that must be returned into the breathing circuit without endangering the patient. Some analysers use room air to calibrate or to keep the measuring chamber clean. Returning this sample flow into the breathing system leads to the accumulation of nitrogen in a closed circuit. Main-stream analysers do not withdraw a sample. Thus, they are preferable for routine clinical use with low-flow techniques. However, they do not allow for the measuring of all gases and vapours of interest, and their presence at the Y-piece may be cumbersome.

Denitrogenation is essential if we want to use the full anaesthetic potential of nitrous oxide and if we want to prevent the accumulation of nitrogen. If we assume a "normal" patient, the behaviour of nitrogen is predictable. A patient breathing air at sea level contains 2.7 l of nitrogen. More than half of it, i.e. 1.6 l, resides in the functional residual capacity (FRC), the remainder being dissolved in the tissues. If only the lungs were denitrogenated, theoretically there would be 1.1 l of nitrogen left. Even if this amount were diluted in the total volume of the breathing system plus FRC (6.5 l plus 2.5 l), the maximally attainable nitrogen concentration would be – roughly – 12%. With a circle system it is possible to reduce the end-tidal nitrogen concentration to less than 5% within 5–10 min provided a high flow of fresh gas is used. We use such a period before and after the intubation, but before the administration of a volatile agent. In our experience, the nitrogen concentration is about 3–6% after 1 h of closed-circuit anaesthesia, depending on the body weight and the period used for denitrogenation. This result is very similar to the findings reported by Barton and Nunn [23]. Other gases, such as methane, carbon monoxide and acetone, may accumulate in the system with particular patients [24]. However, no adverse effects have been reported.

3. *Low-flow techniques prevent the rapid change in the concentration of volatile anaesthetic when requested.*

Using a high flow of fresh gas permits a rapid change in the inspiratory concentration of a volatile anaesthetic agent, for instance, to hasten the induction or emergence processes. Figure 3 illustrates the time course of anaesthetic induction with

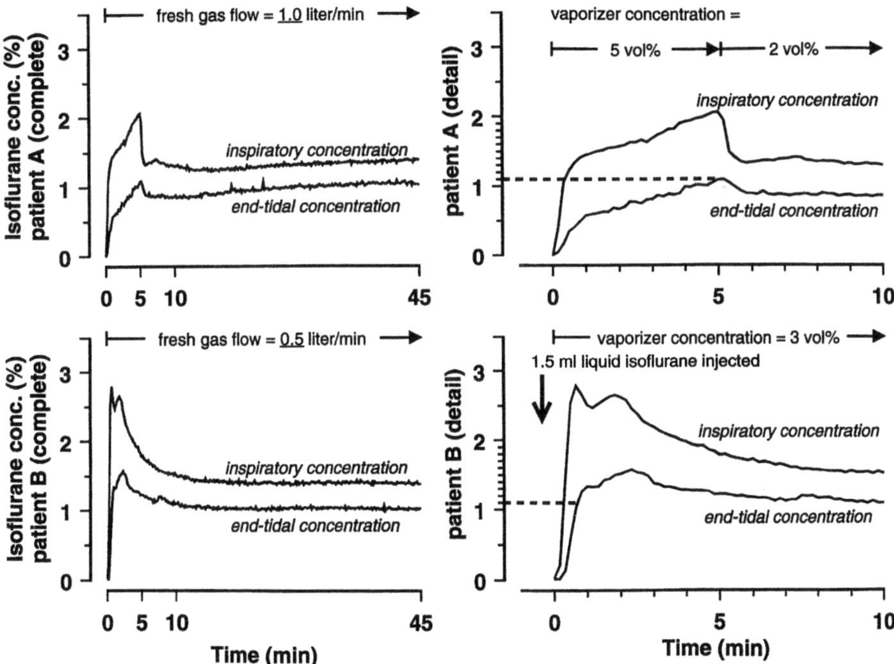

Fig. 4. Comparison of two approaches to the delivery of isoflurane under low-flow conditions. *Patient A* is a 51-year-old woman (weight, 58 kg; height, 1.64 m). *Patient B* is a 65-year-old man (weight, 78 kg; height, 1.74 m). Note the difference in the rate of rise of the alveolar concentrations because of the injection of a single bolus of liquid isoflurane into the expiratory limb of the circle system of patient B. Isoflurane was measured by respiratory mass spectrometry (CaSE, QP 9000, England)

1 l/min as fresh gas flow. In the case of enflurane, it takes 17 min to establish an alveolar concentration of 1.1% (0.65 MAC). This slow rise is due to the ratio of anaesthetic administered and that taken up by the subject. The amount of inhalation anaesthetic delivered to a circle system is determined by the product of the fresh-gas flow and the concentration of the agent in the fresh gas. During the early stages of anaesthesia the uptake rate of enflurane is high and cannot be matched by the limited amount of anaesthetic delivered by a conventional vaporizer in low-flow circumstances. If we used a high flow of fresh gas during the early stages of anaesthesia, we would mimic the theoretical concept of "priming" the breathing system and the FRC of the patient. However, the use of injections of liquid volatile anaesthetic into a closed system is the more rational approach to rapidly attaining the desired alveolar concentrations. This approach is illustrated in Fig. 4.

Figure 4 compares two approaches to the delivery of a volatile anaesthetic under low-flow conditions. We used isoflurane as an example. The figure's upper half illustrates the use of a vaporizer (Ohmeda, Tek 5) outside the circle. The lower half shows the combined use of a single bolus injection of isoflurane and the same

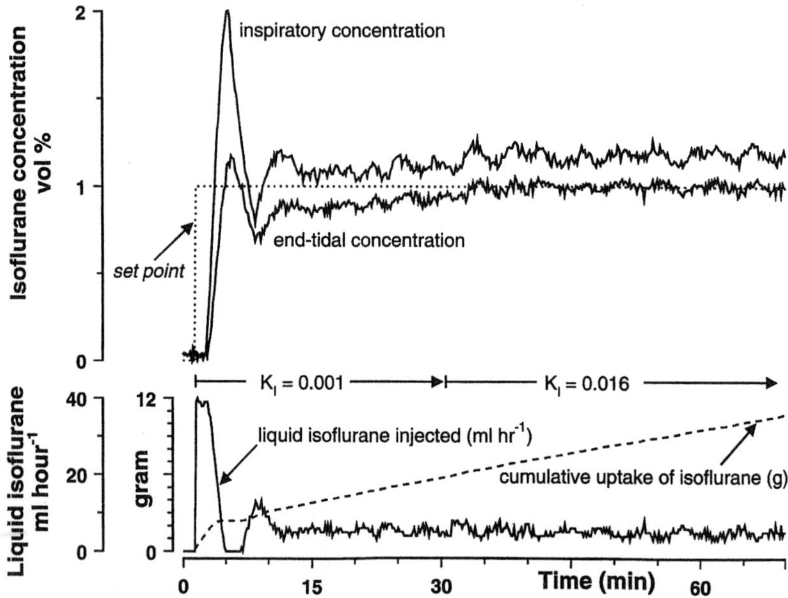

Fig. 5. Feedback-controlled closed-circuit isoflurane anaesthesia in a 21-year-old male patient (weight, 85 kg; height 1.88 m). The integral constant K_I is increased to augment the impact of the integral element in the "proportional-integral" scheme of the controller. Thereafter, the end-tidal concentration matches the set point value

vaporizer. Despite the greater body weight, the lower fresh-gas flow and the lower vaporizer concentration, an alveolar concentration of 1.1% is reached within 1 min in patient B versus 5 min for patient A. This illustrates that the wash-in of isoflurane is remarkably accelerated if we "prime" the circle system plus the FRC by injecting 1.5 ml of liquid isoflurane. In doing so, we administer 300 ml of pure isoflurane vapour into the 9-l volume of our anaesthetic breathing system (6.5 l, as measured by helium dilution) plus the FRC (roughly 2.5 l, under the conditions of general anaesthesia). Figure 4 illustrates that a reliable gas analyser puts the anaesthesiologist in real control of various, flexible approaches to the administration of low-flow or closed-circuit anaesthesia.

Figure 5 shows that an automated feedback-controlled delivery system is capable of rapidly attaining and maintaining the target value for the end-tidal isoflurane concentration. The feedback controller is based on a "proportional-integral" scheme (PI controller). The error signal, i.e., the difference between the measured end-tidal concentration and the set point (Fig. 2), is passed to two feedback-control elements. The first element is the proportional term, the second the integral term. The sum of these elements forms the output of the controller, i.e., the amount of isoflurane delivered to the closed system per unit of time. The proportional term is directly proportional to the error signal, while the second term relates to the integral of the error signal. Each term needs one constant. These constants can be determined empirically, or by computer simulation, or by combining the two approaches. We found out both constants during successive simulation runs of our clinically validated model. In Fig. 5, we used a conservative value of the integral constant to start with. Consequently, the control is mainly proportional and the actual concentration fluctuates just below the set point. Increasing the constant 16-fold yields a close agreement between the actual and the desired end-tidal concentration.

The closed-loop control system provides accurate control of anaesthetic input to the closed circuit. It automatically alters the supply of isoflurane to meet the patient's uptake from minute to minute. Integrating the uptake yields the cumulative uptake (Fig. 5). The exact dose of the potent inhalation anaesthetic is therefore known while clinical anaesthesia is provided with a closed system. Thus, closed-loop control of closed-circuit anaesthesia is the rational direction of the future to implement quantitative anaesthesia.

By diverting gases through a charcoal filter placed in the inspiratory limb of the breathing system, the inspired concentration of a volatile anaesthetic agent approaches zero within a few breaths without disturbing closed-circuit conditions [25]. Charcoal efficiently removes the inhalation anaesthetics, but not nitrous oxide [26, 27]. Fifty grams of charcoal completely absorb 2000 ml of halothane vapour, i.e., about 10 ml of liquid halothane. The charcoal can be reactivated by autoclaving [28].

Conclusions

Based on the material presented, we conclude that:

1. There are no differences in the monitoring aspects of the different breathing systems; each type should be adequately monitored whatever the fresh-gas flow.
2. In comparison to high-flow nonrebreathing systems, closed-circuit and low-flow breathing systems are less easily controlled with the technology commonly used in the anaesthesia systems of today.
3. There is a close relationship between the controllability and the engineering aspects of breathing systems.
4. Although the concentrations of volatile anaesthetic agents in a closed circuit can be predicted with known and clinically acceptable accuracy, they should be monitored because of intra- and interindividual variability in anaesthetic uptake.
5. The control of a closed-circuit breathing system can be optimized by a closed-loop control system; ample effort is required to provide the engineering to incorporate the appropriate sensors and effectors into the control system.

References

1. Cooper JB, Newbower RS, Long CD, McPeek B (1978) Preventable anesthesia mishaps – a human factors study. Anesthesiology 49:399–406

2. Ernst EA, MacKrell TN, Pearson JD, Cutter G, Wagenknecht L (1987) Patient safety: a comparison of open and closed anesthesia circuits. Anesthesiology 67:A474
3. Hamilton WK (1964) Nomenclature of inhalation anesthetic systems. Anesthesiology 25:3–5
4. Aldrete JA (1984) A practical perspective on low, minimal and closed-system anesthesia. Acta Anaesthesiol Belg 34:251–256
5. Foldes FF, Ceravolo AJ, Carpenter SL (1952) The administration of nitrous-oxide anesthesia in closed system. Ann Surg 136:978–981
6. Virtue RW (1974) Minimal-flow nitrous oxide anesthesia. Anesthesiology 40:196–198
7. Leuenberger M, Feigenwinter P, Zbinden AM (1992) The gas leakage of seven anaesthesia circle systems. Eur J Anaesthesiol 9:121–127
8. Morrison JL (1994) FDA Anesthesia apparatus checkout recommendations 1993. ASA Newslett 58:25–26
9. Ghani AG (1984) Fresh gas flow affects minute volume during mechanical ventilation. Anesth Analg 63:619–625
10. Aldrete JA, Adolph AJ, Hanna LM, Farag HA, Ghaemmaghami M (1989) Fresh gas flow rate and I:E ratio affect tidal volume in anaesthesia ventilators. In: van Ackern K, Frankenberger H, Konecky E, Steinbereithner (eds) Quantitative anaesthesia. Anaesthesiology and intensive care medicine, vol 204. Springer, Berlin Heidelberg New York, pp 72–80
11. Eger EI, Ethans CT (1968) The effect of inflow, overflow and valve placement on economy of the circle system. Anesthesiology 29:93–100
12. Zbinden AM, Feigenwinter P, Hutmacher M (1991) Fresh gas utilization of eight circle systems. Br J Anaesth 67:492–499
13. Hayes JK, Westenskow DR, East TD, Jordan WS (1984) Computer-controlled anesthesia delivery system. Med Instrum 18:224–231
14. Ritchie RG, Ernst EA, Pate BL, Pearson JP, Sheppard LC (1990) Automatic control of anesthetic delivery and ventilation during surgery. Med Prog Technol 16:61–67
15. Westenskow DR, Wallroth CF (1990) Closed-loop control for anesthesia breathing systems. J Clin Monit 6:249–256
16. Lin CT (1980) Assessment of vaporizer performance in low-flow and closed circuit anesthesia. Anesth Analg 59:359–366
17. Zbinden AM, Frei F, Westenskow DR, Thomson DA (1986) Control of end-tidal halothane concentration. Part A. Anaesthesia breathing system and feedback control of gas delivery. Br J Anaesth 58:555–562
18. Zbinden AM, Frei F, Westenskow DR, Thomson DA (1986) Control of end-tidal halothane concentration. Part B. Verification in dogs. Br J Anaesth 58:563–571
19. Lerou JGC, Dirksen R, Beneken Kolmer HH, Booij LHDJ (1991) A system model for closed-circuit inhalation anesthesia: I. Computer study. Anesthesiology 75:345–355
20. Lerou JGC, Dirksen R, Beneken Kolmer HH, Booij LHDJ Borm GF (1991) A system model for closed-circuit inhalation anesthesia. II. Clinical validation. Anesthesiology 75:230–237
21. Lerou JGC, Vermeulen PM, Dirksen R, Booij LHDJ, Borm GF (1993) The predictive performance of a system model for enflurane closed-circuit inhalational anesthesia. Anesthesiology 79:932–942
22. Westenskow DR, Jordan WS, Hayes JK (1983) Uptake of enflurane: a study of the variability between patients. Br J Anaesth 55:595–601
23. Barton F, Nunn JF (1975) Totally closed circuit nitrous/oxide anaesthesia. Br J Anaesth 47:350–357
24. Morita S, Latta W, Hambro K, Snider MT (1992) Accumulation of methane, acetone, and nitrogen in the inspired gas during closed circuit anesthesia. Anesth Analg 64:343–347
25. Ernst EA (1982) Use of charcoal to rapidly reduce alveolar anesthetic concentration while maintaining a closed circuit. Anesthesiology 57:343

26. Romano E, Pegoraro M, Vacri A, Pecchiari C, Auci E (1992) Low-flow anaesthesia systems, charcoal and isoflurane kinetics. Anaesthesia 47:1098–1099
27. Kim BM, Sircar S (1977) Adsorption characteristics of volatile anesthetics on activated carbons and performance of carbon canisters. Anesthesiology 46:159–165
28. Capon JH (1974) A method of regenerating activated charcoal anaesthetic absorbers by autoclaving. Anaesthesia 29:611–614
29. Ernst EA, MacKrell TN, Pearson JD, Cutter G, Wagenknecht L (1987) Patient safety: a comparison of open and closed anesthesia circuits. Anesthesiology 67:A474

II Assessment and Evaluation of Signals and Measurements

b) Therapeutic Monitoring of Patients

Does the EEG Measure Therapeutic Opioid Drug Effect?*

V. Billard and S.L. Shafer

Introduction

In this chapter we discuss the extent to which the EEG reflects therapeutic opioid drug effect. For the hypnotics, the EEG has been used to control the depth of anesthesia via closed-loop administration. These systems will be discussed in the chapters by Professors Schwilden [1, 2] (median frequency) and Kenny (auditory-evoked potentials). That computerized systems are able to satisfactorily administer hypnotics based on direct feedback from EEG-derived measures suggests that the EEG is, in fact, a very reasonable measure of hypnotic drug effect. Thus, we will focus here on the EEG as a measure of the therapeutic effect of opioids.

Anesthesiologists titrate drugs to a perceived level of anesthetic depth, which is generally defined by responsiveness to noxious stimulation. Patient responses to noxious stimulation include movement (used in the definition of MAC), hemodynamic response (heart rate or blood pressure), and autonomic responses such as sweating, tearing, flushing. In the unparalyzed patient, movement is usually considered the best sign of anesthetic depth, while hemodynamic responsiveness to noxious stimulation is often used to assess anesthetic depth in the paralyzed patient.

Opioids produce many effects on the body, including relief of pain, depressed sensorium, miosis, respiratory depression, and nausea. Anesthesiologists use opioids primarily for their attenuation of pain and decreased level of consciousness. During general anesthesia, the analgesic component of opioids can be thought of as attenuating the afferent noxious stimulus, while the narcosis caused by opioids contributes to the reduction in level of consciousness. As we will see, the EEG effect of opioids is a profound effect whose concentration-response relationship is in a similar range to the concentration-response relationship for depression of consciousness. The analgesic concentration-response range for opioids occurs well below the EEG concentration-response range but has a constant relationship to the IC_{50} of EEG depression.

---

* Supported, in part, by the Merit Review Program of the Department of Veterans Affairs.

The EEG as a Measure of Opioid Drug Effect

Ausems et al. examined the probability of response to noxious stimulation during an anesthetic consisting of alfentanil with 70% N_2O as a function of the steady-state plasma alfentanil concentration [3]. Their data, shown in Fig. 1, provide a clinical quantitation of opioid effect. Figure 1 shows the probability of no response (Y axis $= 1 = 100\%$) as a function of the plasma alfentanil concentration. In Ausems' study the response to intubation was the most difficult to block with alfentanil, i.e., intubation was the most noxious stimulus. Lower plasma alfentanil concentrations were required to block the response to skin incision than the response to intubation, and still lower levels were required to block the response to skin closure. Thus, Ausems and colleagues were able to provide a clinically relevant method of quantitating opioid drug effect.

Unfortunately, clinical observations, such as of patient responsiveness, have rather low resolution as measures of opioid drug effect. For example, there is usually only one intubation per patient, only one skin incision, and only one skin closure. Thus, data must be gathered from many patients and pooled to permit analysis. Complex analysis of pooled data may then be necessary to separate intraindividual and interindividual variability. Additionally, the infrequent nature of most clinical observations does not permit detailed measurement of the time course of drug effect. Thus, clinical observations such as response to a noxious stimulus may not be adequate for pharmacodynamic modeling.

Clinical observations also have shortcomings as measures of anesthetic depth. The most commonly accepted measurement of anesthetic depth, movement response to noxious stimulation, is available only retrospectively, i.e., after the time

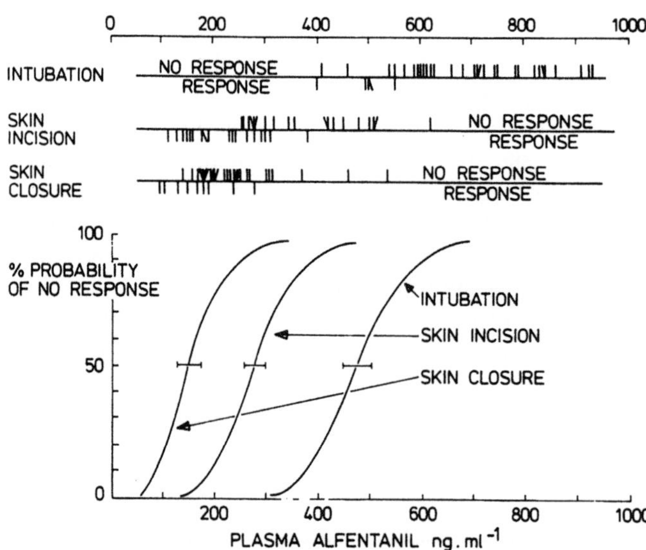

Fig. 1. The probability of no response to three clinically relevant stimuli as a function of plasma alfentanil concentration. (From [3])

when the information would have been most valuable (prior to the stimulus). Measuring response to noxious stimulation also requires exploring the edge of the therapeutic window, and thus may expose the patient to unnecessarily light anesthesia. Finally, the movement response is not available in paralyzed patients, and the measures that are available, such as blood pressure and heart rate, may not predict awareness. Thus, clinical measures have shortcomings both as measures of drug effect and as measures of anesthetic depth.

To address these shortcomings of clinical measures, investigators have turned to the EEG as a continuous, sensitive, and high-resolution measure of opioid drug effect. The EEG effects of opioids are dramatic. Alfentanil transforms the EEG from the high-frequency, low-voltage pattern associated with wakefulness (Fig. 2) to a low-frequency, high-voltage pattern characteristic of deep opioid narcosis (Fig. 3). This change is dose dependent and has been correlated with plasma opioid concentration [4–6]. Since plasma opioid concentration correlates with anesthetic depth during N_2O-opioid anesthesia [3], it is reasonable to anticipate that the EEG

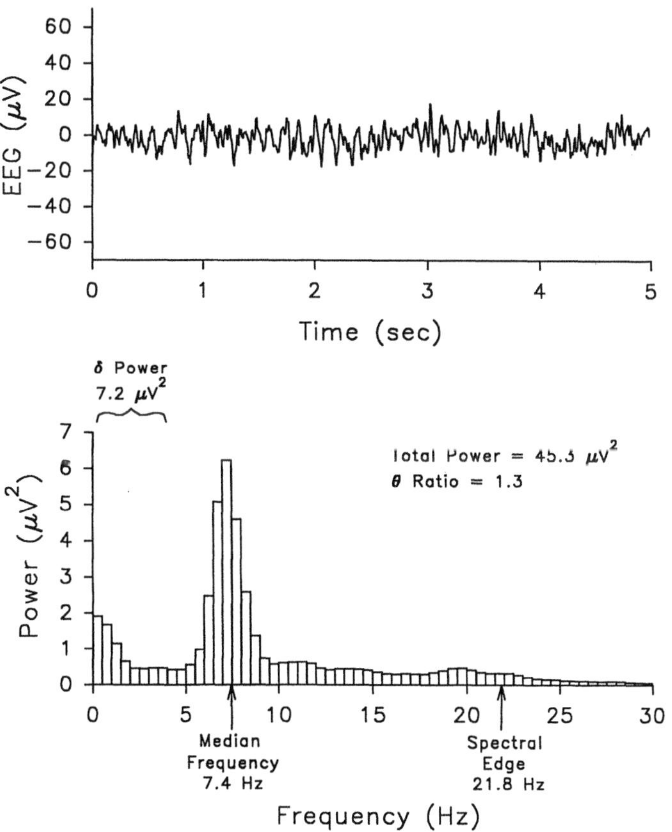

Fig. 2. Five seconds of normal EEG and the histogram showing the underlying frequencies. Several simple measures of the EEG spectrum are noted

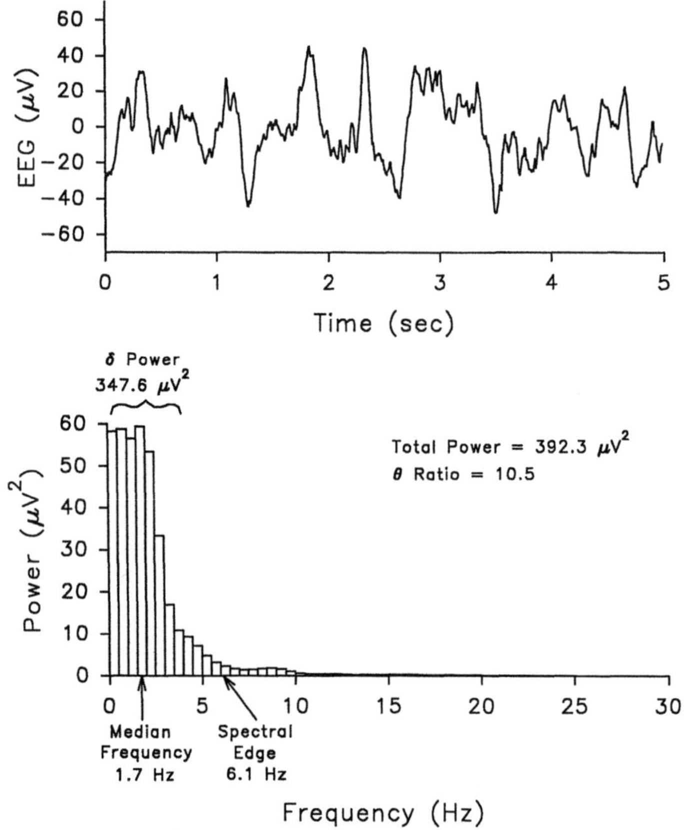

Fig. 3. Five seconds of EEG showing maximal opioid drug effect and the histogram showing the underlying frequencies. The simple measures of drug effect all reflect the increasing power, and shift to lower frequencies, that can be seen in the raw waveform

can be used as a sensitive measure of anesthetic depth, which has been suggested by many investigators [7–11].

To quantitate opioid effect with the EEG, the EEG waveform is chopped up into segments of fixed length, called epochs. Figure 2 shows a 5-s epoch from an awake subject. Each epoch is then processed into the spectrum of frequencies present in the waveform. This is often done using Fourier analysis, although other techniques are available. The histogram in Fig. 2 shows the frequencies present in the pictured EEG waveform. The bimodal pattern of the frequencies is common in awake individuals. To quantify drug effect, it is then necessary to identify a single parameter which describes some characteristic of the EEG spectrum. Five such parameters are shown in Fig. 2. The total power is the combined power in all frequencies, the delta power is the power in the delta band, the median frequency is the frequency at which half of the power is higher and half lower, the spectral edge is the frequency at which 95% of the power is at lower frequencies, and the theta ratio is the ratio of the total power from 2–7 Hz divided by the total power from 5–7 Hz.

The 5-s epoch in Fig. 3 shows profound alfentanil drug effect on the EEG. The power in the waveform has increased dramatically, and there has been a shift towards lower frequencies. These changes are summed up in the five individual parameters. The total power, delta power, and theta ratio have increased, while the median frequency and spectral edge have decreased. Of these five parameters, the spectral edge has proved to be the most useful measure of opioid drug effect [4–6].

Using spectral edge, it is possible to quantitate the EEG changes during and following opioid infusions, and to model those changes as a function of the opioid concentration at the site of drug effect. The model usually takes the form of the "Hill" equation:

$$EEG\ Effect = E_o + \frac{E_{max}C_e{}^\gamma}{IC_{50}{}^\gamma + C_e{}^\gamma}$$

where E_0 is the baseline EEG effect, E_{max} is the maximum possible EEG change from baseline, C_e is the effect site (or steady state) opioid concentration, IC_{50} is the opioid concentration associated with 50% of the maximum response, and γ is the steepness of the concentration-response relationship. C_e is determined by "effect site modeling," and represents the convolution of the plasma opioid concentration over time with the disposition function of the effect site, $k_{e0}\ e^{-k_{e0}t}$. The effect-site concentration is the same as the concentration in the plasma at steady state that would produce a given drug effect. This model produces a sigmoidal relationship that quantitates the effect of opioids on the EEG. We will explore how this quantitation relates to the opioid therapeutic window.

The EEG vs Clinical Measures of Opioid Drug Effect

Figure 4 superimposes the EEG quantitation of opioid effect, as determined by Scott and Stanski [5] with the clinical quantitation of opioid effect reported by Ausems et al. [3]. For alfentanil, there is very little EEG effect below 300 ng/ml. This means that the EEG does not provide information within the therapeutic range of concentrations for skin closure, and cannot provide assurance that the concentrations are sufficiently low at the conclusion of an anesthetic to permit adequate ventilation. However, we can infer that if an opioid EEG effect is present towards the conclusion of an anesthetic, then the patient is very likely overdosed on an opioid, and the infusion should be discontinued.

The range of the EEG response to alfentanil is very well positioned relative to skin incision. Presuming that the anesthesiologist desires a *95% probability* of no response to skin incision, the data of Ausems et al. suggest that a concentration of 350–400 ng/ml will be required. This concentration falls within the early portion of the linear segment of the alfentanil-EEG response relationship, permitting accurate interpretation of the EEG relative to anesthetic depth.

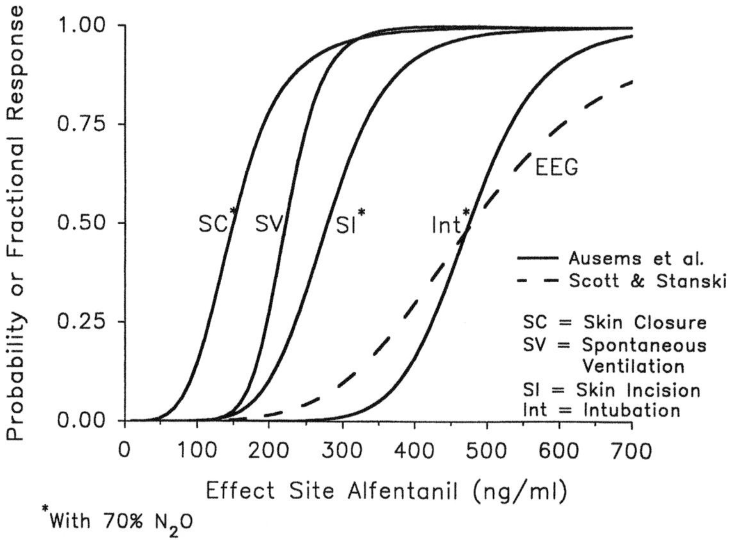

Fig. 4. The EEG effect of alfentanil, as reported by Scott and Stanski [5], superimposed on the clinical measures of alfentanil drug effect reported by Ausems et al. [3]

The therapeutic range for intubation corresponds well to the linear portion of the EEG response curve, suggesting that if alfentanil were administered until a nearly maximal EEG effect was observed, the patient would be unlikely to respond to intubation. These results suggest that the EEG can be used as a measure of opioid effect in the range of concentrations associated with clinically deep anesthesia. They also suggest that the EEG measures an alfentanil effect more profound than either moderate analgesia or ventilatory depression.

This conclusion is supported by comparing the EEG effect of opioids reported by Scott and Stanski with the opioid concentrations necessary for "adequate anesthesia," as determined by Shafer et al. for patients undergoing intra-abdominal procedures [12]. In Fig. 5 we again see that the EEG is associated with deep opioid anesthesia. However, if the clinical goal is to have *at least* a 65% likelihood of adequate anesthesia, then the range of 65–100% "adequate anesthesia" as defined by Shafer and colleagues falls squarely within the linear portion of the EEG, suggesting clinical utility of the EEG as a measure of opioid drug effect in assuring adequate anesthesia.

So far we have considered the alfentanil therapeutic range for anesthesia in the presence of nitrous oxide. Figure 6 compares the EEG response to alfentanil with the alfentanil concentrations required for cardiac surgery without nitrous oxide or a potent volatile anesthetic, (but with a benzodiazepine preanesthetic medication) as reported by Hug et al. [13]. Although the previous graphs suggested that the EEG effect of opioids correlated with profound levels of opioid drug effect, the plasma alfentanil concentrations required for cardiac surgery without concurrent administration of N_2O or a potent vapor are far in excess of the alfentanil

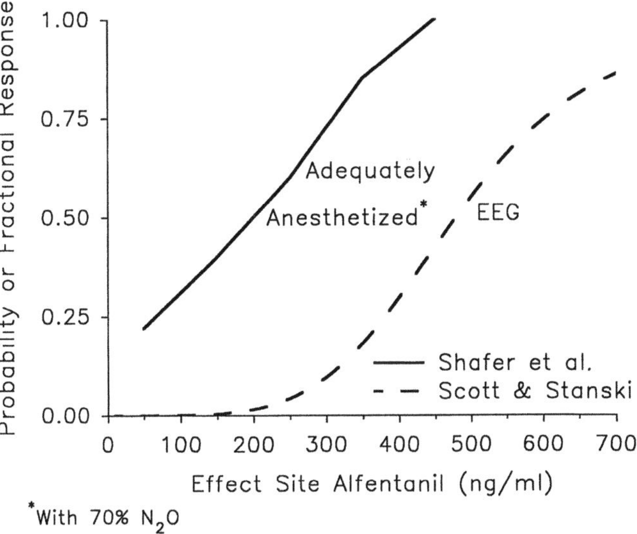

Fig. 5. The EEG effect of alfentanil, as reported by Scott and Stanski [5], superimposed on the concentrations required for adequate anesthesia, as reported by Shafer et al. [12]

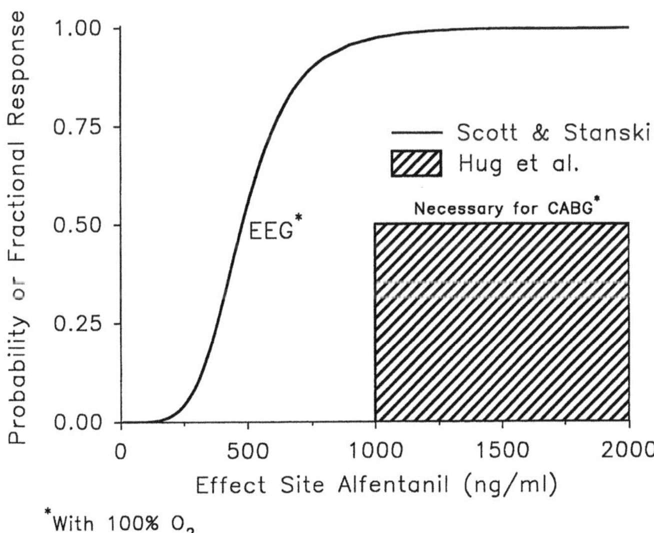

Fig. 6. The EEG effect of alfentanil, as reported by Scott and Stanski [5], superimposed on the alfentanil concentrations necessary for anesthesia in cardiac surgical patients, as reported by Hug et al. [13]

concentrations that produce maximum EEG effect. Even here, the EEG may provide useful therapeutic information, because if a submaximal EEG response is seen, then the patient is likely underanesthetized when a "cardiac" technique is being used.

Is There an Optimal EEG for Opioids?

We have used the spectral edge to describe the opioid effect on the EEG and have related EEG response as measured by spectral edge to opioid drug concentration. Up to this point, we have discussed the EEG response in terms of a fraction of maximal response. This raises two issues. First, the spectral edge is an ad hoc measure of EEG response, in that it represents an intuitively useful summary of the changes that can be visually observed in the EEG, but has no particular reason to be an optimal measure of opioid effect on the EEG. Second, there is nothing in the analysis presented so far about whether the EEG response to the pure μ agonists is uniform.

We have recently addressed these questions using a new statistical technique, semilinear canonical correlation (SCC). SCC is a technique to define an EEG parameter that *optimally* (in some sense) correlates with effect-site drug concentration. In our first study with SCC we analyzed the EEG recorded from 15 individuals receiving an alfentanil infusion [14]. The data were divided into an eight-patient "learning" set and a seven-patient "test" set. We applied the technique of SCC (the details of which we will not address here) to the eight patients in the learning set and derived an EEG parameter which optimally correlated with effect-site alfentanil concentration. We then examined the performance of this EEG parameter, called the "log powers canonical variate," in the seven patients in the test set. As can be seen in Fig. 7, the EEG correlated extremely well in the best and median cases. In the worst case, there was still a clear relationship between the EEG and the effect-site alfentanil concentration (C_E).

Figure 8 shows the performance of spectral edge in the seven-patient test set. In the best and median cases, spectral edge performed as well as the log powers canonical variate. However, there was virtually no relationship between the spectral edge and effect-site alfentanil concentration in the worst cases. We also examined the performance of total power, delta power, median frequency, and theta ratio. Each of these performed well in a few cases, but performed more poorly overall than spectral edge. Thus, the log powers canonical variate proved to be unusually robust, in that, at best, it correlated with effect-site alfentanil concentration as well as any other EEG parameter and, at worst, it still demonstrated a reasonable concentration-response relationship. Thus, we have reason to believe that SCC is a superior method for quantitating opioid effect on the EEG.

The log powers canonical variate was derived as a measurement of alfentanil drug effect. In our second study we tested whether the log powers canonical variate is, in fact, a generalized measure of opioid drug effect. We examined the correla-

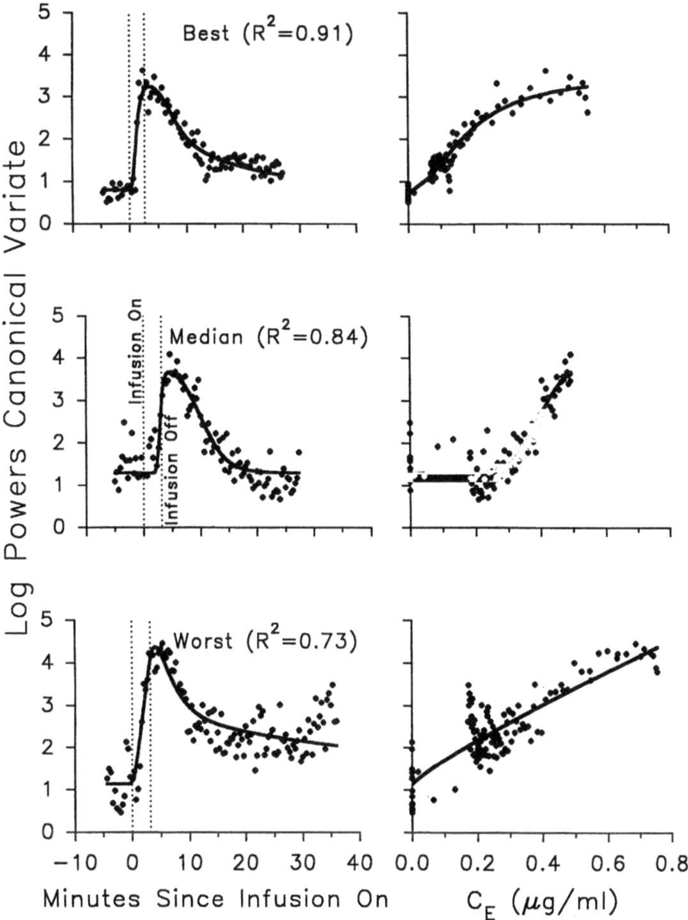

Fig. 7. The *best, median,* and *worst* correlations between the log powers canonical variate and effect-site alfentanil concentration (C_E), demonstrating a reasonable concentration-response relationship in the very worst case

tion between the log powers canonical variate and the effect-site concentration for four additional opioids: fentanyl, sufentanil, trefentanil, and remifentanil. In each case, the log powers canonical variate provided a better correlation with the effect-site concentration than any previously defined measure of opioid drug effect. Thus, our data suggest that the log powers canonical variate is a generalized measure of opioid effect on the EEG. Moreover, this same study shows that the EEG, as "optimally" (in some sense) measured by the log powers canonical variate, is the same for any pure μ agonist.

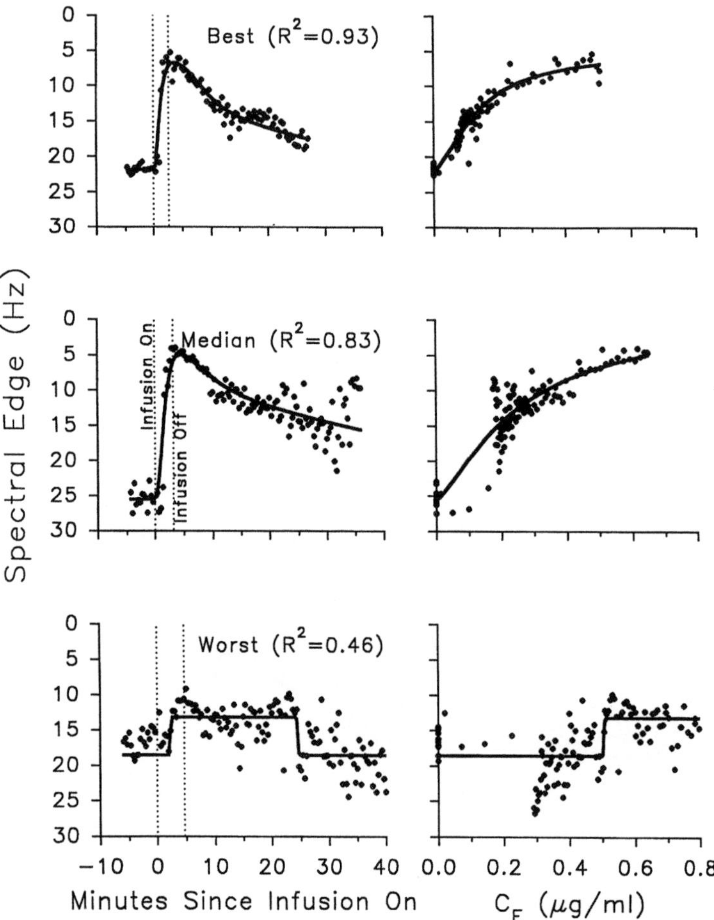

Fig. 8. The *best*, *median*, and *worst* correlations between spectral edge and effect-site alfentanil concentration, demonstrating the potential for breakdown of spectral edge as a measure of opioid effect in some individuals

Generalized Correlation of Opioid Concentration-EEG Effect with Opioid Concentration-Therapeutic Effect Relationships

The EEG has been used to quantitate the opioid effect of fentanyl, alfentanil, and sufentanil [4–6]. When plotted on a common linear axis, as shown in Fig. 9, the EEG effect for sufentanil appears to be almost vertical, suggesting a very steep concentration-response relationship, while the EEG effect of alfentanil looks more flat, suggesting a more graded response. This is an artifact of the linear scale. However, this artifact has occasionally caused investigators to erroneously conclude that more potent drugs are less safe because of a "steeper" concentration-

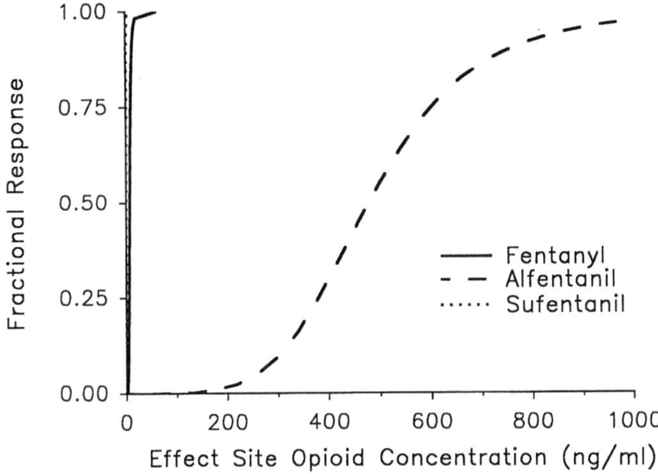

Fig. 9. The EEG effects of fentanyl [5], alfentanil [5], and sufentanil [6] plotted on a linear concentration axis, inappropriately suggesting intrinsic differences in the concentration-vs response relationship beyond a mere difference in potency

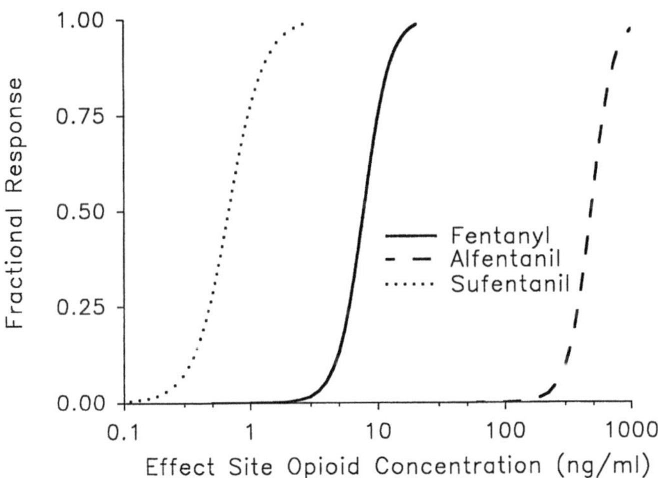

Fig. 10. The EEG effects of fentanyl, alfentanil, and sufentanil shown in Fig. 9, plotted on a log concentration axis, demonstrating that, in terms of relative proportions, the concentration-effect relationships for the three opioids are identical

response relationship and narrower therapeutic window (references are mercifully omitted, but will be provided upon request).

If we plot the response on a scale of log concentration vs EEG response, we can see that the opioid concentration vs EEG effect relationships for fentanyl, alfentanil, and sufentanil are nearly parallel, as shown in Fig. 10. Plotting concentration vs effect relationship for drugs of differing potencies on a logarithmic scale is more rational than plotting on a linear scale, because it shows the relationship between concentration and effect as a fraction of the concentration itself. For example, the peak EEG effect for sufentanil occurs at a concentration about four-fold higher than the concentration at minimum EEG effect, a relationship also true for fentanyl and alfentanil. Thus, the log scale in Fig. 10 permits us to examine the relative potency of the opioids in a more clinically relevant manner than the linear scale shown in Fig. 9.

Since the opioid concentration vs effect relationship, when plotted on a logarithmic scale, appears to be parallel for the three opioids, this suggests that it is appropriate to consider the EEG as a generalized measure of opioid drug effect, and to think of opioid concentration in terms of the IC_{50} of the opioid concentration-EEG effect relationship. As can be seen in Fig. 11, the opioid concentration-EEG effect relationships for fentanyl, alfentanil, and sufentanil are nearly identical when the concentration is expressed as a fraction of the IC_{50}. For each drug, concentrations associated with 20% response are approximately half of the concentrations associated with an 80% response.

Shafer and Varvel recently conducted an extensive review of the pharmacodynamic literature for fentanyl, alfentanil, and sufentanil to determine the therapeutic window of each opioid for induction with thiopental, induction with nitrous oxide, maintenance with isoflurane/nitrous oxide, and maintenance with nitrous oxide only [15]. In this analysis they also reviewed the literature reporting the opioid concentration which would assure adequate ventilation on emergence from anesthesia. Recent work on depression of the MAC of desflurane by fentanyl [16], of isoflurane by fentanyl [17], of isoflurane by sufentanil [18], and

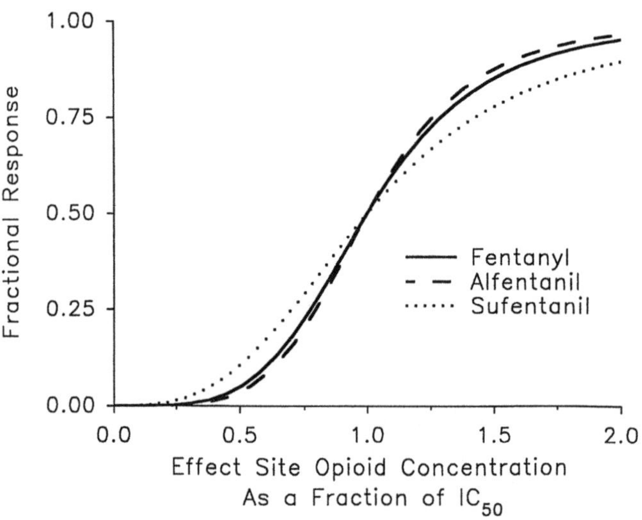

Fig. 11. The same EEG effects as shown in Fig. 9, but plotted as a fraction of the IC_{50}, demonstrating that the EEG effect of opioids is consistent for these three pure μ agonists

the Cp_{50} of fentanyl with nitrous oxide [19] have confirmed these ranges for therapeutic opioid effect.

The concentration ranges reported by Shafer and Varvel are shown in Fig. 12 for sufentanil, fentanyl, and alfentanil as rotated histograms. The bars reflect the therapeutic opioid concentration ranges associated with different drug combinations commonly used in anesthetic practice. The lower graph shows the curves that relate opioid drug concentration to the EEG effects of each opioid, when given to experimental subjects receiving only the opioid and breathing oxygen. The upper histogram (reflecting clinical practice) and lower graph (reflecting scientific results) are linked by effect-site opioid concentration, the X axis for both graphs. Since the EEG in the lower graph shows the opioid concentration-EEG response relationship in the absence of additional drugs, it should not be interpreted as showing the EEG response to the polypharmacy represented by the histograms. However, the effects of nitrous oxide on the EEG are minimal, and so, for techniques in which only nitrous oxide is administered, the EEG effect shown in the lower graph may correspond to the expected EEG during clinical anesthesia.

Figure 12 shows that the relationship between the EEG, as a measure of potency, and the therapeutic windows for different anesthetic techniques is consistent for sufentanil, fentanyl, and alfentanil. Opioid concentrations that produce a moderate EEG response are appropriate for induction if thiopental is used. However, if the patient is to be induced and intubated with just an opioid and nitrous oxide, then the EEG must be at nearly maximal effect. The opioid concentrations necessary for maintenance are those that produce mild EEG depression if a potent vapor and nitrous oxide are also used. However, in the absence of a potent vapor,

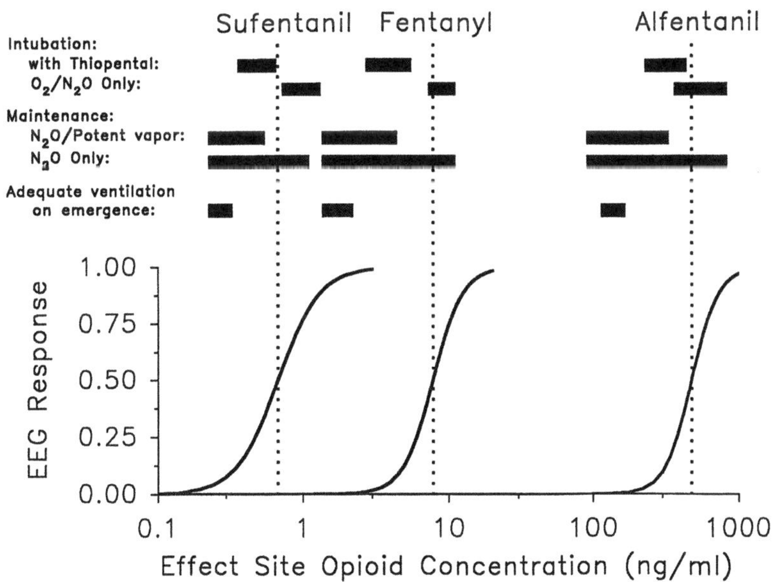

Fig. 12. The therapeutic ranges for sufentanil, fentanyl, and alfentanil, as reviewed by Shafer and Varvel [15], plotted against the EEG effects reported by Scott and Stanski [5, 6]

there is a very wide therapeutic window for the maintenance opioid concentration that covers the range of EEG response. Adequate spontaneous ventilation at the conclusion of an anesthetic requires an opioid concentration below the concentration that produces an opioid EEG effect.

The EEG in Opioid Drug Development

Figure 12 suggests a general correlation between the IC_{50} of the opioid concentration-EEG response relationship and the therapeutic window of opioid concentration for different techniques. Such a correlation is shown in Fig. 13. We can now see the "clinical meaning" of the EEG for opioids: for any pure μ agonist, the therapeutic window for each anesthetic technique will be a constant fraction of the IC_{50}, as determined by scientific studies in which the EEG is recorded under experimental conditions. Thus, while the EEG is not a measure of analgesia, ventilatory depression, or even a direct measure of cortical depression, the concentration at which each of these opioid effects occurs can be determined from the IC_{50} of the EEG response.

We have used the relationship shown in Fig. 13 to assist in the early development of novel opioids. We conducted an early phase-I pharmacokinetic/pharmacodynamic (PK/PD) study of the experimental opioid trefentanil [20]. From this analysis, we identified the IC_{50} of the EEG response to trefentanil, as shown in the lower graph in Fig. 14. From our knowledge of the IC_{50} of the EEG response we

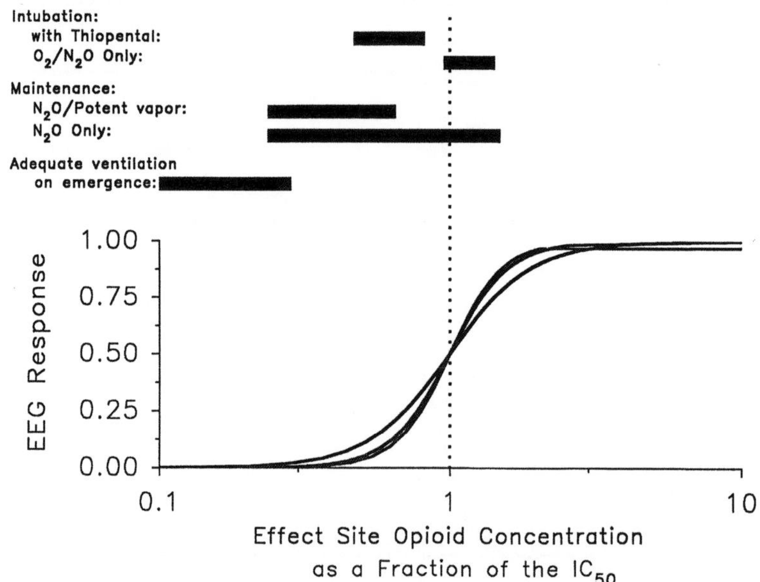

Fig. 13. The therapeutic ranges for any pure μ agonist, plotted as a fraction of the IC_{50} of the opioid. The *line graph* shows the overlapping concentration-EEG response relationships for fentanyl, alfentanil, and sufentanil on this scale (same as Fig. 11)

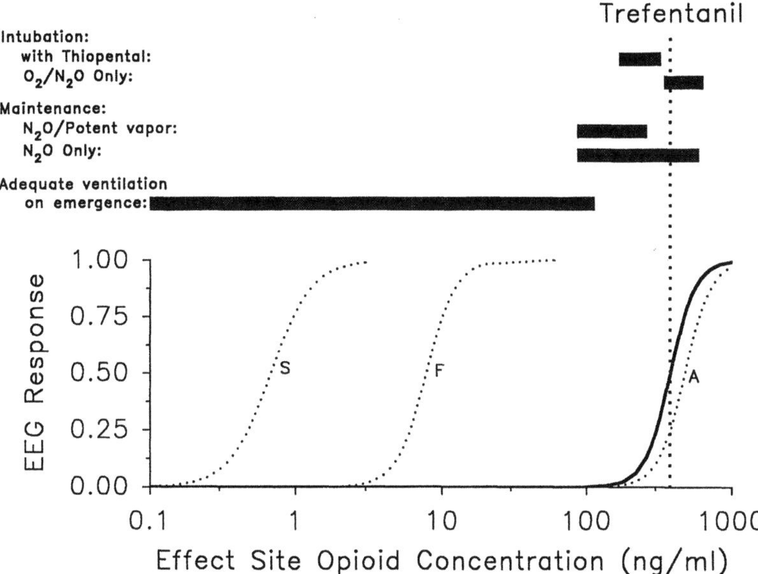

Fig. 14. The therapeutic ranges for trefentanil for different therapeutic techniques, as computed based only on knowledge of the trefentanil IC_{50} and the common opioid fingerprint shown in Fig. 13

were able to characterize the expected therapeutic windows for trefentanil for different anesthetic techniques, shown in the upper histogram in Fig. 14.

From the same study we also determined the pharmacokinetics of trefentanil, and k_{e0}, the rate constant that characterizes the disequilibrium between plasma and effect-site trefentanil concentration. By combining the PK/PD model of trefentanil with the therapeutic windows shown in Fig. 14, we were able to compute theoretically optimal trefentanil dosing regimens required for different anesthetic techniques without ever having administered an anesthetic with trefentanil. This analysis permitted the pharmaceutical company, Ohmeda Pharmaceutical Products, to design subsequent phase-I, -II, and -III studies around nearly optimal trefentanil dosing regimens. Thus, early use of PK/PD modeling in drug development, based on the EEG response, improved the efficiency of the development process. Glaxo, Inc. also incorporated a high-resolution PK/PD EEG response study of remifentanil into their early phase-I drug-development program, and used the resulting pharmacokinetic and pharmacodynamic model to develop theoretically optimal dosing regimens for their subsequent clinical trials.

Future Directions

It would appear that the quantitation of opioid effect using the EEG falls within a clinically useful range. However, there are two major issues which need to be resolved before an EEG measure of opioid drug effect has clinical utility:

1. The EEG effects reported are those of the opioid in an unpremedicated patient breathing oxygen. The clinical reality is polypharmacy, and each CNS depressant contributes to the EEG response. For example, thiopental given for induction will cause burst suppression of the EEG for a few minutes, eliminating the EEG as a measure of opioid drug effect prior to intubation.
2. The correlation of the EEG to drug concentration is scientifically interesting, but clinically of little use. The correlation of the EEG to *anesthetic depth* is the clinically important application of EEG technology. This requires calibrating the EEG against movement, the most commonly accepted measure of anesthetic depth. Ideally, a measure of the EEG can be found which predicts movement regardless of the anesthetic technique.

Both of these issues have been addressed in a remarkable study by Aspect Medical Systems, a biomedical development company in Framingham, MA. Conventional computerized EEG analyses, including those described above, are based upon Fourier analysis, but the phase information within the EEG is ignored. Bispectral analysis of the EEG is a new technique, based on Fourier analysis, which integrates the frequency, amplitude, and phase information within the EEG into the analysis. In their study, Aspect Medical demonstrated that the EEG bispectrum appears to measure the level of hypnosis. When this information is combined with knowledge of the patient's effect-site opioid concentration (developed through PK/PD modeling of the opioid administration), a nearly ideal measure of anesthetic depth emerges. This measure of anesthetic depth has been prospectively tested in clinical settings with representative polypharmacy and has been found to be robust. Because these results are presently awaiting peer review, we cannot offer greater detail about the results from Aspect Medical's trials in this forum. However, it is our belief that the unique measures of anesthetic depth developed by Aspect Medical may offer true integration of the EEG as a measure of CNS state into the clinical practice of anesthesia.

In summary, the EEG is a powerful method for quantitating opioid drug effect. It has the advantages of providing a continuous, high-resolution measure of drug effect. Clinical measures have also been used to quantitate opioid response, and the opioid concentration-EEG effect window overlaps clinically determined therapeutic windows in potentially useful ways. The EEG is a measure of profound opioid drug effect. Thus, moderate analgesia and ventilatory depression are achieved at opioid concentrations that have minimal effect on the EEG. The EEG reaches maximum effect at opioid concentrations below the therapeutic range required for an opioid/oxygen "cardiac" anesthetic. Despite these limitations in signal range, the EEG has potential use as an intraoperative measurement of opioid drug effect.

The EEG is also an excellent measure of opioid potency, being precise, accurate, and reproducible. As such, it may be more useful than clinically based measures of opioid potency. The relative potency between opioids developed from EEG analysis appears to be the same as the relative potency determined from clinical measures. This has important implications for drug development.

Finally, new techniques, including bispectral analysis and semilinear canonical correlation, may improve the quantitation of opioid drug effect and the application of the EEG to measurement of anesthetic depth.

References

1. Schwilden H, Schuttler J, Stoeckel H (1987) Closed-loop feedback control of methohexital anesthesia by quantitative EEG analysis in humans. Anesthesiology 67:341–347
2. Schwilden H, Stoeckel H, Schuttler J (1989) Closed-loop feedback control of propofol anaesthesia by quantitative EEG analysis in humans. Br J Anaesth 62:290–296
3. Ausems ME, Hug CC, Stanski DR, Burm AGL (1986) Plasma concentrations of alfentanil required to supplement nitrous oxide anesthesia for general surgery. Anesthesiology 65:362–373
4. Scott JC, Ponganis KV, Stanski DR (1985) EEG quantitation of narcotic effect: the comparative pharmacodynamics of fentanyl and alfentanil. Anesthesiology 62:234–241
5. Scott JC, Stanski DR (1987) Decreased fentanyl/alfentanil does requirement with increasing age: a pharmacodynamic basis. J Pharmacol Exp Ther 240:159–166
6. Scott JC, Cooke JE, Stanski DR (1991) Electroencephalographic quantitation of opioid effect: comparative pharmacodynamics of fentanyl and sufentanil. Anesthesiology 74:34–42
7. Dutton RC, Smith WD, Smith NT (1990) Does the EEG predict anesthetic depth better than cardiovascular variables? Anesthesiology 73:A532 (abstract)
8. Dutton RC, Smith WD, Smith NT (1991) EEG prediction of awareness during anesthesia with combinations of isoflurane, fentanyl, and N_2O. Anesthesiology 75:A448 (abstract)
9. Long CW, Shah NK, Loughlin C, Spydell J, Bedford RF (1989) A comparison of EEG determinants of near-awakening from isoflurane and fentanyl anesthesia. Spectral edge, median power frequency, and delta ratio. Anesth Analg 69:169–173
10. Sidi A, Halimi P, Cotev S (1990) Estimating anesthetic depth by electroencephalography during anesthetic induction and intubation in patients undergoing cardiac surgery. J Clin Anesth 2:101–107
11. Smith NT, Westover CJ jr, Quinn M, Benthuysen JL, Dec Sliver H, Sanford TJ jr (1985) An electroencephalographic comparison of alfentanil with other narcotics and with thiopental. J Clin Monit 1:236–244
12. Shafer A, Sung ML, White PF (1986) Pharmacokinetics and pharmacodynamics of alfentanil infusions during general anesthesia. Anesth Analg 65:1021–1028
13. Hug CC jr Hall RI, Angert KC, Reeder DA, Moldenhauer CC (1988) Alfentanil plasma concentration v. effect relationships in cardiac surgical patients. Br J Anaesth 61:435–440
14. Gregg KM, Varvel JR, Shafer SL (1992) Application of semilinear canonical correlation to the measurement of opioid drug effect. J Pharmacokinet Biopharm 20:611–635
15. Shafer SL, Varvel JR (1991) Pharmacokinetics, pharmacodynamics, and rational opioid selection. Anesthesiology 74:53–63
16. Sebel PS, Glass PS, Fletcher JE, Murphy MR, Gallagher C, Quill T (1992) Reduction of the MAC of desflurane with fentanyl. Anesthesiology 76:52–59
17. McEwan AI, Smith C, Dyar O, Goodman D, Smith LR, Glass PS (1993) Isoflurane minimum alveolar concentration reduction by fentanyl. Anesthesiology 78:864–869
18. Brunner MD, Braithwaite P, Jhaveri R, McEwan AI, Goodman DK, Smith LR, Glass PS (1994) MAC reduction of isoflurane by sufentanil. Br J Anaesth 72:42–46
19. Glass PS, Doherty M, Jacobs JR, Goodman D, Smith LR (1993) Plasma concentration of fentanyl, with 70% nitrous oxide, to prevent movement at skin incision. Anesthesiology 78:842–847
20. Lemmens, HJM, Dyck JB, Shafer SL, Stanski DR (1994) Pharmacokinetic/dynamic modeling in drug development: application to the investigational opioid trefentanil. Clin Pharmacol Ther (in press)

Somatosensory Evoked Potentials: Objective Measures of Antinociception in the Anesthetized Patient?

E. Kochs

Introduction

The most critical problems in pain research and clinical practice are the quantitation of nociception and the subjective experience of pain. From a physiologic point of view, pain is a consequence of the activation of nociceptive afferents and neural activity induced by noxious stimuli. The increased nociceptive signal transmission induces changes in brain electrical activity which may be assessed by physiologic measures. One of these neurophysiologic measures is the somatosensory evoked potential (SEP). SEPs reflect changes in brain electrical activity induced by electrical, mechanical, thermal, chemical, or tactile stimulation of peripheral neves. SEPs represent the activities of a rather large number of subcortical and cortical neural generators and are widely used as objective measures of sensory function [56]. The evoked cerebral potential reflects activation of specific afferent sensory systems. However, the evoked response is not specific for a unique stimulus modality. The early SEP components show peak latencies of less than 80 ms. They are separated into early farfield potentials with origins in subcortical structures (e.g., spinal cord, brain stem, thalamus) and early nearfield potentials generated by stimulus-induced summated postsynaptic activity of cortical neurons [22] (Fig. 1). Late SEP components with peak latencies of 80 ms or more may coincide with cognitive signal recognition or magnitude estimation [3, 4, 11, 12, 14–17]. They can best be recorded over the vertex. Both early and late SEPs reflect activity in large myelinated peripheral nerve fibers which activate the dorsal column [23]. Usually, for perioperative monitoring early nearfield potentials are recorded. They show very low variability across subjects and may be used for diagnostic procedures when impairment of afferent sensory pathways is assumed.

Generally, electrical stimulation of peripheral nerves is performed using surface electrodes. The electrical stimulus predominantly activates fast-conducting myelinated nerve fibers ($A\alpha$- and $A\beta$-fibers) with conduction velocities of 50 m/s or more. In addition, electrical nociceptive stimulation activates small $A\delta$- and C-fibers with conduction velocities between 0.5 and 30 m/s. All changes in brain electrical activity following noxious stimulation are delayed in comparison to the activation of large myelinated fibers. However, it has to be remembered that experimentally induced pain may differ fundamentally from clinical pain experienced by a patient [3]. For perioperative monitoring the most commonly

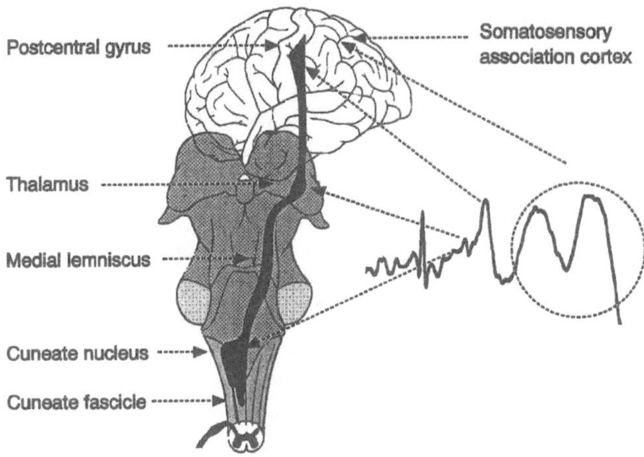

Fig. 1. Afferent pathways and relay stations for somatosensory evoked responses. Farfield potentials are generated in the *cuneate fascicle, cuneate nucleus, medial lemniscus,* and *thalamus.* Early cortical nearfield potentials are generated in the *postcentral gyrus,* while later components (*circle*) may have origins in various association areas

stimulated nerves are the median and ulnar nerves at the wrist, the peroneal nerve at the leg, and the tibial nerve at the ankle. The voltages generated are one order of magnitude lower than those of the spontaneous EEG. Electrical signals from various parts of the central nervous system (CNS) may also interfere with EEG and SEP recordings. Impairment of small peripheral nerve fibers or of the anterolateral spinothalamic tract cannot be assessed by SEPs [41].

Nociception is the result of changes in neuronal activity of a highly specialized sensory system which principally can be measured using neurophysiologic methods [21, 28]. Nocicpetors are known to respond to mechanical, thermal, and chemical forms of energy, and any of these stimulus modalities may be employed. Nociception is transmitted by low-conducting myelinated afferents (Aδ units). However, natural stimuli are not as easily controlled as electrical stimuli. It is generally assumed that weaker electrical stimuli excite mechanoreceptive afferent nerve fibers, whereas thinner nociceptive units are recruited when the stimulus strength is increased [28]. To overcome the unnatural throbbing character of electrical stimuli, a percutaneous electrical stimulation technique has been developed. With this method the dynamic range from nonpainful to painful stimuli is smaller than with transcutaneous electrical stimulation [5]. This technique probably excites a spectrum of nerve fibers similar to that excited by traditional forms of transcutaneous stimulation.

Even when nerve stems are stimulated, the lack of selectivity of electrical stimuli results in some ambiguity: (a) some nocicpetors may have fast-conducting and therefore thick myelinated afferents; (b) a part of the thin nerve fibers may not be nociceptive; and (c) the higher stimulus levels needed to stimulate nociceptors may result in recruitment of units with lower thresholds [28]. For the investigation of nociceptive reactions, the most suited model is the so-called phasic or acute pain in response to short and well-defined stimuli, which should activate specifically or at least predominantly the nocicpetors. Since all nocifensive reactions to repeated pain stimuli exhibit a certain amount of variance, averaging techniques must be applied. From this it follows that the experimental pain stimulus should be reproducible and certainly painful, but barely "noxious" in order to avoid tissue damage.

Even though early SEPs are not specific for nociceptive signal transmission, they have been used for assessment of depth of anesthesia. For intraoperative SEP recording following upper limb stimulation, usually the negative deflection with a latency of approximately 20 ms (N20) is evaluated. This component represents the first major early thalamocortical SEP, which is best recorded at the postcentral cortex contralateral to the stimulation site. Using noncephalic reference, a widespread bilateral component N18 may be distinguished from the later N20. The N18 component appears to be generated below the thalamus, whereas the N20 seems to be generated in the thalamus or by thalamic-cortical radiation [19]. The N20 is followed by a contralateral positivity with varying latency (P23–P27). Using neck recordings with noncephalic reference a spinal nearfield component N13 may be detected. This SEP component is distinct from the P15 component, which is recorded with frontal reference. The neck N13 potential is generated below the foramen magnum. It most probably reflects initial intraspinal postsynaptic activity generated in neurons of the dorsal horn. The P14 farfield potential is generated above the foramen magnum between the lower medulla and the thalamus, probably by the afferent volley in the medial lemniscus. The difference between the major cervical SEP N13 and the first negative thalamocortical peak N20 recorded over the scalp represents the CCT (central conduction time), which is the time interval for the evoked response to travel through the intracranial portion of the somatosensory pathway. Depending on the filter settings and electrode locations, the CCT of healthy subjects is 5.8 ± 0.5 ms. The CCT has been show to correlate with critical levels of brain perfusion [29] and is subject to changes in body temperature and drug effects [37]. Intraoperative SEP monitoring is used increasingly to improve monitoring of neural tracts at risk during surgical procedures. Changes in SEP latencies and waveforms may indicate impaired transmission in the pathway monitored. In addition to SEP changes due to surgical trauma and cerebral hypoxia/ischemia or in physiologic variables, SEPs are also modulated by anesthetic drugs. For the interpretation of a modulation of the nociceptive system the effects of centrally acting drugs on the SEP have to be known.

Effects of Anesthetics

The effects of anesthetics on spinal, subcortical, and cortical SEP have been studied over the past 20 years. Because the effects of anesthetic drugs on SEP are mostly not agent specific and predictable, monitoring of early cortical SEP has been advocated for assessment of depth of anesthesia [50]. Spinal and subcortical SEP components appear to be very robust against the effects of anesthetics. SEPs with latencies >20 ms with origins in thalamocortical or corticocortical projection systems are subject to the effects of intravenous hypnotics, inhalational anesthetics, and, to a lesser degree, narcotic analgesics. With the exception of etomidate, dose-dependent decreases in amplitude and increases in latencies have been found for almost all anesthetics [35, 44]. Later cortical SEPs may be completely abolished. However, SEPs may still be recorded in the presence of complete suppression of spontaneous brain electrical activity [24]. Etomidate has been shown to increase early cortical SEP amplitudes and latencies [33, 39]. The increase in amplitude probably indicates suppression of inhibitory neural mechanisms in thalamo-cortical pathways [33]. It has been suggested that the amplitude-enhancing effect of etomidate may be beneficial for intraoperative monitoring in patients with small SEP amplitudes [36]. With an intravenous anesthetic technique for hypnotics the early cortical SEP component may be used for intraoperative monitoring. The effect of hyponotics on polysynaptic SEP components with latencies of 25 ms or more is variable. They may be suppressed with higher doses. Subcortical SEP components are not significantly affected by hypnotics.

The effect of volatile anesthetics on spinal and subcortical SEPs is variable. Halothane administration does not result in changes of spinal SEP [2]. Animal studies have shown that isoflurane and enflurane may increase the N13 peak latency and decrease the interval between the N14 peak and the P14 peak of median nerve SEPs [57]. However, in human beings no significant changes in latencies of subcortical SEPs have been found [49, 53]. Increasing concentrations of volatile anesthetics depress cortical SEPs and increase latencies [45, 46, 53, 54]. With respect to the early cortical component N20/P25, enflurane produces the greatest depressing effect. Later SEP components are most susceptible to the effects of halothane. Recent data suggest that sevoflurane given at increasing concentrations has effects on median nerve SEPs similar to those of isoflurane [43].

The changes on upper or lower extremity SEPs induced by narcotic analgesics are smaller compared with the effects of intravenous or inhalational anesthetics. Opioid-activated spinal pathways apparently do not interfere with transmission of afferent impulses resulting from stimulation of peripheral somatic nerves. Early cortical SEP components are slightly depressed by bolus doses of narcotic analgesics [39]. An opioid-based anesthetic technique allows adquate SEP signal acquisition in most instances.

The effects of anesthetics on spinal, subcortical, and cortical SEP have been studied over the past 20 years. Because the effects of anesthetic drugs on SEP are mostly not agent specific and predictable monitoring of early cortical SEP has been advocated for assessment of depth of anesthesia [50].

It has been proposed that SEPs reflect the analgesic rather than the hypnotic action of anesthesia [55]. This would be consistent with the finding that nitrous oxide depresses SEP more profoundly than volatile anesthetics when given at equipotent doses, and that, in comparison to narcotic analgesics, hypnotics such as etomidate and propofol without analgesic potency fail to depress the SEP response. However, few data are available on the effects of noxious stimulation on median or tibial nerve somatosensory evoked potentials. In anesthetized patients a decrease in latency and an increase in amplitude of the first negative peak of the early cortical SEP induced by skin incision was found [51]. In contrast, no SEP changes were observed during the stimulatory response induced by tracheal intubation. It is unclear if the type of noxious stimulation may play a role for the SEP response. Further evidence for the usefulness of SEP monitoring for assessment of nociception has been given in another study [25]. Significant reductions in cortical SEP amplitude (N100) were observed during anesthesia with propofol and nitrous oxide. During surgery (tract of the mesentery) the amplitude was increased again towards baseline values. From these findings it can be concluded that the offset of the anesthetic-induced depressant effects on SEPs are most likely related to noxious stimulation when depth of anesthesia is inadequate in relation to the intensity of the surgical stimulus. The mechanisms for an increase in early cortical SEP amplitudes following noxious stimulation are unclear. The SEP N20 component has its origin in the thalamocortical radiation and in the primary sensory cortex, reflecting the synchronized postsynaptic activity of pyramid cells in area 3. The P25 and N35 SEP components are probably generated in area 1, which receives input from thin axons of the thalamus. These SEP components most probably reflect corticocortical activity in the sensory cortex.

In spite of the observation that SEP may change following noxious stimulation in anesthetized patients, these changes appear to be unspecific. In addition, they have not yet been quantitated with respect to nociceptive signal transmission or the effects of analgesic treatments. The most important reasons why early SEP components have not been used for assessment of nociception are as follows: Early components show a very low signal-to-noise ratio, such that up to 1000 stimuli have to be applied to extract early potentials from the spontaneous EEG, excluding the use of painful stimuli. In addition, slow conduction velocities are typical for nociceptive afferents. The earliest brain potential in response to a noxious stimulus would coincide with the EEG response to secondary signal processing of simultaneously co-activated fast-conducting Aβ-fibers.

Nocieptive signals are transmitted through slowly conducting peripheral axons, Aδ- and C-fibers. From this it can be concluded that experimental pain stimuli evoke cerebral potentials with latencies ranging up to several hundred milliseconds. There is increasing evidence that, in contrast to early SEPs, the amplitudes of late cortical event-related SEPs during painful laboratory stimulation relate to the individual pain relief [3, 6, 11, 12, 15, 16, 18, 20] after administration of narcotic analgesics. These pain-related SEPs have been used for assessment of analgesic drug effects of nonsteroidal anti-inflammatory drugs and narcotic analgesics. Drug-induced changes in SEP components have often been considered evidence of their nociceptive background. However, electrical median or posterior tibial nerve stimulation used for intraoperative SEP monitoring stimulates not only Aδ- and C-fibers, but also thick myelinated nerves not involved in nociceptive transmission. Therefore, specific pain models developed for pain research in humans have been used for the assessment of analgesic treatment.

Even though late SEPs hold promise for assessment of functional changes in the nociceptive system, these SEP components have not been rigorously studied for intraoperative monitoring. One reason may be that they are almost completely depressed by virtually all anesthetics. In addition, the late components are unspecific and show a large variability in latencies within and between subjects [3]. They most probably reflect secondary signal processing of the received information, such as stimulus recognition, magnitude estimation, quality of sensation induced by the stimulus, e.g., painfulness, or the cortical initiation of movements in reaction to a stimulus. Typically, late SEPs show a negativity at 140 ms and a positivity at 240 ms. In pain research, late SEP components have been shown to correlate to the intensity of painful stimuli. However, late SEPs are modulated by the experimental surrounding, background noise, stress situations, stimulus expectancy, vigilance level, and habituation [27, 47].

Techniques most often used for stimulation of pain-related SEPs include electrical tooth pulp stimulation, intracutaneous electrical stimulation, radiant heat stimuli by an infrared CO_2 laser, and stimulation of the nasal mucosa by CO_2. Using tooth pulp electrical stimulation, SEPs were compared with stimulus strength and pain intensity [17]. Late SEP amplitudes, but not latencies, were related to changes in stimulus intensity and subjective pain ratings. From this it was concluded that the responses reflected sensory processing rather than only sensory transmission. Cerebral potentials in response to electrical stimuli have been investigated extensively because the stimulus is easy to control [5, 6, 11, 52]. However, electrical stimuli excite afferent pathways in an unnatural, synchronized manner. In addition, almost all peripheral nerve fibers are recruited by electrical stimuli [28]. Intracutaneous electrical stimulation tries to overcome some shortcommings of transcutaneous stimulation. With this method, electrical stimuli become less throbbing and more stinging. Because electrical stimuli may recruit non-nociceptive nerve fibers, there may be some ambiguity in the interpretation of pain-related SEPs. Heat stimuli applied to the skin by contact-free CO_2-laser radiation pulses simultaneously activate both Aδ- and C-fibers which terminate in the most superficial skin layers [7]. Correspondingly, two SEP waveforms may be observed which are related to different pain sensations. Significant correlations between SEP amplitudes elicited by laser heat stimulation and pain estimates have been found in various studies [3, 7, 12]. Chemical drugs may also be used for nociceptive stimulation. Recent studies suggest that polymodal nociceptors in the nasal mucosa can be stimulated by well-defined CO_2 application in a continuous air stream [31]. CO_2 excites afferent units in the nasal mucosa that are capsaicin sensitive [28, 31]. The CO_2 stimulus probably acts by quickly lowering the tissue pH. With this technique, amplitudes of event-related cerebral potentials as well as subjective pain experience have been shown to be significantly changed by CO_2 stimulus intensity. Others methods for studying pain-related cerebral potentials include mechanical and cold stimuli.

Carefully controlled laboratory studies with healthy volunteers have shown that amplitudes of late SEPs elicited by short noxious stimuli are correlated with the intensity of pain sensation [6, 13, 30, 40]. There is increasing evidence that SEP amplitudes following thermal [7, 13], intracutaneous [5, 30, 34], and tooth pulp stimulation decrease as perceived pain is relieved by analgesic treatment.

Objective electrophysiologic measures of drug-induced analgesia have been given for acetylsalicylic acid [7, 10, 17, 32], flupirtine [9], paracetamol, lidocaine [1, 42], metamizol [48], nitrous oxide [16], morphine [1], fentanyl [15, 26, 34], pentazocine [9, 32], tilidine [8], and alfentanil [26]. The N150/P250 amplitude following electrical stimulation has been shown to be highly correlated to subjective pain sensation [6, 11, 12]. From these findings it was concluded that late cortical SEPs and subjective pain ratings will be at least partially redundant sources of information, and under certain conditions both measures may be substituted for each other. However, it has also been shown that decreases in SEP and pain ratings were not exactly synchronous. These findings indicate that SEP amplitudes and pain reports may represent two different central effects of narcotic analgesics. In spite of these unsolved problems relating changes in SEP to analgesic treatment, the paradigms used in experimental pain research have been successfully transferred to the clinical setting [34]. In anesthetized patients (0.8% halothane in 66% nitrous oxide) no cortical SEP components to intracutaneous electrical stimuli could be recorded. After withdrawal of nitrous oxide, late SEPs similar in waveform to control data were noted. In contrast, EEG and auditory evoked responses were unchanged. It was concluded that changes in pain-related SEPs correlated with analgesic treatment. The applicability of the electrophysiologic technique of intracutaneous stimulation is supported by its intraindividual reliability and its consistency with previous reports on the sensitivity to analgesic treatment effects [8, 11].

Habituation and changes in vigilance are known to affect evoked cortical responses. Therefore, randomization of stimulus conditions with respect to intensity and interstimulus intervals has been shown to be of importance in order to minimize habituation and sensibilization effects [6]. The high and constant individual level of arousal is reflected in unchanged SEPs and pain ratings in subjects without analgesic treatment. The fairly constant threshold intensities of electrical pain stimuli are a particular advantage of the intracutaneous stimulus technique, which can be employed in the operating room. A close correlation between verbal pain ratings and late SEPs in unanesthetized patients does not prove that late SEP are pain specific. Even when carefully controlled, it is difficult to decide whether the decrease in SEP amplitude is due to a specific analgesic drug effect or to changes in vigilance. This holds especially true during anesthesia, because almost all centrally acting drugs tend to decrease late SEPs. The differentiation between pain relief and decrease in vigilance constitutes a basic problem in pain research. In the spontaneous EEG decreased cortical arousal is reflected in a reduction of alpha-activity and an increase in theta- and delta-activity. Drowsiness and narcotic analgesics have been shown to alter spontaneous EEG to a similar degree [38]. Therefore, from the spontaneous EEG it appears to be impossible to differentiate between analgesic drug effects and changes in vigilance. In this situation, pain-related SEPs may help to separate analgesic from unspecific hypnotic treatment effects. The dose-dependent decrease in SEP amplitudes following administration of analgesics indicate that cortical SEPs following specific sensory stimulation reflect attenuation of nociceptive transmission, even in anesthetized patients when no subjective pain report is available. The narcotic, in contrast to the hypnotic, effects may be simultaneously assessed by EEG measures.

Late SEP components have been shown to be sensitive to analgesic drugs. From this it was concluded that nociception and pain experience may be assessed objectively by pain-related cerebral potentials.

Summary

Early farfield and cortical nearfield SEPs may be used for intraoperative monitoring when neural tracts are at risk by the surgical procedure or following central nervous system injury. All cortical SEPs are depressed in a graded, mostly dose-dependent manner by almost all anesthetics, however, to a different degree. Early cortical SEPs may be recorded during general anesthesia, especially when an intravenous anesthetic technique is used. Both early and late cortical SEPs show unspecific changes to noxious stimulation. However, late SEPs have been shown to change in relation to the intensity of a painful stimulus. In addition, in awake volunteers a close correlation to subjective pain experience has been shown in many studies. From this it may be concluded that late cortical SEPs hold promise for assessment of analgesic treatment effects. This has already been shown in some clinical studies. Further studies using specific pain stimuli, such as radiant laser heat stimuli, have to elaborate if late SEPs may be recorded in anesthetized patients and if the SEP changes induced by noxious stimulation are related to the analgesic state.

References

1. Arendt-Nielsen L, Oberg B, Bjerring P (1990) Laser-induced pain for quantitative comparison of intravenous regional anesthesia using saline, morphine, lidocaine, or prilocaine. Reg Anaesth 15:186–193
2. Baines DB, Whittle IR, Chaseling RW, Overton JH, Johnson IH (1985) Effect of halothane on spinal somatosensory evoked potentials in sheep. Br J Anaesth 57:869–899
3. Bromm B (1984) The evoked cerebral potential and pain. In: Fields HL, Dubner R, Cervero F (eds) Pain measurement in man. Elsevier, Amsterdam, pp 397–408
4. Bromm B (1994) Central evoked brain potential as overall control of afferent systems. In: Schulte am Esch J, Kochs E (eds) Central nervous system monitoring. Springer, Berlin Heidelberg New York, pp 115–126
5. Bromm B, Meier W (1984) The intracutaneous stimulus: a new pain model for algesimetric studies. Meth Find Exp Clin Pharmacol 6:405–410
6. Bromm B, Scharein E (1982) Principal component analysis of pain-related cerebral potentials to mechanical and electrical stimulation in man. Electroencephalogr Clin Neurophysiol 53:305–329
7. Bromm B, Treede RD (1991) Laser-evoked cerebral potentials in the assessment of cutaneous pain sensitivity in normal subjects and patients. Rev Neurol 147:625–643
8. Bromm B, Meier W, Scharein E (1983) Antagonism between tilidine and naloxone on cerebral potentials and pain ratings in man. Eur J Pharmacol 87:431–439

9. Bromm B, Ganzel R, Herrmann WM, Meier W, Scharein E (1986) Pentazocine and flupirtine effects on spontaneous and evoked EEG activity. Neuropsychobiology 16: 152–156

10. Bromm B, Rundshagen I, Scharein E (1991) Central analgesic effects of acetylsalicylic acid in healthy man. Arzneim Forsch Drug Res 11:1123–1129

11. Buchsbaum MS, Davis GC, Naber D, Pickar D (1983) Pain enhanced naloxone-induced hyperalgesia in humans as assessed by somatosensory-evoked potentials. Psychopharmacology 79:99–103

12. Carmon D, Dotan Y, Sarne Y (1978) Correlation of subjective pain experience with cerebral evoked responses to noxious thermal stimulations. Exp Brain Res 33:445–453

13. Carmon A, Friedman Y, Coger R, Kenton B (1980) Single trial analysis of evoked potentials to noxious thermal stimulation in man. Pain 8:21–32

14. Chapman CR, Benedetti C (1979) Nitrous oxide effects on cerebral evoked potentials to pain: partial reversal with a narcotic analgesic. Anesthesiology 51:135–138

15. Chapman CR, Chen ACN, Colpitts YM, Martin RW (1981) Sensory decision theory describes evoked potentials in pain discrimination. Psychophysiology 18:114–120

16. Chapman CR, Colpitts YM, Benedetti C, Butler S (1982) Event-related potential correlates of analgesia; comparison of fentanyl, acupuncture and nitrous oxide. Pain 14:327–337

17. Chatrian GE, Canfield RC, Knauss TA, Lettich E (1975) Cerebral responses to electrical tooth pulp stimulation. Neurology (Minneapolis) 25:745–757

18. Chen ACN, Chapman CR (1980) Aspirin analgesia evaluated by event-related potentials in man: possible central action in brain. Exp Brain Res 39:359–364

19. Chiappa KH, Choi SK, Young RRG (1980) Short-latency somatosensory evoked potentials following median nerve stimulation in patients with neurological lesions. In: Desmedt JE (ed) Clinical uses of cerebral, brainstem and spinal somatosensory evoked potentials, vol 7. Prog Clin Neurophysiol, Karger, Basel, pp 264–281

20. Chen ACN, Treede RD, Bromm B (1986) Modulation of pain-evoked cerebral potentials by concurrent subacute pain. In: Bromm B (ed) Pain measurement in man. Neurophysiological correlates of pain. Elsevier, Amsterdam, pp 301–310

21. Chudler EH, Dong WK (1983) The assessment of pain by cerebral evoked potentials. Pain 16:221–244

22. Creutzfeldt O (1983) Cortex cerebri. Springer, Berlin Heidelberg New York

23. Desmedt JE (1989) Somatosensory evoked potentials in neuromonitoring. In: Desmedt JE (ed) Neuromonitoring in surgery. Elsevier, Amsterdam, pp 1–20

24. Drummod JC, Todd MM, Hoi Sang U (1985) The effect of high-dose sodium thiopental on brain stem auditory and median nerve somatosensory evoked responses in humans. Anesthesiology 63:249–254

25. Freye E, Hartung Schenk GK (1989) Somatosensory-evoked potentials during block of surgical stimulation with propofol. Br J Anaesth 63:357–359

26. Hill HF, Chapman CR, Saeger LS, Bjurstrom R, Walter MH, Schoene RB, Kippes M (1990) Steady-state infusions of opioids in humans. II. Concentration-effect relationships and therapeutic margins. Pain 43:69–79

27. Hillyard SA (1978) Sensation, perception and attention: analysis using ERPs. In: Callaway E, Tueting P, Koslow SH (eds) Event-related brain potentials in man. Academic, London, pp 223–321

28. Handwerker HO, Kobal G (1993) Psychophysiology of experimentally induced pain. Physiol Rev 73:639–671

29. Hume AL, Cant BR (1978) Conduction time in central somatosensory pathways in man. Electroencephalogr Clin Neurophysiol 69:277–286

30. Joseph J, Howland EW, Wakai R, Backonja M, Baffa O, Potenti FM, Cleeland CS (1991) Late pain-related magnetic fields and electric potentials evoked by intracutaneous electric finger stimulation. Electroencephalogr Clin Neurophysiol 80:46–52

31. Kobal G (1985) Pain-related electrical potentials of the human nasal mucosa elicited by chemical stimulation. Pain 22:151–163
32. Kobal G, Hummel C, Nuernberg B, Brune K (1990) Effects of pentazocine and acetylsalicylic acid on pain-rating, pain-related evoked potentials and vigilance in relationship to pharmacokinetic parameters. Agents Actions 4:342–359
33. Kochs E, Treede RD, Schulte am Esch J (1986) Increase of somatosensory evoked potentials during induction of anaesthesia with etomidate. Anaesthesist 35:359–365
34. Kochs E, Treede RD, Schulte am Esch J, Bromm B (1990) Modulation of pain-related somatosensory evoked potentials by general anesthesia. Anesth Analg 71:225–230
35. Kochs E, Bischoff P (1994) Anesthesia and somatosensory evoked responses. In: Schulte am Esch J, Kochs E (eds) Central nervous system monitoring. Springer, Berlin Heidelberg New York, pp 146–175
36. Koht A, Schultz W, Schmidt G, Schramm J, Watanabe E (1988) The effects of etomidate, midazolam and thiopental on median nerve somatosensory evoked potentials and the additive effects of fentanyl and nitrous oxide. Anesth Analg 67:435–441
37. Markand ON, Warren CH, Moorthey SS, Stoelting RK, King RD (1984) Monitoring of multimodally evoked potentials during open heart surgery under hypothermia. Electroencephalogr Clin Neurophysiol 59:432–439
38. Martin WR, Kay DC (1977) Effects of analgesics and antagonists on the EEG. In: Longo VG (ed) Handbook of electroencephalography and clinical neurophysiology, vol 7C. Elsevier, Amsterdam, pp 97–109
39. McPherson RW, Sell B, Traystman RJ (1986) Effects of thiopental, fentanyl, and etomidate on upper extremity somatosensory evoked potentials in humans. Anesthesiology 65:584–589
40. Miltner W, Johnson R jr, Braun C, Larbig W (1989) Somtasensory event-related potentials to painful and non-painful stimuli: effects of attention. Pain 38:303–312
41. Namerow NS (1969) Somatosensory evoked responses following cervical cordotomy. Bull Los Angeles Neurol Soc 34:184–188
42. Nielsen JC, Arendt-Nielsen L, Bjerring P, Carlsson P (1991) Analgesic efficacy of low doses of intravenously administered lidocaine on experimental laser-induced pain: a placebo-controlled study. Reg Anaesth 16:28–33
43. Nishiyama Y, Ito M (1993) Effects of isoflurane, sevoflurane and enflurane on median nerve somatosensory evoked potentials in humans. Jpwn J Anesth 42:339–343
44. Nuwer MR (1986) Evoked potential monitoring in the operating room. Raven, New York
45. Pathak KS, Ammadio M, Kalamchi A, Scoles PV, Shaffer JW, Mackay W (1987) Effects of halothane, enflurane, and isoflurane on somatosensory evoked potentials during nitrous oxide anesthesia. Anesthesiology 66:753–757
46. Peterson DO, Drummond JC, Todd MM (1986) Effects of halothane, enflurane, isoflurane and nitrous oxide on somatosensory evoked potentials in humans. Anesthesiology 65:35–40
47. Picton TW (ed) (1989) Human event-related potentials. Elsevier Science, Amsterdam (Handbook of electroencephalography and clinical neurophysiology, vol 3)
48. Rhodewald P, Neddermann E (1988) Dose-dependence of the analgesic action of metamizol. Anaesthesist 37:150–155
49. Samara SK, Vanderzant CW, Domer PA, Sackellares J (1987) Differential effects of isoflurane on human median nerve somatosensory evoked potentials. Anesthesiology 66:29–35
50. Sebel PS, Heneghan CP, Ingram DA (1985) Evoked responses – a neurophysiological indicator of depth of anesthesia? (editorial) Br J Anaesth 57:841–842
51. Sebel PS, Withington PS, Rutherford CF, Markman K (1988) The effect of tracheal intubation and surgical stimulation on median nerve somatosensory evoked potentials during anaesthesia. Anaesthesia 43:857–860

52. Sitaram N, Buchsbaum MS, Gillin JC (1977) Physostigmine analgesia and somatosensory evoked responses in man. Eur J Pharmacol 42:285–290
53. Thiel A, Russ W, Kafurke H, Hempelmann G (1987) The effects of enflurane and isoflurane on somatosensory evoked potentials after stimulation of the median nerve. Anaesth Intensivther Notfallmed 22:159–165
54. Thiel A, Russ W, Hempelmann G (1988) Evoked potentials and volatile anaesthetics. Klin Wochenschr 66[Suppl XIV]:11–18
55. Thornton C (1991) Evoked potentials in anaesthesia. Eur J Anaesth 8:89–107
56. Treede RD, Kief S, Hölzer T, Bromm B (1988) Late somatosensory cerebral potentials in response to cutaneous heat stimuli. Electroencephalogr Clin Neurophysiol 70:429–441
57. Vandesteene A, Nogueira MC, Mavroudakis N, Defevrimont M, Brundo E, Zegers de Beyl D (1991) Topographic analysis of the effects of isoflurane anesthesia on SEP. Electroencephalogr Clin Neurophysiol 88:77–81

Do Auditory Evoked Potentials Assess Awareness?

D. Schwender, S. Klasing, C. Madler, E. Pöppel, and K. Peter

Components of Auditory Evoked Potentials

The auditory evoked potentials (AEP) consist of a series of positive and negative waves that represent processes of transduction, transmission, and processing of auditory information from the cochlea to the brain stem, the primary auditory cortex, and the frontal cortex. Figure 1 shows an idealized waveform of an auditory evoked potential depicted on a semilogarithmic time base [1]. The early peaks of the potential, the brain-stem auditory evoked potentials, are generated in the cochlear nerve and relays of the brain-stem. They reflect successful stimulus transduction and primary stimulus transmission [2]. The mid-latency auditory evoked potentials occur 10–100 ms post-stimulus. These early cortical waves originate from overlapping activation within different structures of the primary auditory cortex and reflect primary cortical processing of auditory stimuli [2–4]. Finally, late-latency auditory evoked potentials depict the neuronal activity of association cortices in the frontal cortex. They reflect the process of emotional stimulus evaluation and cognitive analysis of the auditory information [5].

The brain-stem auditory evoked potentials remain stable during general anesthesia [6–8]. Late-latency auditory evoked potentials are highly variable in awake subjects and rely strongly on the processes of attention and orientation to the stimulus [5]. In contrast, the mid-latency auditory evoked potentials are interindividually stable [2]. Recordings of mid-latency auditory evoked potentials therefore offer the best opportunity for monitoring auditory information processing in the primary auditory cortex during general anesthesia.

Figure 2 shows an original tracing of an auditory evoked potential of an awake patient. Five (V) belongs to the brain-stem-generated potentials, which demonstrates that auditory stimuli were correctly transduced. NA, PA, NB, P1 are the mid-latency auditory evoked potentials and are generated in the primary auditory cortex of the temporal lobe [2–4]. Mid-latency auditory evoked potentials in the awake state have high peak-to-peak amplitudes and a characteristic periodic wave form.

AEP During Anesthesia

General anesthesia with a number of general anesthetics – for example, the volatile anesthetics halothane, enflurane, isoflurane or the intravenously administered

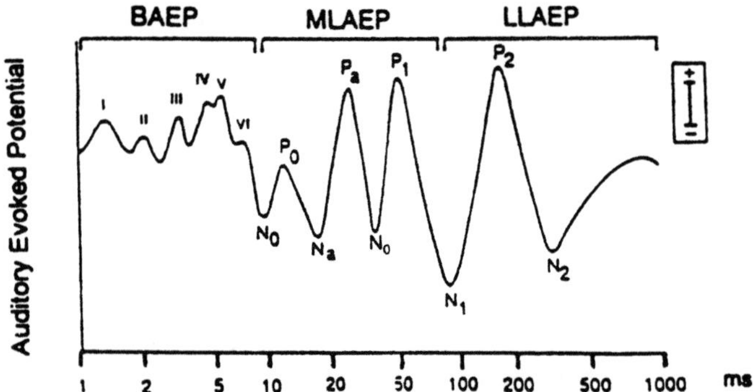

Fig. 1. Auditory evoked potential. *BAEP*, Brain-stem auditory evoked potentials; *MLAEP*, mid-latency auditory evoked potentials; *LLAEP*, late-latency auditory evoked potentials. (From [1])

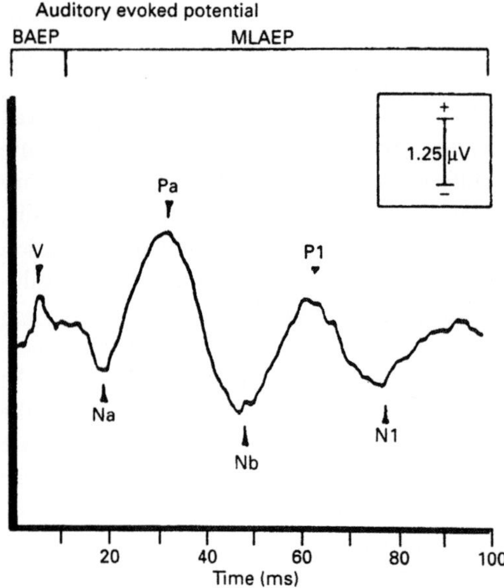

Fig. 2. Auditory evoked potential of an awake patient. (From [18])

anesthetics propofol, etomidate, and althesin – suppress mid-latency auditory evoked potentials dose dependently. This means that with increasing end-expiratory concentrations or increasing blood levels of these general anesthetics, dose-dependent increases in latencies of the MLAEP peaks and decreases in amplitudes can be observed [6–11].

Figure 3 demonstrates such a dose-response relation between volatile anesthetics and mid-latency AEPs [6]. Mid-latency AEPs were recorded under increasing concentrations of isoflurane. In the upper trace one can see the AEP of the awake patient with high amplitudes and a characteristic periodic waveform. Under

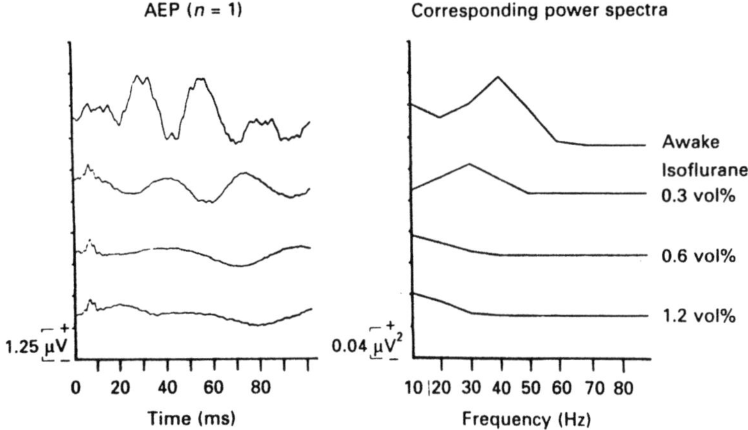

Fig. 3. Auditory evoked potentials under increasing end-expiratory concentrations of isoflurane. (From [6])

increasing end-expiratory concentrations of isoflurane the brain-stem AEPs do not change in latency or amplitude compared with the awake state. In contrast, MLAEP peaks show a clear dose-dependent increase in latencies and a decrease in amplitudes. Under surgical anesthesia with 1.2 vol% in the last tracing, mid-latency AEPs are nearly completely suppressed.

This dose-dependent depression of mid-latency AEPs, i.e., the suppression of the early cortical potentials under a number of general anesthetics, raises the question of whether mid-latency AEPs can measure the "depth of anesthesia" and indicate intraoperative awareness. In this context the following questions are particularly important:

1. Is there any relation between mid-latency auditory evoked potentials and intraoperative wakefulness or awareness?
2. Is intact primary cortical information processing, as indicated by mid-latency auditory evoked potentials, a prerequisite for postoperative recall of intraoperative events?

AEP During Thiopental Bolus Injection

In a first step we did a very simple experiment [12]. We gave our patients thiopental for induction of general anesthesia. After loss of consciousness the patient's lungs were ventilated via facemask until the first purposeful movement of the limbs appeared. Then a second bolus of thiopental was given and routine general anesthesia was maintained according to normal anesthetic practice. Auditory evoked potentials were recorded when the patient was awake, online at the start of the first thiopental injection, and up to 8 min there after.

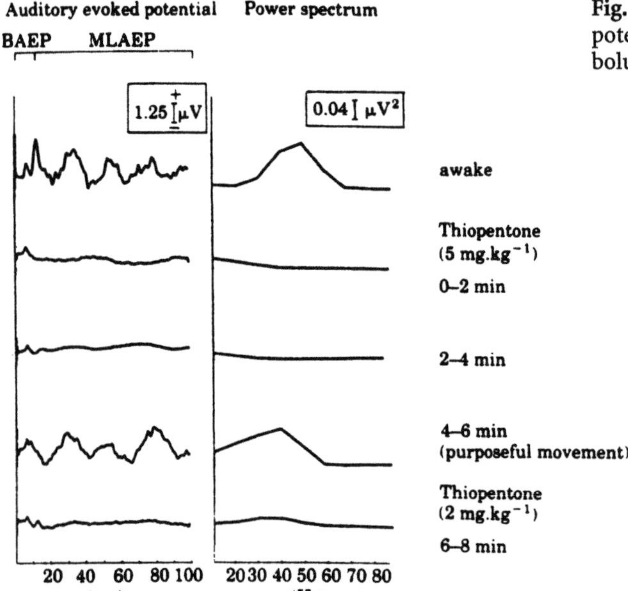

Fig. 4. Auditory evoked potentials during thiopental bolus injection. (From [12])

Figure 4 shows a typical AEP recording during the experiment. In the upper trace one can see the AEP of the awake patient. The brain-stem response can be identified easily; mid-latency AEPs have high amplitudes and a characteristic periodic waveform. After injection of thiopental the brain-stem response can be identified, as in the awake state. In contrast, mid-latency AEPs are severely attenuated or abolished. With the purposeful movement 4–6 min after injection, mid-latency AEP amplitudes increase and peak latencies return to the values of the awake patients, as demonstrated in the fourth trace of this recording. In the last recording a second thiopental bolus injection again leads to a significant increase in latencies and a decrease in amplitudes of mid-latency AEPs. This means that when mid-latency AEPs were suppressed no motor signs of wakefulness were observed. In contrast, when mid-latency AEPs were preserved as in the awake state, patients showed purposeful movements as a clinical sign of decreasing central anesthetic action.

AEP During Cesarean Section

To investigate the relation between mid-latency AEPs and intraoperative awareness we recorded mid-latency AEPs during elective cesarean section under general anesthesia [13]. Twenty patients were included in the study. Intraoperatively purposeful movements of the head and the limbs, eye opening, and other facial movements were interpreted as signs of intraoperative wakefulness. They were recorded as spontaneous movements during the surgical procedure and after

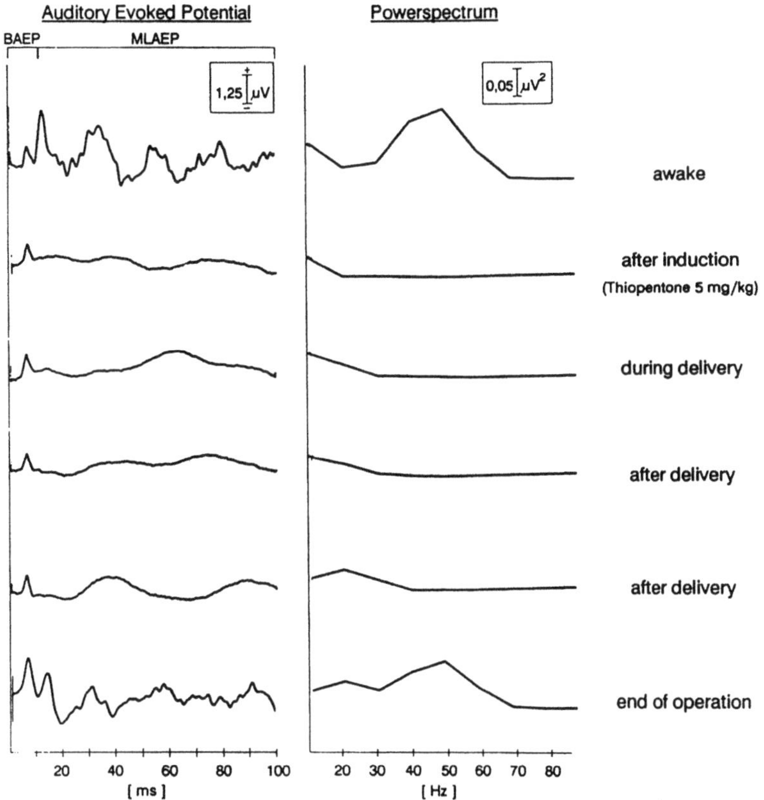

Fig. 5. Auditory evoked potentials during cesarean section: adequate anesthesia

presentation of one of two audiotapes (tape A: sound of a crying baby, tape B: classical music) which were presented in a double-blind randomized order after delivery of the baby. Postoperatively, the patients were interviewed to evaluate intraoperative dreams, hallucinations, and detailed reports of intraoperative events. Auditory evoked potentials were recorded in the awake state and during the entire surgical procedure.

Figure 5 shows an original tracing of AEPs during cesarean section under adequate general anesthesia. This patient showed no spontaneous or provoked purposeful movements and had no recall of intraoperative events. In the upper trace is the AEP of the awake patient. Brain-stem AEPs can be identified easily; mid-latency AEPs show high amplitudes and a characteristic periodic waveform. During general anesthesia in this patient brain-stem AEPs appear as in the awake state. In contrast, mid-latency AEPs are severely attenuated or completely suppressed. At the end of anesthesia, during recovery in the last tracing, mid-latency AEPs reestablished high amplitudes and the periodic waveform, as in the awake state.

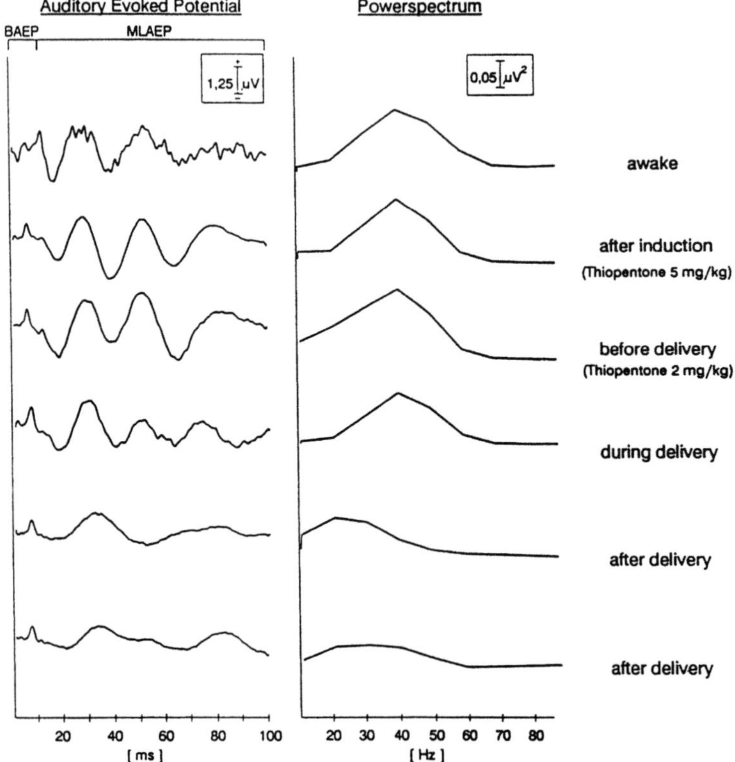

Fig. 6. Auditory evoked potentials during cesarean section: intraoperative wakefulness

Different are the auditory evoked potentials in a patient with apparent signs of inadequate anesthesia during cesarean section in Fig. 6. This patient showed repeated purposeful movements intraoperatively and recalled surgical manipulations postoperatively in detail. In the upper trace is the AEP of the awake patient. It is characterized by high amplitudes and a periodic waveform. During general anesthesia, before and during delivery in this patient, mid-latency AEPs are recorded similar to those in the awake state. The high amplitudes and the periodic waveform are preserved. This is also true after a second thiopental bolus injection. Following delivery, when anesthesia is deepened by adding a volatile anesthetic, mid-latency AEPs are reduced in amplitude and increased in latency. Four purposeful movements were observed after presentation of the sound of a crying baby (tape A) but only one after classical music (tape B). This observation underlines the importance of the emotional significance of the intraoperatively presented stimulus.

The interindividual grand averages recorded after the audiotape presentation are presented in Fig. 7. After tape presentations which were not followed by purposeful movements, mid-latency AEPs were suppressed. In contrast, when

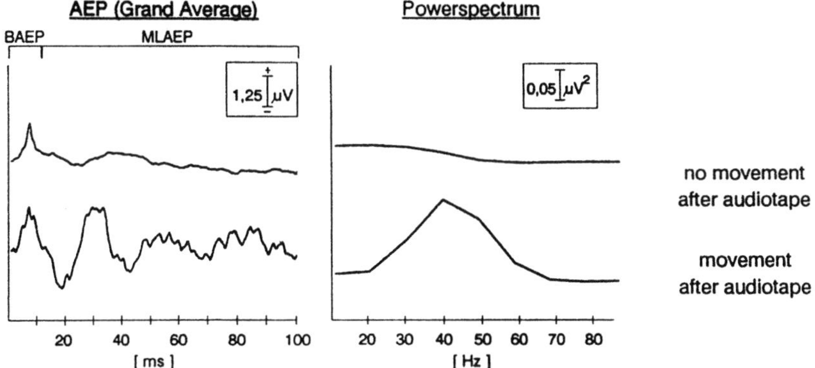

Fig. 7. Auditory evoked potentials (grand averages) during cesarean section, following audiotape presentation

purposeful movements followed the audiotape presentation, mid-latency AEPs had high amplitudes and peak latencies were in the normal range, as in the awake patients.

One important question which may follow from these data is: What is the relation between mid-latency auditory evoked potentials and postoperative recall of intraoperative events? What is a sensitive method for detecting recall of intraoperative events postoperatively? A successful registration retention and retrieval of auditory information has as its prior condition an intact auditory stimulus processing as well as an intact memory system.

Explicit and Implicit Memory Sytems

An often-used taxonomy of memory in cognitive science is the distinction between explicit and implicit memory [14, 15]. Explicit memory is the deliberate active and conscious recollection of an experience in time and space, for example, episodes in a human life. In contrast, implicit memory remembers passively and unconsciously in an associative or semantic context without being related to time and space, for example, knowledge about the language and the world.

An impressive example which demonstrates differences between explicit and implicit memory systems is an experiment made by Claparede 90 years ago [16]. He welcomed amnesic patients holding a needle between his fingers, which was naturally a very unpleasant experience for the patients. The following day the patients did not remember ever having met Claparede. Nevertheless, they refused to shake hands with him, stating that hands sometimes may contain pins. This experiment clearly demonstrates the existence of the two distinct memory systems. The patients of Claparede were able to recollect the previous experience implicitly without having any explicit memory of the circumstances in which they had gained the information.

How can these findings be transferred to the situation of general anesthesia? A recall of intraoperative events occasionally occurs after cardiac surgery.

AEP and Explicit and Implicit Memory During Cardiac Surgery

We therefore investigated the postoperative memories of 45 patients who underwent elective cardiac surgery [17]. For maintanance of general anesthesia all patients received high doses of opioid analgesia using fentanyl. Additionally, they received either the benzodiazepine flunitrazepam (ten patients, group 1), the volatile anesthetic isoflurane (ten patients, group 2), or propofol (ten patients, group 3); 15 patients served as a control group (group 4).

After sternotomy an audiotape was presented to the patients of groups 1, 2, and 3, which included an implicit memory task. Besides positive suggestions for the perioperative course, the story of Robinson Crusoe was told in a short version and the patients received the suggestion to remember Robinson Crusoe when they were asked about their associations to the code word "Friday" postoperatively. Three to five days after the operation the patients were asked about their recall of intraoperative events and about their associations to "Friday". All experimental evaluations were conducted under double-blind conditions; i.e., neither the patients nor the interviewer knew which anesthetic had been employed, or if an audiotape had been presented or not. Auditory evoked potentials were recorded awake and during general anesthesia before and after the tape presentation.

In the postoperative interview none of patients was able to explicitly recollect intraoperative events. Some patients stated hearing voices or noise, but these perceptions could not definitely be related to the intraoperative situation. Typical associations to the code word "Friday" were "approaching weekend", "last working day of the week", or "fish for lunch or dinner". These statements were also given by patients who then spontaneously remembered Robinson Crusoe. Typical reproductions of the story of Robinson Crusoe were as follows: "When you say Friday I have to think of an island and the story of Robinson Crusoe, but I think this has nothing to do with your question." Another typical answer was: "When you say Friday, I remember that when I was a child, we used to play on a little island in a river near my parents' home. We called that place Robinson Island." It is interesting to note that all patients with implicit memory strongly denied that their associations had anything to do with information heard during anesthesia.

There were no implicit memories in patients belonging to the control group. One patient of the propofol group and one patient of the isoflurane group made the expected association between Friday and Robinson Crusoe. In contrast, five of ten patients of the flunitrazepam-fentanyl group remembered the key word Robinson Crusoe when asked about an association to the code word Friday.

Figure 8 shows auditory evoked potentials of the patients without implicit memory, in the upper part the isoflurane and in the lower part the propofol group. All upper traces show the AEPs of the awake patients. Brain-stem potentials can be

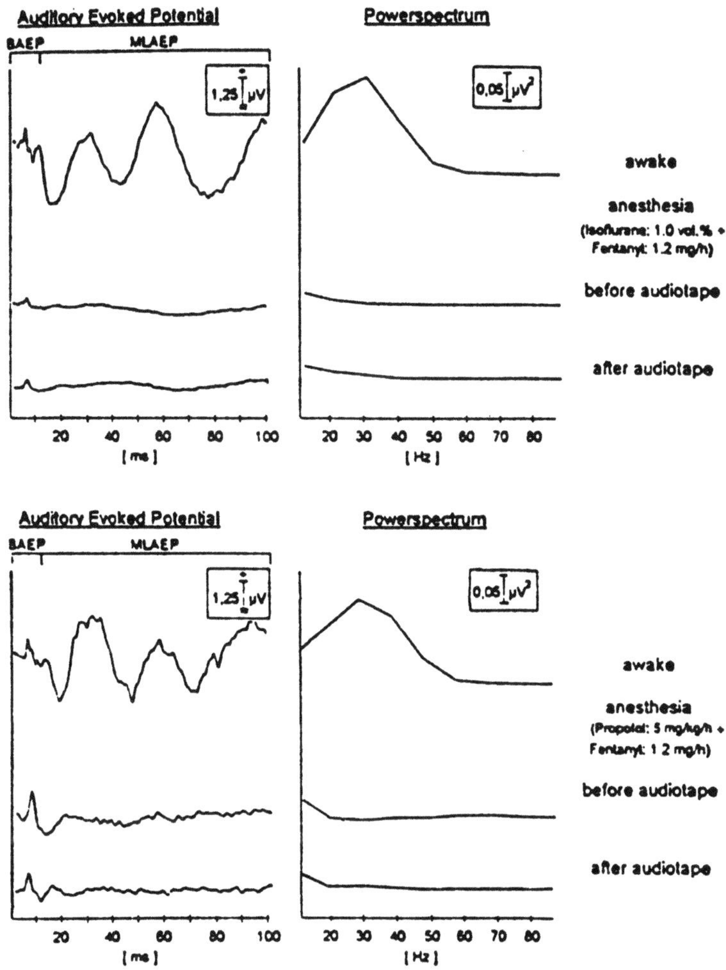

Fig. 8. Auditory evoked potentials during cardiac surgery: no implicit memory postoperatively. (From [17])

identified easily; mid-latency potentials show high amplitudes and the periodic waveform. During general anesthesia in these patients brain-stem potentials can be identified as in the awake state. In contrast, mid-latency potentials show markedly increased latencies and decreased amplitudes, or are even suppressed completely.

A different picture is presented by the mid-latency AEPs of the patients of the flunitrazepam-fentanyl group who remembered Robinson Crusoe implicitly after the operation, as demonstrated in Fig. 9. Again, the upper traces show the AEPs of the awake patients, characterized by high peak-to-peak amplitudes. During general anesthesia, before and after the audiotape was presented to these patients,

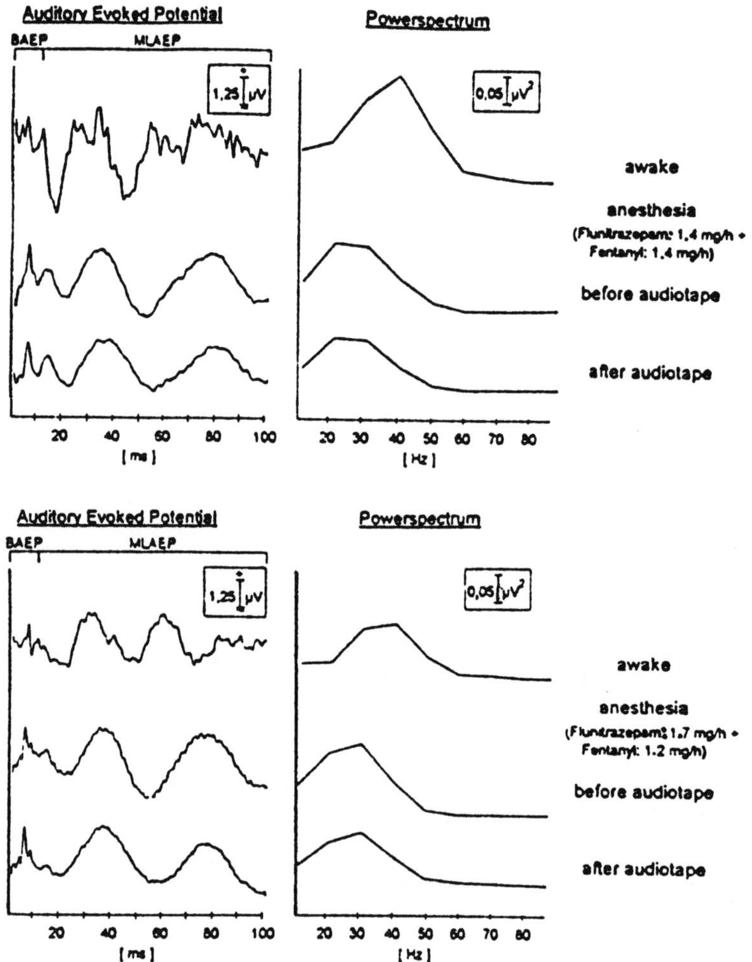

Fig. 9. Auditory evoked potentials during cardiac surgery: implicit memory postoperatively. (From [17])

mid-latency AEPs were recorded similar to those in the awake state. The high amplitudes are preserved. This means that the electrophysiological conditions of primary cortical processing of auditory stimuli are at least partly preserved.

Conclusions

A number of general anesthetics, e.g., halothane, enflurane, isoflurane, propofol, etomidate, and althesin, suppress mid-latency auditory evoked potentials dose dependently. Therefore, MLAEP offer a good opportunity to monitor central cortical effects of general anesthetics.

Mid-latency auditory evoked potentials are suppressed after thiopental bolus injections. With decreasing anesthetic effects of thiopental with the first purposeful movement, MLAEP reestablish high peak-to-peak amplitudes, as in the awake state.

Mid-latency auditory evoked potentials recorded during cesarean section correlate with intraoperative motor signs of wakefulness and, in some patients, with explicit recall of surgical manipulations. Auditory information, as demonstrated in cardiac patients, can be processed during general anesthesia and remembered postoperatively by an implicit memory function.

We found a close correlation between implicit memory and mid-latency auditory evoked potentials. No implicit memory was detected when mid-latency AEPs were suppressed. Implicit memory was observed when mid-latency AEPs and primary cortical processing of auditory stimuli where at least partly preserved.

Further studies will have to determine threshold values of the different AEP parameters for intraoperative wakefulness and explicit and implicit recall of intraoperatively presented information for the different commonly used anesthetics. On the basis of these results, one may decide whether auditory evoked potentials are a valuable method for monitoring what is currently known as "depth of anesthesia."

References

1. Schwender D, Klasing S, Madler C, Peter K, Pöppel E (1993) Mid-latency auditory evoked potentials and cognitive function during general anesthesia. Int Anesthesiol Clin 31:89–106
2. Picton TW, Hillyard SA, Krausz HI, Galambos R (1974) Human auditory evoked potentials. I. Evaluation of components. Electroencephalogr Clin Neurophysiol 36:179–190
3. Deiber MP, Ibanez V, Fischer C, Perrin F, Mauguière F (1988) Sequential mapping favours the hypothesis of distinct generators for Na and Pa middle latency auditory evoked potentials. Electroencephalogr Clin Neurophysiol 71:187–197
4. Scherg M, von Cramon D (1986) Evoked dipole source potentials of the human auditory cortex. Electroencephalogr Clin Neurophysiol 65:344–360
5. Picton TW, Hillyard SA (1974) Human auditory evoked potentials. II. Effects of attention. Electroencephalogr Clin Neurophysiol 36:191–199
6. Madler C, Keller I, Schwender D, Pöppel E (1991) Sensory information processing during general anaesthesia: effect of isoflurane on auditory evoked neuronal oscillations. Br J Anaesth 66:81–87
7. Thornton C, Heneghan CP, James MF, Jones JG (1984) Effects of halothane or enflurane with controlled ventilation on auditory evoked potentials. Br J Anaesth 56:315–323
8. Thornton C, Heneghan CP, Navaratnarajah M, Bateman PE, Jones JG (1985) Effect of etomidate on the auditory evoked response in man. Br J Anaesth 57:554–561
9. Thornton C, Newton DE (1989) The auditory evoked response: a measure of depth of anaesthesia. In: Jones JG (ed) Clinical anesthesiology, vol 3. Bailliere Tindall, London, pp 559–585
10. Thornton C, Heneghan CP, Navaratnarajah M, Jones JG (1986) Selective effect of althesin on the auditory evoked response in man. Br J Anaesth 58:422–427

11. Thornton C, Konieczko KM, Knight AB et al (1989) Effect of propofol on the auditory evoked response and oesophageal contractility. Br J Anaesth 63:411–417
12. Schwender D, Klasing S, Madler C, Pöppel E, Peter K (1994) Mid-latency auditory evoked potentials and purposeful movements after thiopental bolus injection. Anaesthesia 49:99–104
13. Schwender D, Klasing S, Madler C, Pöppel E, Peter K (1994) Mid-latency auditory evoked potentials and wakefulness during caesarean section. Eur J Anaesth (in press)
14. Schacter DL (1987) Implicit memory: history and current status. J Exp Psychol 13:501–518
15. Kihlstrom JF (1987) The cognitive unconscious. Science 237:1445–1452
16. Claparede E (1911) Recognition et moiite. (Reprinted 1951 as Recogniton and "meness". In: Rappaport D (ed) Organizations and pathology of thought. Columbia University Press, New York). Arch Psychol 11:79–90
17. Schwender D, Kaiser A, Klasing S, Peter K, Pöppel E (1994) Mid-latency auditory evoked potentials and explicit and implicit memory in patients undergoing cardiac surgery. Anesthesiology 80:493–501
18. Schwender D, Haessler R, Klasing S et al (1994) Mid-latency auditory evoked potentials and circulatory response to loud sounds. Br J Anaesth 72:307–314

Should Neuromuscular Transmission Be Monitored Routinely During Anaesthesia?

J. Viby-Mogensen

Traditionally, anaesthetists evaluate the effect of neuromuscular blocking agents clinically: we observe the fasciculations following injection of succinylcholine, the movements of the reservoir bag, the spontaneous movements of the patient, head lift, etc.

Over the past decade or so there has been an increasing understanding of the necessity of a more objective assessment of neuromuscular function during anaesthesia, and many anaesthetists today use nerve stimulators routinely whenever neuromuscular blocking drugs are used. Other anaesthetists, however, never use a nerve stimulator; they consider it unnecessary and time consuming. They simply feel they do quite well without it—so why go to the trouble? Who is right? Is neuromuscular monitoring essential? Or is it unnecessary, time consuming and of only academic interest?

Let us have a look at the arguments for routine monitoring. Figure 1 is a diagrammatic illustration of the changes in response to train-of-four (TOF) nerve stimulation during a nondepolarizing neuromuscular blockade. By using a nerve stimulator during *the induction phase* it is possible to judge the sensitivity of the individual patient to the muscle relaxant used. Also, it may be a help in finding the optimal time for tracheal intubation. Most importantly, the nerve stimulator gives you the possibility at an early stage to diagnose an abnormal response to the muscle relaxant, i.e. an abnormal sensitivity to succinylcholine or mivacurium caused by an abnormal plasma cholinesterase activity. Further, the nerve stimulator may guide you in treating the abnormal response [1, 2].

During the *period of intense block* (no response to TOF nerve stimulation, Fig. 1), the use of a nerve stimulator allows you to quantitate the degree of block by using the post-tetanic count (PTC) method [3, 4]. Figure 2 illustrates that during very intense blockade, there is no response to either tetanic or post-tetanic stimulation. However, when the very intense blockade dissipates and before the first response to TOF stimulation reappears, the first response to the post-tetanic twitch stimulation occurs. The main application of PTC is in evaluating the degree of neuromuscular block when there is no reaction to TOF nerve stimulation, as may be the case after injection of a large dose of a nondepolarising neuromuscular blocking drug (Figs. 2 and 3). However, the PTC can also be used whenever sudden movements must be eliminated (e.g., during ophthalmic surgery). To ensure paralysis of the diaphragm and elimination of bucking and coughing, neuromuscular blockade of the peripheral muscles should be so intense that no response to post-tetanic twitch stimulation can be elicited (PTC = 0) [4].

During *surgical block* you can keep your patient exactly at the degree of block that is necessary for smooth surgical intervention, and thereby avoid unnecessary deep neuromuscular block. This has several advantages: it is easier to discover

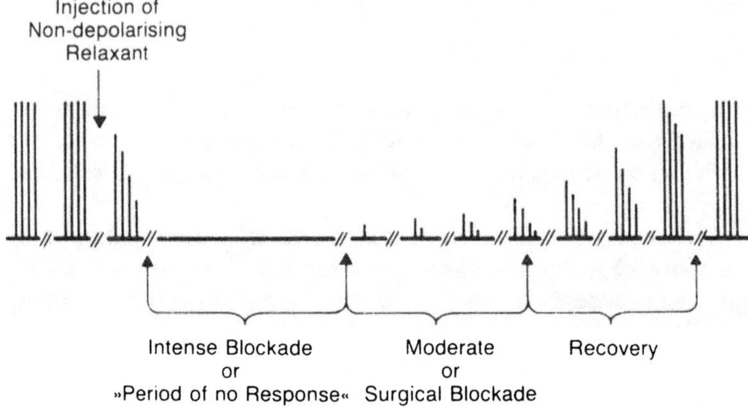

Fig. 1. Changes in response to train-of-four nerve stimulation during nondepolarizing neuromuscular blockade

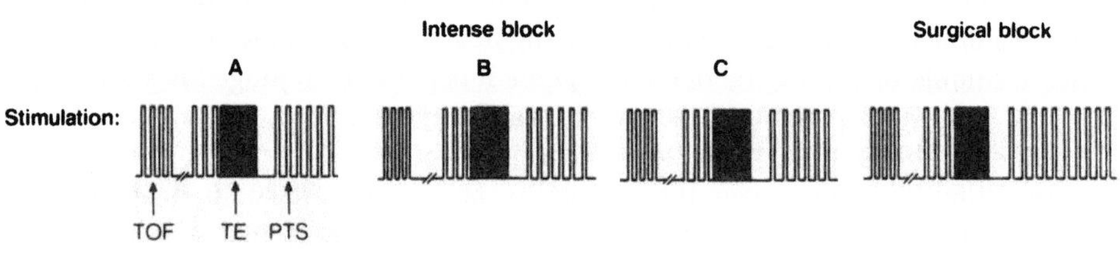

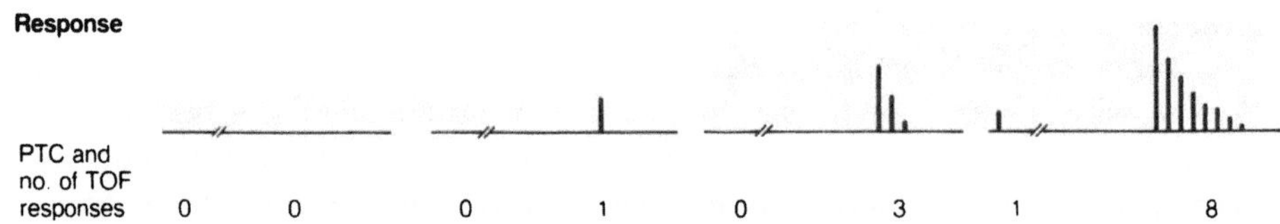

Fig. 2. Pattern of electrical stimulation and evoked muscle responses to train-of-four (*TOF*) nerve stimulation, 50-Hz tetanic nerve stimulation for 5 s (*TE*), and 1.0-Hz post-tetanic twitch stimulation (*PTS*) during four different levels of nondepolarising neuromuscular blockade. During very intense blockade of the peripheral muscles (*A*), no response to any of the forms of stimulation occurs. During less pronounced blockade (*B and C*) there is still no response to TOF stimulation, but post-tetanic facilitation of transmission is present. During surgical block, the first response to TOF appears and post-tetanic facilitation increases further. The post-tetanic count (*PTC*, see text) is 1 during intense block (*column B*), 3 during less intense block (*column C*), and 8 during surgical block. (From [15])

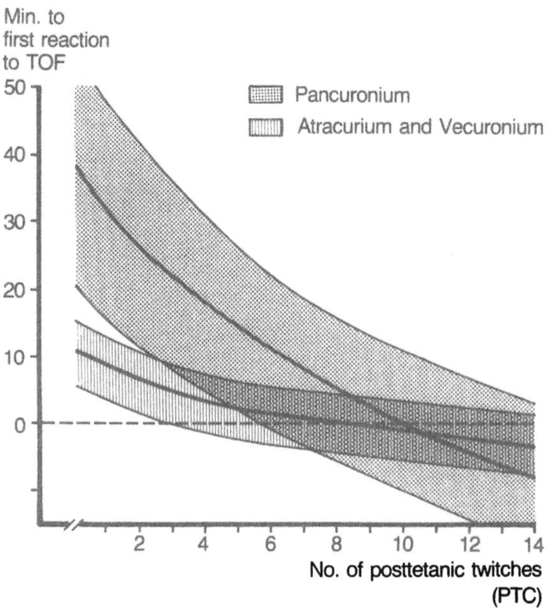

Fig. 3. Relationship between time to the first reaction to train-of-four (*TOF*) nerve stimulation and the number of post-tetanic twitches, i.e., the post-tetanic count (*PTC*) during intense blockade caused by pancuronium, atracurium and vecuronium. Mean curves and 95% prediction regions are shown. (From [15])

awareness, which is not least important during total intravenous anaesthesia. If the patient is not totally paralysed, he or she is able to perform spontaneous movements, for instance with the fascial muscles, if he or she wakes up during the procedure. Also, reversal can often be initiated earlier and is more likely to be sufficient in a short time. Antagonism of a nondepolarising neuromuscular block should not be initiated before obvious clinical signs of returning neuromuscular function are present, or at least two, and preferably three or four, responses to TOF stimulation can be felt.

By using a nerve stimulator during *the recovery phase*, it is possible to ensure that a patient does not regain consciousness at a time when he or she is still paralysed. This may seem banal, but judging from my more than 20 years of experience with a referral center for prolonged responses to succinylcholine, it is still a problem [5]. Even today some patients experience the trauma of their lifetime, when they wake up after surgery totally or partially paralysed.

Probably the most important advantage of the use of a nerve stimulator is that it makes it possible to objectively measure the degree of reversal, thereby excluding the problems of residual neuromuscular block in the recovery room. During recovery from neuromuscular blockade, the degree of residual block can be evaluated from the responses to TOF nerve stimulation. However, without recording equipment, it is not possible by visual or tactile means to evaluate the TOF response with sufficient certainty to exclude shallow degrees of residual neuromuscular block [6]. With double-burst stimulation (DBS), as opposed to TOF stimulation, it is easier to "feel" fade in the response (Figs. 4 and 5). DBS was developed with the specific aim of allowing manual (tactile) detection of small amounts of residual neuromuscular blockade under clinical conditions [7, 8]. In

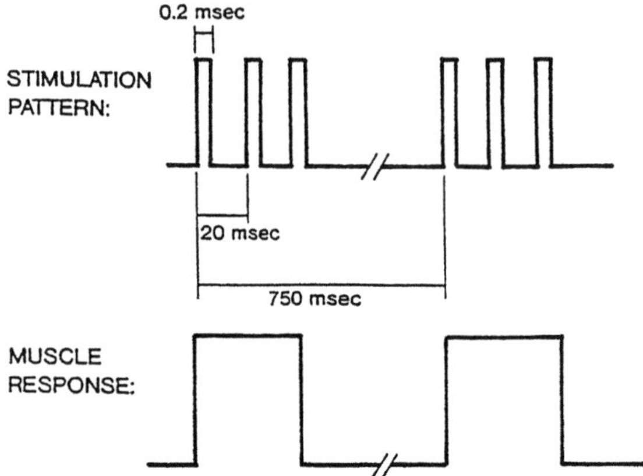

Fig. 4. Stimulation pattern of $DBS_{3,3}$ and the corresponding response of the muscle. $DBS_{3,3}$, Three impulses in each of the two tetanic bursts

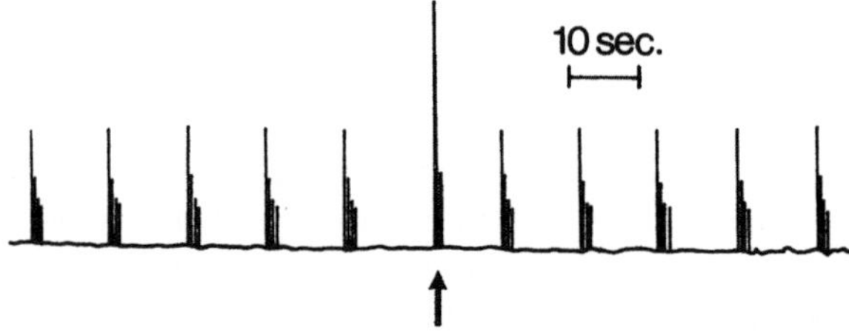

Fig. 5. Mechanical twitch recording of a $DBS_{3,3}$ (*at arrow*). Notice that the degree of fade in the DBS response corresponds to the degree of fade in the TOF response

the nonparalysed muscle the response to DBS is two short muscle contractions of equal strength. In partially paralysed muscle, the second response is weaker than the first (i.e., the response fades). Measured mechanically, the TOF ratio correlates closely with the DBS ratio. During recovery and immediately after surgery, tactile evaluation of the response to DBS is superior to tactile evaluation of the response to TOF stimulation. Thus, absence of fade in the response to DBS means that severe residual neuromuscular blockade does not exist.

Now some anaesthetists would probably claim that they can achieve all of the above without a nerve stimulator. They may be correct, but if so, at least residual neuromuscular block should not be a problem. However, many studies have documented that residual neuromuscular blockade is frequent in patients in the recovery room after surgery [9–12]. The incidence range is 20–50% following the use of the longer acting agents (i.e., dTC and pancuronium) and 4–10% after use of the intermediate acting agents (i.e., atracurium and vecuronium). By postoperative manual evaluation of the response to DBS or the use of a TOF guard, the problem of residual block can be minimized or even eliminated [13, 14].

At a meeting in Montreal in 1992, held in celebration of the introduction of curare into clinical anaesthesia 50 years earlier, Professor Cecil Gray said: "There is no finer recipe for disaster than to allow patients to leave the operating theatre with any residual curarization." I would like to make his words mine! Today we do have the means of avoiding residual neuromuscular blockade in the recovery room, and I see no reason why we should not use these means. The answer to the question in the title of this presentation is: Yes, judging from available data on the frequency of residual block in the recovery room, it does seem essential to monitor neuromuscular function during routine anaesthesia involving muscle relaxants.

References

1. Viby-Mogensen J (1981) Succinylcholine neuromuscular blockade in subjects homozygous for atypical plasma cholinesterase. Anesthesiology 55:429
2. Østergaard D, Jensen FS, Jensen E et al (1993) Mivacurium-induced neuromuscular blockade in patients with atypical plasma cholinesterase. Acta Anaesthesiol Scand 37:314
3. Viby-Mogensen J, Howardy-Hansen P, Chræmmer-Jørgensen B et al (1981) Posttetanic count (PTC): a new method of evaluating an intense non-depolarizing neuromuscular blockade. Anesthesiology 55:458
4. Fernando PUE, Viby-Mogensen J, Bonsu AK et al (1987) Relationship between posttetanic count and response to carinal stimulation during vecuronium-induced neuromuscular blockade. Acta Anaesthesiol Scand 31:593
5. Jensen FS, Viby-Mogensen J (1995) Plasma cholinesterase and abnormal reaction to succinylcholine: twenty years' experience with the Danish Cholinesterase Research Unit. Acta Anaesthesiol Scand 39:150
6. Viby-Mogensen J, Jensen NH, Engbæk J et al (1985) Tactile and visual evaluation of the response to train-of-four stimulation. Anesthesiology 63:440
7. Engbæk J, Østergaard D, Viby-Mogensen J (1989) Double-burst stimulation (DBS): a new pattern of nerve stimulation to identify residual neuromuscular block. Br J Anaesth 62:274
8. Drenck NE, Ueda N, Olsen NV et al (1989) Manual evaluation using double-burst stimulation: a comparison with train-of-four. Anesthesiology 70:578
9. Viby-Mogensen J, Chræmmer-Jørgensen B, Ørding H (1979) Residual curarization in the recovery room. Anesthesiology 50:539
10. Lennmarken C, Löfström B (1984) Partial curarization in the postoperative period. Acta Anaesthesiol Scand 28:260
11. Beemer GH, Rozental P et al (1986) Postoperative neuromuscular function. Anesth Intensive Care 14:41
12. Bevan DR, Smith CE, Donati F (1988) Postoperative neuromuscular blockade: a comparison between atracurium, vecuronium and pancuronium. Anesthesiology 69:272
13. Jensen E, Viby-Mogensen J, Bang U (1988) The accelograph: a new neuromuscular transmission analyzer. Acta Anaesthesiol Scand 32:49
14. Mortensen CR, Berg H, El-Mahdy A, Viby-Mogensen J (1995) Perioperative monitoring of neuromuscular function using acceleromyography prevents residual block following pancuronium. Acta Anaesthesiol Scand (accepted for publication)
15. Viby-Mogensen J (1994) Neuromuscular monitoring. In: Miller RD (ed) Anesthesia, 4th edn. Churchill Livingstone, Edinburgh

III Control and Automation of Artificial Ventilation

Pulmonary Function and Ventilatory Patterns During Anaesthesia

P. König, F. Donald, and P.M. Suter

Introduction

Respiratory function is significantly altered when a patient undergoes surgery and anaesthesia. Alterations occur in both the physical properties of the inhaled gases such as temperature, viscosity and humidity and in the characteristics of the upper and lower airways. Endotracheal intubation or the application of a face mask alter both the anatomical dead space and the airway resistance, as does decreased ciliary motility and the resultant decreased clearance of mucus from the airways. Decreased ciliary motility is caused by a number of factors including the use of inhaled anaesthetic agents, decreased temperature and humidity of inspired gases, increased fractional inspired oxygen concentration and the presence of an endotracheal tube [1–4].

Intrapulmonary gas exchange may be directly influenced by anaesthesia itself, by the position of the patient on the operating table (knee-chest, lithotomy, lateral) and by intraoperative blood loss and/or fluid replacement. In each case impaired gas exchange is related to alterations in pulmonary ventilation/perfusion (V/Q) ratios. Intraoperative modifications can lead to diminished respiratory function in the postoperative period and may contribute to postoperative respiratory-related morbidity and mortality. Indeed, atelectasis following abdominal surgery was described by Pasteur as long ago as 1910 [5], and in 1933, Beecher demonstrated the importance of a decrease in lung volume as a cause of respiratory insufficiency following laparotomy [6].

Intraoperative ventilation in its various forms may be used to attenuate some of the above-mentioned modifications. In this way V/Q ratios may be normalised or even improved during anaesthesia. This would be of particular importance where there is a pre-existing V/Q mismatch, e.g., during surgery for lung disease. However, the ventilatory mode chosen must also take into account the type of surgery involved. For instance, abdominal surgery requires the use of muscle relaxants to allow proper surgical access, and in this case controlled positive-pressure ventilation becomes necessary. Certain thoracic operations are facilitated by one-lung ventilation, and surgical access for operations involving the airways may be improved by the use of jet ventilation.

The following discussion will consider the character and causes of intraoperative modifications in pulmonary perfusion and ventilation, changes in V/Q ratios, with particular reference to the diminution in functional residual capacity (FRC) in the perioperative period and, finally, the ways in which ventilation may be manipulated to minimise these changes.

Intraoperative Alterations in Pulmonary Perfusion

The main energy source for the pulmonary circulation is the kinetic energy generated by the right ventricle, which acts in opposition to a hydrostatic gradient. Thus, gravitational forces have a major influence on the distribution of pulmonary perfusion. Under normal physiological conditions 55% of pulmonary blood flow goes to the right lung and 45% to the left. This distribution ratio is not altered by a change in position from the upright to the supine position. However, in the lateral position upper lung blood flow is decreased by 40%; i.e., in the right lateral position the left lung will receive only 19% of pulmonary blood flow.

Intrapulmonary and intrathoracic pressures have both direct and indirect effects on pulmonary blood flow. Pulmonary capillary flow is directly influenced by intra-alveolar pressure changes, but pleural pressure and pulmonary interstitial pressures have negligible effects on hilar and intraparenchymatous vessels, respectively. However, elevated pulmonary interstitial pressures lead to areas of atelectasis in dependent parts of the lung, which will in turn result in reflex hypoxic pulmonary vasoconstriction (HPV).

Thus, it seems that it is at the level of intra-alveolar pressures that ventilation may influence V/Q ratios. This has been very well explained by J.B. West [19] in his description of the four zones of the lung (Fig. 1). Zone 1 is equivalent to dead space, since alveolar pressure (P_A) is greater than pulmonary artery pressure (P_{pa}), prohibiting blood flow. Under normal physiological conditions this zone is practically nonexistent, but during anaesthesia positive-pressure ventilation increases P_A whilst relative hypovolaemia and the use of negatively inotropic anaesthetic agents tend to decrease P_{Pa}, such that zone 1 may increase in size. In zone 4 interstitial pressure (P_{ISF}) is greater than pulmonary venous pressure (P_{pv}), which is in turn greater than P_A. Thus blood flow is dependent on the difference between P_{pa} and P_{ISF}. If interstitial pressure is increased by volume overload, increased hydrostatic pressure (e.g., Trendelenburg position) or pulmonary venous occlusion, then interstial oedema will tend to develop. This, in turn, will lead to alveolar collapse and areas of shunt.

Thus, in order to minimise the increase in zone 1 it would be preferable to maintain spontaneous ventilation, avoiding the use of positive pressure and subsequent increases in P_A. In reality, this is not always possible, but it is important to monitor intratracheal pressure and to keep it as low as possible in order to avoid excessive increases in P_A. The shunt effect produced in zone 4 is probably best treated by the use of positive end-expiratory pressure (PEEP), although this does not seem to prevent the formation of atelectasis [7].

The Four Zones of the Lung

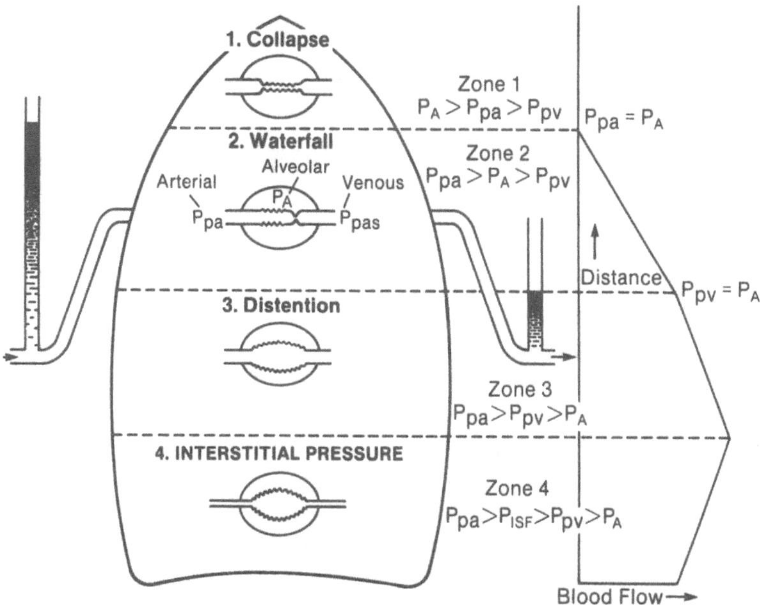

Fig. 1. Distibution of blood flow in the upright lung. In *zone 1* alveolar pressure (P_A) exceeds pulmonary artery pressure (P_{pa}), so no flow occurs. In *zone 2* P_{pa} exceeds P_A, which in turn exceeds pulmonary venous pressure (P_{pv}). Blood flow is dependent on the P_{pa}-P_A difference. In *zone 3* P_{pv}, is greater than p_A, and it is the P_{pa}-P_{pv} difference which determines blood flow. Finally, in *zone 4* pulmonary interstitial pressure (P_{ISF}) is increased, and it is the arterial-interstitial pressure difference which determines blood flow. (Reprinted with permission of the publisher from [19])

Hypoxic Pulmonary Vasoconstriction

Hypoxic pulmonary vasoconstriction consists of a constriction of the pulmonary arterioles which occurs in response to alveolar hypoxia. It is an important clinical entity, as it allows a diminution by approximately 50% of blood flow in areas which are poorly ventilated, e.g., areas of atelectasis or the nonventilated lung during one-lung ventilation. Vascular tone seems to be regulated by chemical mediators which are formed by the metabolism of arachidonic acid: vasodilatory prostaglandins or vasoconstrictory leukotrienes. It is possible that the metabolism of the cells of the vessel walls is directly influenced by the level of oxygenation.

The ventilatory mode chosen probably has little or no direct influence on HPV but may have indirect effects by means of alveolar oxygenation or haemodynamic variations. The pulmonary vessels have scant musculature, and any increase in P_{pa} will tend to cause vasodilation and, at least partially, overcome HPV.

The halogenated inhalational anaesthetic agents inhibit HPV, whilst intravenous agents have little effect [8]. However, the deterioration in gas exchange seen during anaesthesia results mainly from the modifications in inotropism and pulmonary vascular tone caused by these agents, and not from their effect on HPV.

PEEP and Intrapulmonary Pressure

PEEP increases intra-alveolar and intrathoracic pressures with subsequent modifications of capillary flow and venous return. Excessive PEEP may cause the foramen ovale, which is patent in 20% of the population, to open, thereby increasing the shunt effect.

Intraoperative Ventilatory Modifications

During spontaneous respiration the distribution of ventilation is determined by gravity through its effect on pulmonary compliance and intrapleural pressure. The base of the lung receives more of the ventilation than the apex, such that the distribution of ventilation parallels that of perfusion. In the upright position the right lung receives 53% of the ventilation and the left 47%, and, as for perfusion, this distribution is not affected by adoption of the supine position. However, in the supine or lateral positions the viscera cause an elevation of the dependent part of the diaphragm, such that during inspiration there is greater diaphragmatic excursion in this region. This, in turn, leads to improved ventilation of the dependent part of the lung. In the right lateral position, during spontaneous respiration, the right lung receives 60% of ventilation and the left 40%, whilst in the left lateral position the distribution is 47% to the right lung and 53% to the left (Fig. 2).

The introduction of positive-pressure ventilation considerably modifies the above situation. The influence of gravity is now minimal and the movement of the diaphragm is passive, with the viscera presenting an obstacle to this movement. Thus ventilation is preferentially distributed to the upper part of the lung. In the right lateral position both lungs now receive 50% of the ventilation and in the left lateral position the right lung receives 68% and the left 32%. The mediastinum is an additional weight on the dependent lung in the lateral position. Taking into consideration the above, we can see that general anaesthesia with controlled positive-pressure ventilation will have entirely different effects on gas exchange than a spinal or epidural anaesthestic with the patient breathing spontaneously.

The Effect of PEEP on Ventilation

The use of PEEP will accentuate the effect of positive-pressure ventilation with an increase in alveolar pressure, which may lead to an increase in zone 1 and thus in dead space volume.

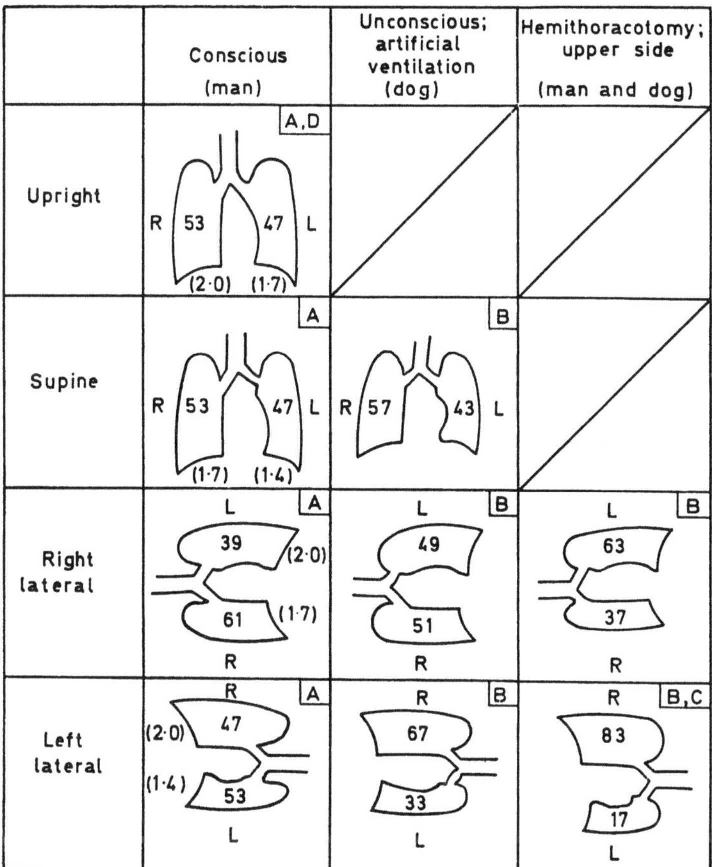

Fig. 2. Relative distribution of inspired gas between the two lungs. The *numbers inside the lungs* represent the percentage total ventilation and those *in parentheses* the lung volume in litres. *A, C* and *D* are human lungs, whilst *B* refers to canine lungs. (Reprinted with permission of the publisher from [20])

Positive-Pressure Ventilation with Open Pleural Cavity

In this context, the upper lung receives almost all the ventilation (Fig. 2), as there is practically no resistance to its expansion. Since the lower lung receives more of the blood flow than the upper, there is V/Q mismatching and the dependent parts of the lower lung will be susceptible to the development of interstitial oedema (West's zone 4). This will be of particular importance where there is fluid overload or obstruction to pulmonary blood flow causing pulmonary hypertension, e.g., by the presence of surgical instruments in the thorax. In order to attenuate this problem the use of a double-lumen endotracheal tube allows selective application of PEEP to the dependent lung. P_A becomes greater than P_{ISF} and prevents the formation of zone-4 areas.

Changes in Functional Residual Capacity with Anaesthesia and Muscle Paralysis: Impact on V/Q Ratios

It would seem from the above discussion of the effects of positive-pressure ventilation on the distribution of ventilation and perfusion within the lung that spontaneous respiration is always to be preferred. However, this is not entirely true, as anaesthesia also causes a deterioration in V/Q ratios by modifying lung volumes, and only the use of positive-pressure ventilation can overcome these modifications and improve gas exchange. Certain terms pertaining to lung volumes will now be defined.

Functional residual capacity (FRC) is the volume of gas in the lungs at the end of a normal expiration, i.e., at the point at which the forces tending to expand and retract the thoracic cage are in equlibrium. The closing capacity (CC) is the point at which small airways start to close during expiration. The small airways are held open during expiration by the radial forces of the pulmonary parenchyma, which are directly related to pulmonary volume. These forces are opposed by the positive pleural pressure during expiration. Thus, the small airways are particularly prone to collapse in the dependent part of the lung, where pleural pressure is at its greatest. Since these are the more well perfused areas, this increases the shunt effect [7]. This phenomenon is more marked when radial forces are diminished, as in emphysema, or when there is an increase in airway resistance, as in chronic bronchitis.

Residual volume (RV) is the volume of gas in the lungs at the end of a forced expiration. The closing volume (CV) is the difference between the CC and the RV. It is usually expressed as a percentage of the vital capacity (VC).

Figure 3 shows how the CC may be measured using a bolus of tracer gas such as xenon 133. In young, healthy people the CC is smaller than FRC, but tobacco smoking, obesity, increasing age and the supine position will all tend to increase it. At 40 years of age the CC and the FRC are approximately equal in the supine position but at 65 years of age they are equal only when the patient is standing up. This implies that for a 40-year-old patient in the supine position the tidal volume (V_T) does not encroach on the CC, assuming FRC does not change. Thus there will be no closure of the small airways and no heterogenicity of ventilation. However, the 65-year-old patient will have a V_T which encroaches on the CC and this will lead to modifications of V/Q ratios and subsequent impairment of gas exchange.

Hence, it would seem that in terms of anaesthesia it is important to know, for each patient, the relationship between the V_T and the CC as well as that between the FRC and the CC. However, V_T and FRC are significantly altered, both by anaesthesia itself and by muscle paralysis, such that alterations in V/Q ratios are seen even in young, healthy patients [18].

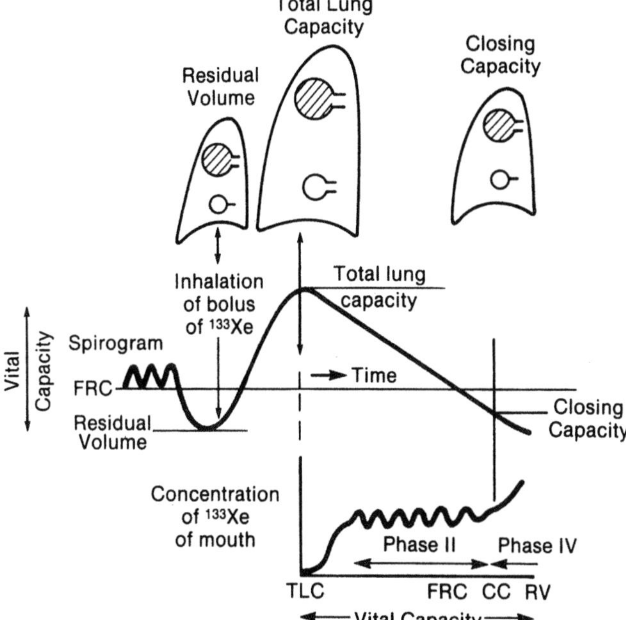

Fig. 3. Measurement of closing capacity using a tracer gas. A bolus of tracer gas is inhaled near residual volume and is distributed only to nondependent alveoli whose air passages are still open. During expiration the concentration of tracer gas is constant after dead space gas is washed out, and starts to rise when there is once again closure of dependent airways. (Reprinted with permission of the publisher from [19])

Changes in Lung Volumes During Anaesthesia

Tidal Volume

V_T can vary enormously during spontaneous ventilation. During light anaesthesia hyperventilation may occur, and in the presence of large amounts of anaesthetic gases or opioids respiration may become very superficial with small V_T. During controlled ventilation V_T is predetermined.

Functional Residual Capacity

Functional residual capacity is reduced during anaesthesia. The induction of anaesthesia in itself causes a reduction of approximately 15% (0.5l) in the FRC. This is the case for both controlled and spontaneous ventilation but is not seen in awake patients undergoing controlled ventilation [9]. The reduction in FRC is not immediately reversible at the end of anaesthesia and must be taken into consideration when planning postoperative respiratory therapy.

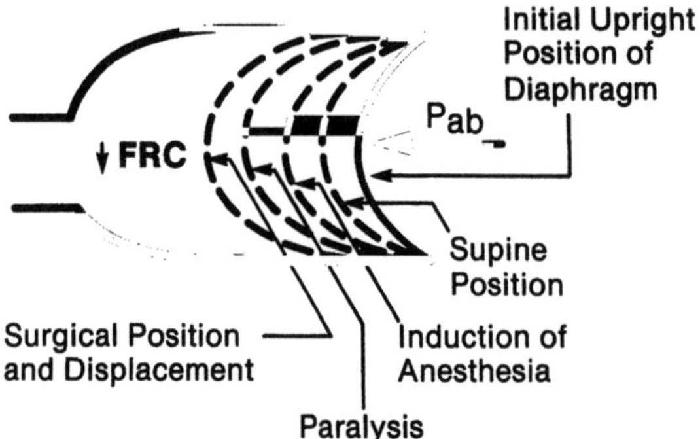

Fig. 4. Anaesthesia and surgery may cause progressive cephalad displacement of the diaphragm. This results in decreased functional residual capacity (*FRC*). P_{ab}, Pressure of abdominal contents. (Reprinted with permission of the publisher from [19])

There is a further reduction in FRC due to the adoption of the supine position which is estimated at 0.8 l. This is caused by upward movement of the diaphragm under the weight of the abdominal contents but is offset by the increased force of contraction of the diaphragm due to its being under tension. Muscle paralysis removes the beneficial effect of this upward excursion and allows it to become even greater [Fig. 4].

In summary, anaesthesia significantly reduces FRC, such that V_T may encroach on CC, causing disturbances of the V/Q ratio. Controlled ventilation can increase V_T but may also further diminish FRC. The use of PEEP can increase FRC and thus improve gas exchange in both the intra- and postoperative periods.

Table 1 summarises the various respiratory modifications which occur during anaesthesia and the implications of these modifications for the anaesthetist. A brief commentary is given regarding the choice of anaesthetic technique in each case.

Frequently Used Mechanical Ventilatory Patterns

Despite the numerous changes in respiratory physiology which occur during anaesthesia and the varying surgical requirements, the pattern of mechanical ventilation used is remarkably constant. A mechanical ventilator causes active inflation of the lungs using positive pressure, whilst deflation or exhalation is passive. The time allowed for exhalation is usually twice that for inflation, i.e., the inspiratory: expiratory (I:E) ratio is 1:2. This ratio may be altered, for example, in patients with obstructive pulmonary disease where more time is needed for exhalation. In this case the I:E ratio could be 1:4. Inverse ratio ventilation (I:E ratio 1.1:1) is rarely used in anaesthesia, although it is seen in the intensive care setting. Inspiratory time is thus longer than expiratory time, allowing an inspiratory pause which may improve oxygenation in much the same way as PEEP.

Table 1. Changes in ventilation/perfusion (V/Q) ratios induced by anaesthesia – implications for the anaesthetist

Anaesthetic	Changes in perfusion	Changes in ventilation	Changes in V/Q by changes in FRC	Comments
Regional anaesthesia + spontaneous ventilation	Hypovolaemia, vasoplegia, increase in West zone 1	Increase in dead space by increase in West zone 1	Decrease in FRC due to supine position	Decreased FRC necessitates increased FiO_2 above 40 years of age
General anaesthesia + spontaneous ventilation	Interaction between anaesthetic agents and HPV	Changes in tidal volume according to depth of anaesthesia	Decreased FRC due to 1. supine position 2. gen. anaesth.	Only for patients under 40 years of age undergoing short operations 1. FiO_2 30–40% 2. Assisted ventilation to maintain tidal volume
General anaesthesia + controlled ventilation + muscle relaxation	Interaction between anaesthetic agents and HPV	Nondependent zones preferentially ventilated, increased dead space Dependent zones poorly ventilated, shunt effect	Decreased FRC due to 1. supine position 2. gen. anaesth. 3. muscle relax.	1. Increase in tidal volume to prevent small airway closure 2. PEEP to increase FRC 3. FiO_2 30–40%

V_T is increased during controlled ventilation from the normal $7\,\text{ml}/\text{kg}^{-1}$ during spontaneous ventilation to approximately $10\,\text{ml}/\text{kg}^{-1}$. Respiratory frequency is generally kept constant at 10–12 breaths/min, such that minute volume is increased. Increasing both tidal and minute volume counteracts the effect of increased dead-space volume by increasing alveolar ventilation.

PEEP is also used as an adjunct to mechanical ventilation during anaesthesia. Its major effect is to reverse decreases in FRC, such that the latter is larger than CC and small airway closure is minimised. A disadvantage of PEEP is that it increases intratracheal pressure and may lead to barotrauma. This is of particular importance in lungs with low compliance, e.g., fibrotic or oedematous lungs. In these cases the ventilatory pattern must be adjusted to achieve maximum oxygenation within acceptable pressure limits. V_T will often need to be decreased, with a concomitant increase in frequency to maintain minute volume. High-frequency ventilation, which is described below, may be seen as a similar process carried to greater extremes.

High-Frequency Ventilation in Anaesthesia

We will now consider the use of high-frequency ventilation (HFV) in anaesthesia.

Definition

HFV encompasses three classes of ventilation, i.e., high-frequency positive-pressure ventilation (HFPPV), high-frequency jet ventilation (HFJV) and high-frequency oscillation (HFO). The three groups are divided according to ventilatory frequency. HFPPV uses respiratory rates between 60 and 120 breaths per minute (bpm), HFJV 120–300 bpm and HFO 300–3000 bpm. However, as Mapleson et al. point out in their editorial [10], the separation is based essentially on the type of ventilator used. HFV may be described as ventilation with a respiratory rate greater than 60–80 bpm, although mechanisms of gas exchange may not begin to alter until frequencies of 120–180 bpm have been reached [10]. In the following discussion only HFJV will be considered.

Respiratory Effects

HFJV involves the use of very small tidal volumes of the order of 1–3 ml/kg body wt., which means that the tidal volume is equal to, or less than, the physiological dead space. Effective gas exchange obviously does take place in spite of this apparent paradox, but, as mentioned above, the mechanisms are not the same as for conventional positive-pressure ventilation. It is not within the scope of this article to develop this subject, but for a brief overview the reader is directed to a review of HFV by B.E. Smith [11].

Peak airway pressure is lower during HFJV than during conventional positive-pressure ventilation. Mean airway pressure is variable according to lung compliance and respiratory frequency but also tends to be lower with HFJV.

Haemodynamic Effects

The feasibility of HFV was first demonstrated as far back as 1915 [12], but it was in 1969 that Oberg and Sjostrand used the technique in order to avoid cardiovascular variations during the respiratory cycle [13]. Since then, many papers have been published concerning the haemodynamic effects of HFJV.

In the presence of normal cardiovascular function the cardiac output is regulated primarily by the venous return. During positive-pressure ventilation the increase in intrathoracic pressure tends to diminish venous return and hence cardiac output, especially in the presence of hypovolaemia. As mentioned above, mean airway pressures are probably slightly lower during HFJV than during conventional positive-pressure ventilation, but in spite of this, no real evidence of less decrease in cardiac output related to the use of HFJV has been found in patients with normal cardiac function. However, in studies using animal models of cardiac insufficiency increases in thoracic pressure seem to improve left ventricular (LV) function [14]. This is thought to be due to a diminution in the LV transmural pressure gradient, which dereases wall stress. The use of HFV synchronised to the cardiac cycle would seem to be of particular interest in this field. An increase in intrathoracic pressure timed to occur at the moment of aortic valve opening may cause afterload reduction and improve LV function [15].

Uses in Anaesthesia

HFJV is used in anaesthesia for laryngeal and tracheal surgery and for endoscopy of the upper and lower respiratory tract. Gunta et al. [16] reported a series of 300 patients in whom HFJV had been used both in these situations and for thoracic surgery. Adequate gas exchange can be achieved with the use of fine catheters as opposed to traditional endotracheal tubes, and this is obviously an advantage when the airway is also the operative site. The authors point out that in the particular case of tracheal stenosis HFJV cannot be used until after resection of the stenosed area, as before this, expiration would be hindered. However, during reconstruction it allows excellent surgical access.

The small tidal volumes used in HFJV decrease movement of the operative field in thoracic, abdominal and neurosurgery, which may be advantageous especially in the case of microsurgery.

The fact that HFJV is not more widely used in anaesthesia is probably due to a number of factors. Firstly, the gas is delivered at a pressure of 25–400 kPa with a flow rate of up to 30 l/min. Hence, it would be very easy to inject large amounts of gas into the tissues in a very short space of time if the catheter were to become displaced [17]. Sensitive pressure alarms and a system to automatically stop gas insufflation are needed to avoid this problem. Secondly, there is the problem of monitoring expired carbon dioxide tension. Gunta et al. overcame this problem by using a second catheter, placed slightly distally to the injection catheter, which was able to monitor carbon dioxide tension. The results obtained were compatible with those of concomitant blood gas analysis [16].

In summary, HFJV is widely used for surgery of the respiratory tract but less so in other situations where it might also have a role. The development of synchronised HFV may prove useful in patients with compromised cardiac function, but this remains to be proved. At present, it seems that doubts regarding the safety of utilisation and monitoring of HFJV in the operating theatre are an obstacle to its use.

Conclusion

As can be seen from the above review, there is no one ventilatory mode which is suitable for all types of anaesthesia or all patients. In each case the potential risks and benefits for the patient must be measured against the needs of the surgeon. What is clear is that a sound knowledge of physiology is necessary to be able to make this judgement.

References

1. Forbes AR (1973) Humidity and mucus flow in the intubated trachea. Br J Anaesth 45:874
2. Bang BG, Bang FB (1961) Effect of water deprivation on nasal mucous flow. Proc Soc Exp Biol Med 106:516
3. Hirsch JA, Tokayer JL, Robinson MJ et al (1975) Effect of dry air and subsequent humidification on tracheal mucheal velocity in dogs. J Appl Physiol 39:242
4. Sackner MA, Hirsch J, Epstein S (1975) Effect of cuffed endotracheal tubes on tracheal mucous velocity. Chest 68:774
5. Pasteur W (1910) Active lobar collapse of the lung after abdominal operations: a contribution to the study of postoperative lung complications. Lancet 2:1080–1083
6. Beecher (1933) Effect of laparotomy on lung volume: demonstration of a new type of pulmonary collapse. J Clin Invest 12:651–658
7. Brismer B, Hedenstierna G, Lundquisth et al (1985) Pulmonary densities during anaesthesia with muscular relaxation – a proposal of atelectasis. Anesthesiology 672:422–28
8. Miller RD (1990) Anaesthesia, vol 2, 3rd edn. Churchill Livingstone, Edinburgh, p 1534, Table 50-7
9. Westbrook PR et al (1973) Effects of anaesthesia and muscle paralysis on respiratory mechanics in normal man J Appl Physiol 34:81
10. Mapleson WW et al (1989) High-frequency ventilation (E). Br J Anaesth 63:1–2S
11. Smith BE (1990) High-frequency ventilation: past, present and future? Br J Anaesth 65:130–138
12. Henderson Y, Chillingworth FD, Whitney JL (1915) The respiratory dead space. Am J Physiol 38:i–ii

13. Oberg PA, Sjostrand UH (1969) Studies of blood pressure regulation. 1. Common carotid artery clamping in studies of the carotid sinus baroreceptor control of the systemic blood pressure. Acta Physiol Scand 75:276–282
14. Pinsky MR, Summer WR, Wise RA, Permutt S, Bromberger-Barnea B (1983) Augmentation of cardiac function by elevation of intrathoracic pressure. J Appl Physiol 54:950–955
15. Pinsky MR, Matuschak GM, Bernardi L, Klain M (1986) Hemodynamic effects of cardiac cycle-specific increases in intrathoracic pressure. J Appl Physiol 60:604–612
16. Gunta F et al (1990) Clinical uses of high-frequency jet ventilation in anaesthesia. Br J Anaesth 63:102–106S
17. Smith BE (1990) Developments in the safe use of high-frequency jet ventilation. Br J Anaesth 65:735–736
18. Wahba RWM (1991) Postoperative functional residual capacity. Can J Anaesth 38:384–400
19. Benumof JL (1987) General respiratory physiology and respiratory function during anesthesia. In: Benumof JL (ed) Anesthesia for thoracic surgery. Saunders, Philadephia, pp 40–103
20. Nunn JF (1972) Applied respiratory physiology. Butterworths, London

What Can and What Should Be Controlled During Artificial Ventilation?

H.J. BENDER

Although significant improvements in respiratory monitoring have occurred over the past decade, modern technology has not decreased the incidence of inadvertently low oxygen concentrations; rather, the incidence has increased [20]. Despite the ubiquitous presence of pulse oxymeters in the intensive care unit, it is unclear if they really contribute to clinical decision-making or if they affect patient morbidity or mortality. We have to conclude, therefore, that the management of ventilation can and should be improved. The question whether an automatic control of ventilation based on excellent respiratory monitoring is useful and whether it may improve the safety for artificially ventilated patients should be discussed.

A control system attempts to manage some output based on information provided by an input signal. In this contribution, neither the different kinds of existing controllers nor the possible output signals to a ventilator are discussed; this will be done in one of the following chapters. The purpose here is to evaluate the possible parameters of automatic control of ventilation.

In general, control will be less accurate, or even impossible, if a direct measurement of the controlled variable is not available. Since successful ventilation cannot be represented by a single parameter alone, we have to select those parameters which may be of interest for future control of respiration.

If we were to summarise the features of an ideal monitoring system we could easily draw up a nearly endless list. Some of these features are shown in Table 1. The decisive element for control of a system is finding which monitors derive useful and specific information. Thus the problem is to decide which of the myriad devices used for oxymetry, capnography and pulmonary mechanics are so-called lead monitors, as opposed to lag monitors wasting only precious time [22].

It is well recognised that the most common cause of anaesthesia- and ventilator-related mortality and morbidity is an inadequate delivery of O_2 to the tissues [23]. Consequently, monitoring of oxygen, or more exactly of O_2 delivery, O_2 extraction and O_2 consumption, should be essential for control of ventilation. To guarantee an adequate oxygenation of the tissues we have to monitor oxygen at several sites; ideal would be the continuous monitoring of every step of the so-called O_2 cascade (Fig. 1). This also includes oxygen supply, delivered oxygen content, inspired O_2 concentration, alveolar O_2 concentration, arterial and venous pO_2 and, where possible, the tissue oxygenation.

Table 1. Features of an ideal signal

- Accurate
- Reproducible
- Specific
- Sensitive
- Easy to measure
- Cost-effective
- Lead signal

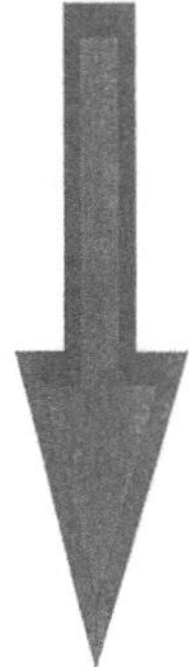

O₂ supply
circuit
airway
alveolor
arterial
capillary
tissue
mixed venous

Fig. 1. Steps in the oxygen cascade

During the past 10 years great advances have been made in our ability to monitor noninvasively and continuously some of these stages of the O₂ cascade. Perhaps the most widely used oxygen monitor in the ICU and the operating theatre is the pulse oxymeter. Pulse oxymeters have allowed us to rapidly recognise hypoxic hypoxaemia in the peripheral arterial circulation. At first sight, pulse oxymetry seems to be an ideal monitor for the control of oxygen uptake and delivery in the blood. Although it is used to measure oxygen uptake and delivery continuously, its further use as an indicator of successful oxygenation during controlled ventilation is restricted.

First, pulse oxymeters are not very sensitive. The measurement of oxyhaemoglobin concentration is inherently related to the exponential nature of the dissociation curve of oxygen and therefore provides no warning until the O₂ tension has fallen below 90 mmHg. This restriction is based on the accuracy of the common oxymeter. In general, they measure arterial oxygen saturation within 95% confidence limits of ±4% when the saturation is above 70% [14]. If we accept these limits, an oxymeter reading of 95% could represent an oxygen tension between 60 mmHg at a saturation of 90% and 160 mmHg at a saturation of 99% (Fig. 2). This is too inaccurate for an exact control algorithm.

Second, pulse oxymeters are not specific. They will not detect any hypoxia as long as the redness of the blood is maintained. Recent investigations show that local anaesthetics, sulphonamides, nitrates, antimalarials and nitroprusside influ-

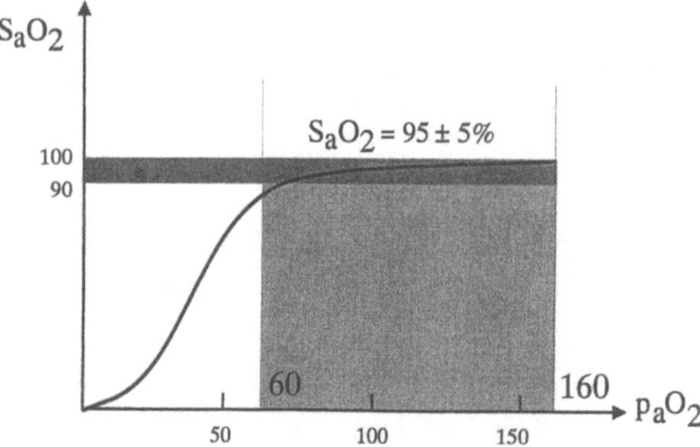

Fig. 2. Sample pulse oxymetry reading

Table 2. Influences on pulse oxymetry

- Methaemoglobin
  nitrates
  sulfonamids
  antimalarials
  local anaesthetics
- Haematocrit
- Low saturation
- Measuring site

ence the accuracy of pulse oxymeters by producing methaemoglobin after administration [19] (Table 2). Furthermore, low haematocrit and low saturation exert a considerable influence on the accuracy of pulse oxymetry [24]. Even the measurement site can influence the response time of this device. Ear probes have proved to give a faster and more accurate response than finger probes [17].

Consequently, though the pulse oxymeter is unsurpassed for the detection of central hypoxaemic hypoxia, under certain conditions it may be misleading. Any other cause of hypoxaemia where the redness of blood is maintained, such as toxic, anaemic or ischaemic hypoxia, cannot be detected. For this reason pulse oxymetry is not acceptable as a control indicator of oxygenation.

Clark electrodes can provide a continuous measurement of O_2 partial pressure in the arterial blood. They determine oxygen tension directly by quenching the fluorescence of an indicator substance caused by oxygen accumulation. The recent development of fluorescent-based probes or optodes located at the tip of a flexible fibre-optic strand are certainly promising. They fit within a 20-gauge arterial cannula and still permit continuous pressure monitoring, continuous flushing of the cannula, and withdrawal of blood samples. But so far they have not gained widespread acceptance because of their price and some other disadvantages. The combined sensor for pH and pCO_2 and the Clark electrode for pO_2 measurement still show a baseline drift, and clotting of the tip requires careful handling by the staff and depends upon haemodynamic stability. The present price is still too high for a routine monitoring sensor.

However, modern technology has provided us with a device to monitor oxygen at a lower level of the O_2 cascade, namely in the airways. Oxygraphy refers to the graphic presentation of the rapidly changing concentration of inhaled and exhaled O_2 during the respiratory cycle. Rapid-response paramagnetic O_2 analysers have been introduced for clinical use. At present, only side-stream rapid-response O_2 monitors are available, but other techniques such as mass, acoustical or Raman spectrometry provide the same data. These data furnish information regarding inspiratory oxygen concentration, end-tidal O_2 and the differences of inhaled and exhaled O_2 in real time. As such, oxygraphy reflects the balance of alveolar O_2 available during inspiration minus the O_2 uptake by pulmonary perfusion. Any significant change in alveolar O_2 supply, diffusion, O_2 uptake, circulation, ventilation or the circuit during the respiratory cycle will be reflected in the O_2 waveform. This measure of the relationship between O_2 supply and demand distinguishes oxygraphy from all other noninvasive monitoring methods.

The oxygram is essentially the mirror image of the capnogram. However, unlike the capnogram, it has more than one normal configuration because the waveform can be influenced by changes in inspired gas concentrations. Normally, during a steady state of ventilation the inspiratory-to-expiratory O_2 difference is 4–5%. After a sudden change in inspired oxygen concentration this difference can actually be larger but will eventually reach the normal value of 5% when a steady state is established (Fig. 3). A value of more than 5% during a steady-state anaesthesia can serve as a faster and even more sensitive indicator of acute hypoventilation than end-tidal CO_2 [2]. A value of more than 5% indicates a body supply-demand imbalance that must be recognised and should be corrected.

Oxygraphic evidence of an O_2 supply-demand mismatch precedes pulse oxymetry and capnographic changes. During manual hypoventilation the inspiratory-to-expiratory O_2 differences increase twofold, while end-tidal CO_2 increases only by 30% [6]. In addition, low end-tidal levels reveal inadequate fresh-gas supplementation. So the inspiratory-to-expiratory O_2 difference provides the earliest warning of the development of an impending hypoxic episode. Based on these advantages, online oxygraphy can be recommended as the most reliable measure for controlling oxygen delivery.

Measurement of oxygen consumption or oxygen extraction has been an invasive procedure so far. The most common technique is the detection of mixed venous oxygen saturation. Mixed venous oxygen saturation is commonly used only as a means of assessing cardiopulmonary status in critically ill patients.

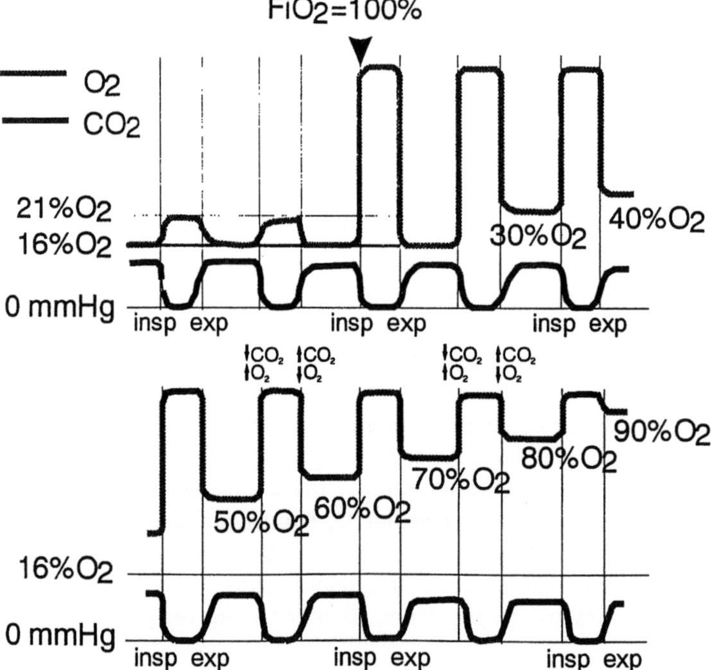

Fig. 3. Oxygraphy during preoxygenation

However, it also represents the end of the oxygen cascade and is therefore important for controlled oxygenation. An advantage of measuring mixed venous rather than arterial saturation is the fact that normal mixed venous saturation values are represented on the steep portion of the O_2 dissociation curve. Therefore, a linear relationship exists between changes in mixed venous oxygen tension and saturation, which is essential for any control.

A disadvantage of mixed venous saturation values is that there are many factors which can influence the degree of saturation. Factors altering mixed venous saturation include O_2 delivery, arterial saturation and haemoglobin, O_2 consumption, influenced, for example, by a weaning trial or temperature, and O_2 extraction. However, if cardiac output, arterial saturation and haemoglobin concentration remain constant, changes in mixed venous saturation should reflect changes in O_2 consumption. One of the most important exceptions is sepsis, where a reduction in tissue oxygenation is associated with an elevated mixed venous saturation. Thus, mixed venous saturation cannot be used as a sole guide to tissue oxygenation or for controlled ventilation, but it provides useful information which should be considered in critically ill patients.

Since its introduction in 1981, capnography has come to be recognised as an extremely valuable method for the continuous monitoring of respiration and circulation in unconscious patients. Recognition of the value of capnography for the detection and prevention of mishaps has grown, to the extent that some of the United States have mandated its use on all intubated patients.

Due to the absence of CO_2 in the inspired gas, there is only one normal capongram, and all variations from the normal pattern indicate some abnormality that must be recognised and corrected if possible [21]. Any factor that impairs the free exhalation of gas, such as a kinked, displaced or otherwise obstructed endotracheal tube, asthma or chronic obstructive pulmonary diseases, will produce a change in the slope of the ascending limb. The angle might vary from about 90° to 160°, depending on the severity of the expiratory obstruction.

An ascending limb with a long rise time and no plateau indicates that exhalation has not been completed before inhalation occurs. It is important to recognise that the value of the end-tidal CO_2 is clinically significant only if a normal plateau is present.

Any significant failure in circulation, such as decreased cardiac output, cardiac arrest or severe hypotension, will decrease the height of the plateau. In a circulatory crisis, if ventilation remains constant, the plateau will fall in proportion to the severity of the event and slowly rise as pulmonary circulation improves. In fact, of all available monitors in use during cardiac arrest, capnography provides the best real-time, continuous information regarding the effectiveness of resuscitation efforts [3].

The descending limb reflects the dynamics of inspiration. If inspiration is prolonged or if there is a leak around the endotracheal tube, the angle of the descending limb and the plateau will be greater than 90° and the descending limb will take a longer time to reach baseline. The baseline will not reach zero if CO_2-containing gases are rebreathed, which will occur if the circuit valves malfunction, if the soda absorber becomes exhausted, or if the inspiratory flow rate is inadequate. On the basis of these multiple advantages, capnography is recommended in many reviews as the leading monitor of respiration, or at least of ventilation [14].

Although pulmonary mechanics seem to be easily, noninvasively and continuously measured, both the basic mechanisms responsible for these effects and their clinical significance remain obscure. True compliance is measured only in static volume-pressure loops, which require about 2 min to be performed. They include much valuable information such as the compliance during inspiration, represented by the slope of the loop, tidal volume and different airway pressures, including the so-called inflection point [5], which can be used for the assessment of PEEP during mechanical ventilation (Fig. 4).

However, spontaneous breaths reduce the reproducibility of the measurements, and a difference of about 30% between each breath may be seen [7]. In patients with high airway resistance expiration may be prolonged, which leads to gas trapping, to an auto-PEEP, and therefore to an underestimation of static compliance by as much as 50% [12]. Also, simple volume measurements may be difficult to obtain due to compressed air in the tubing. In the presence of low compliance, as much as 20% of the intended tidal volume remains in the ventilator circuit at the end of lung inflation, which leads to a measuring error of 20% due to

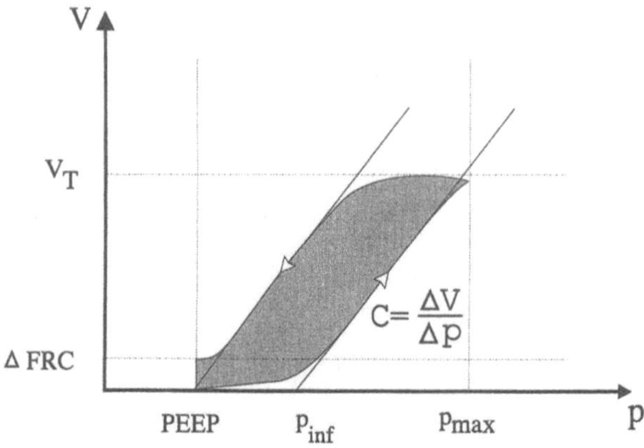

Fig. 4. Static pressure-volume loop. *FRC*, functional residual capacity

the tubing alone [12]. So we have to conclude that the normally employed and almost universally presented pressure-volume diagrams cannot be used for sophisticated control of pulmonary mechanics.

Respiratory mechanic monitoring has recently been improved [2]. Modern technology has made it possible to use monitors in the ICU or even the operating theatre that we know only from the respiratory function lab. On-line spirometry during ventilation has been demonstrated to be a potent tool because it substantially improves the discriminating features of capnography. Side-stream spirometry provides flow-volume and pressure-volume curves, as well as routine spectrometric data such as inspired and expired tidal and minute volume, respiration rate, different airway pressures and breath-to-breath calculated compliance. The percentage of expired volume in 1 s can be presented as a partial estimate of airflow resistance.

Detection of changes in pulmonary mechanics is facilitated by an on-line display of flow-volume and pressure-volume (PV) curves, which show characteristic patterns specific for airway problems. An obstructive pattern is easily identified by observing reduced expiratory flow rate, or reduced tidal volume exhaled in 1 s, represented by the inverse value of the gradient of the loop. Pulmonary parenchymal and/or chest wall problems, on the other hand, are more rapidly identified as compliance changes, which are represented by the slope of a PV loop during inspiration. Therefore, the interpretation of the PV loops requires experience in dealing with such curves before they can be read with confidence [1]. The application of these curves for an automated control remains restricted. Although these limitations may be very severe, static PV loops are believed to be as valuable for monitoring respiratory mechanics as for monitoring controlled ventilation.

Weaning continues to be a problem, sometimes ameliorated by predictions from contemporaneous data [10, 15]. One of these, the work of breathing, is as difficult to measure as compliance or true airway pressure. It can be represented by the area under the inspiratory limb of a PV loop. The differentiation between rib cage movement and lung elastic properties is nearly impossible during spontaneous respiration. Even after extubation the work of breathing is difficult to interpret and may actually be increased or decreased [16]. So we have to realise that no clear prediction of weaning outcome can be derived from the work of spontaneous breathing.

Measuring airway occlusion pressure 100 ms after initiating an inspiratory effort against an occluded airway provides a certain measure of drive. This pressure is regarded as the intention to breathe. Another approach to assessing respiratory drive is to measure the mean inspiratory airflow by calculating the ratio of inspired tidal volume and inspiratory time. Both $P_{0.1}$ and inspiratory airflow may underestimate respiratory drive in the presence of deranged pulmonary mechanics, but an elevated value clearly represents increased drive [4]. Different groups of investigators have reported [9, 13] that an elevated $P_{0.1}$ is predictive of weaning failure, although the line separating success from failure differed among the studies. Montgomery et al. did not find measurement of $P_{0.1}$ to be helpful [8]; in contrast, they found that the patients who failed a weaning trial were less able to increase $P_{0.1}$ during CO_2 stimulation. Therefore, it is currently possible to evaluate neither the site for monitoring inspiratory drive in critically ill patients nor its use for the automated control of weaning.

Inductive plethysmography allows the detection of asynchronous motion, defined as the time lag between the movement of the rib cage and abdomen and paradoxical motion, which means two compartments moving in opposite directions. The employment of these devices, which record motion of the rib cage and abdomen separately, has been considered in several studies to be helpful in the clinical management of weaning trials [11]. Paradoxical abdominal movements, often regarded as a specific indicator of weaning outcome, were found to be a poor predictor of weaning success [18]; this was better predicted by observation of asynchronous motion and an index that quantitates the breath-to-breath variability between the contribution of the rib cage and the abdomen towards the tidal volume as a measure of diaphragmatic failure.

To summarise this review of respiratory monitoring, we conclude that the information on equipment and patient data has expanded enormously in the past 10 years. But the expansion of respiratory monitoring may bring its own pitfalls. Up to now, more monitoring devices, and thus more alarms, have brought more confusion. Given the opportunity, more anaesthetists would vote against them. So the time seems to be ripe for an automated control of ventilation. Perhaps only a computer-controlled respirator can combine monitors correctly so they can give more information than the simple sum. It can be hazardous to us and to our patients if we overlook this information. Perhaps controlled ventilation is the right tool to help us watch the patient rather than the gadgets of monitoring.

References

1. Bardoczky Gl, D'Hollander A (1992) Continuous monitoring of the flow-volume loops and compliance during anaesthesia. J Clin Monit 8:251–252
2. Bardoczky G, De Francquen P, Engelman E, Capello M (1992) Continuous monitoring of pulmonary mechanics with sidestream spirometry during lung transplantation. J Cardio Thorac Anaesth 6:731–734
3. Falk JL, Rackow EC, Weil MH (1988) End-tidal carbon dioxide concentration during cardiopulmonary resuscitation. N Engl J Med 318: 607–611
4. Herrera M, Blasco J, Venegas J, Barba R (1985) Mouth occlusion pressure ($p_{0.1}$) in acute respiratory failure. Intensive Care Med 11:134-139
5. Lemair F, Benito S, Mancebo J (1992) The lung pressure-volume relationship during mechanical ventilation. In: Artigas A, Lemaire F (eds) Adult respiratory distress syndrome. Churchill Livingstone, London, pp 379–384
6. Linko K, Paloheimo M (1989) Inspiratory end-tidal oxygen content difference: a sensitive indicator of hypoventilation. Crit Care Med 17:345–348
7. Marini JJ (1988) Monitoring during mechanical ventilation. Clin Chest Med 9:73–100
8. Montgomery AB, Holle RHO, Neagley SR, Pierson DJ (1987) Prediction of successful ventilator weaning using airway occlusion pressure and hypercapnic challenge. Chest 91:496–499
9. Murciano D, Boczkowski J, Lecocguic Y, Milic-Emili J (1988) Tracheal occlusion pressure: a simple index to monitor respiratory muscle fatigue during acute respiratory failure. Ann Intern Med 108:800–805
10. Nathan SD, Ishaaya AM, Koerner SK, Belman SJ (1993) Prediction of minimal pressure support during weaning from mechanical ventilation. Chest 103:1215–1219
11. Ochiari R, Shimadu M, Takeda J, Iwaq Y (1993) Contribution of rib cage abdominal movement to ventilation for successful weaning from mechanical ventilation. Acta Anaesthesiol Scand 37:131–136
12. Rossi A, Gottfried SB, Zocchi L (1989) Measurement of static lung compliance during mechanical ventilation. The effect of intrinsic PEEP. Am Rev Respir Dis 139:672–677
13. Sassoon CSH, Te TT, Mahutte CK, Light RW (1987) Airway occlussion pressure: an important indicator for successful weaning. Am Rev Respir Dis 135:107–113
14. Severinghaus J, Kelleher J (1992) Recent Developments in pulse oximetry. Anesthesiology 76:1018–1038
15. Strickland JH, Hasson JH (1993) A computer-controlled ventilator weaning system. Chest 103:1220–1226
16. Tobin MJ (1990) Respiratory monitoring. JAMA 264: 244–251
17. Tobin MJ (1990) Respiratory monitoring during mechanical ventilation. Crit Care Clin 6:679–709
18. Tobin MJ, Perez W, Guenther SM (1987) Does rib cage abdominal paradox signify respiratory muscle fatigue? J Appl Physiol 63:851–860
19. Trillo R, Aukburg S (1992) Dapsone-induced methemoglobinemia and pulse oximetry. Anesthesiology 77:594–536
20. Ty Smith N (1993) Monitoring and equipment. Curr Opin Anaesthesiol 6:927–929
21. Weingarten M (1986) Anesthetic and ventilator mishaps: prevention and detection. Crit Care Med 14:1084–1086
22. Weingarten M (1989) Prioritization of monitors for the detection of mishaps. Semin Anaesth 8:1–12
23. Weingarten M (1990) Respiratory monitoring of carbon dioxide and oxygen: a ten-year perspective. J Clin Monit 6:217–225
24. Vegfors M, Lindberg L, Oberg P, Lennmarken C (1992) The accuracy of pulse oximetry at two haematocrit levels. Acta Anaesthesiol Scand 36:454–459

Closed-Loop Control of Artificial Ventilation

D.R. Westenskow

Since 1956, researchers have developed numerous closed-loop controllers to adjust mechanical ventilation [1, 2]. In almost all systems, the end-tidal CO_2 is measured on a breath-to-breath basis and the ventilator's tidal volume or respiratory rate is adjusted using classical PID control. These systems reach the set end-tidal CO_2 in less than 1 min and maintain the end-tidal CO_2 within ± 0.1 vol% of the set point. The variability is less than half that seen during periods of open-loop control [3]. Closed-loop control has also been used to adjust the inspired oxygen concentration to maintain the desired arterial oxygen concentration in neonates [4]. Once again, the closed-loop controller out-performs the human operator.

Closed-loop controllers of ventilation have not found their way into clinical practice. The main reason may be that end-tidal CO_2 does not always reflect arterial CO_2. Following an embolism, a closed-loop controller may reduce ventilation inappropriately. Also, the end-tidal CO_2 measurement may be artifactual (with shallow spontaneous breaths) and ventilation may be reduced inappropriately. Intra-arterial sensors, which measure arterial CO_2 and O_2 directly, are slow to respond and drift considerably. Thus the clinical application of closed-loop control of ventilation has been limited by sensor technology.

Closed-loop control does provide a vitally important function in modern ventilators. Even though the closed-loop control envisioned by Frumin has not been implemented, many of the functions on modern ventilators are possible only because of closed-loop control (Siemens Elema, Solna, Sweden). These functions include numerous ventilatory modes, automatic start-up, inspired oxygen control, minimization of breathing work, and automatic weaning. Ventilators of the future are almost certain to include new modes of operation, which will be possible because of closed-loop control.

Pressure control and volume support modes rely on closed-loop control. The flow control valves which are the heart of many modern ventilators rely on closed-loop control to adjust the flow rate delivered to the ventilator, based on a sensor's measurement of flow. The Siemens 300 Ventilator is a good example (Siemens Elema, Solna, Sweden). In the pressure control and pressure support modes, this ventilator measures airway pressure and, under closed-loop control, adjusts the flow to achieve the desired inspiratory pressure. In the volume support and the pressure-regulated volume control modes, a closed-loop controller measures the delivered tidal volume and adjusts the pressure of the gas delivered. These modern modes of support would not be possible without effective closed-loop controllers.

Automatic control has been used effectively to select appropriate start-up settings for the ventilator [5]. A patient is connected to a ventilator, using the pressure-controlled synchronized intermittent mandatory ventilation mode. The first five breaths are analyzed, and tidal volume, expiratory time constant, and series dead space are measured. A respiratory frequency and tidal volume are calculated to minimize work of breathing, based on an estimate of the patient's size and work of breathing. These automatic settings of tidal volume and respiratory rate, when evaluated in 42 ICU patients, did not differ significantly from those that would have been selected with a nomogram. The advantage that makes this method potentially useful is that the ventilator was set up fully automatically, without the need for manual entry of patients' weight or height.

Closed-loop control has been shown to be effective in automatically weaning patients from ventilatory support. These approaches range from very sophisticated expert systems, which includes hemodynamics and other patient data, to a very simple SIMV reduction scheme [6, 7]. Using the simple approach, a patient begins the weaning process with an SIMV rate of 6/min, pressure support of $20\,cm\,H_2O$, a tidal volume which ranges from 10 to $15\,ml/kg$, and a respiratory rate between 8 and 30 breaths per min. The SIMV rate is reduced by two breaths per min every hour, as long as the patient's parameters remain within the bounds listed above. When the SIMV rate reaches 2 per min, pressure support is reduced by $2\,cm\,H_2O$ each hour, as long as the patient's parameters remain within the tidal volume and respiratory rate bounds. The weaning process is complete when pressure support reaches $5\,cm\,H_2O$. If at any time during the weaning process the parameters fall outside the allowable range, the therapy is increased using the steps specified above, at a rate of once every 5 min. Using this simple scheme, seven of nine patients were weaned in an average time of 18.7 $\pm$ 5.6 h. In the control group, where patients were weaned as judged appropriate by the physician, the average weaning time was 25.6 $\pm$ 5.6 h. The number of arterial blood gases drawn for the closed-loop group was 1.4 $\pm$ 0.7, whereas the control group had 7.2 $\pm$ 4.3. Strickland and Hasson have shown that the computer-directed weaning results in fewer arterial blood gas samples and shorter weaning times [7].

A more clinically based approach to weaning has been taken by East et al. using the Help computer system at the LDS Hospital [8–10]. Protocols for ventilation management were developed by 14 physicians, three nurses, a respiratory therapist, and a Ph.D. scientist. In weekly meetings, these experts reviewed the weaning protocols. They abandoned their personal style in favor of a group consensus. Using a ventilator in the CPPV mode, their rules use measurements of oxygen saturation or arterial oxygen partial pressure to suggest the best change in the level of PEEP or inspired oxygen concentration. The system was used in 111 ARDS patients with arterial-to-alveolar oxygen partial pressure ratios less than 0.2, static compliance less than $50\,ml/cm\,H_2O$, and ARDS risk factors and radiographic evidence of ARDS. Of these critically ill ARDS patients, 62% survived. The survival rate was at least as good as that published for other centers with similarly ill ARDS patients. Of the 11 780 instructions generated during this trial, only 7% were not followed (software errors 0.4%, inappropriate data entry 3.1%, cascading errors 1.1%, logic conflicts 1%, and all other reasons 1%). This success clearly indicates the feasibility of using expert systems to care for critically ill patients.

The rules used in weaning have been implemented in a continuous closed-loop system to control oxygenation [11]. A Hamilton Amedeus ventilator is controlled by an Apple Macintosh SE 30 computer. A Shiley Continucath (Shiley, Irvine, CA) intra-arterial electrode is used to provide continuous measurement of P_aO_2. When tested in dogs, the controller provided an aggressive response to hypoxemia and a more conservative response to hyperoxia and performed well with no hazardous or failure conditions noted.

Closed-loop control has a significant role in mechanical ventilation. It makes possible the modern modes of pressure control, pressure support, and volume support ventilation. Recent work indicates that closed-loop control is effective in setting the initial conditions for ventilation, minimizing the work of breathing and aiding in the weaning process. When sensors to accurately measure arterial CO_2 and oxygen become available, then the closed feedback loops envisioned by pioneers can be implemented.

References

1. Frumin MJ (1957) Clinical use of a physiological respirator producing N_2O amnesia/analgesia. Anesthesiology 18:290–299
2. Frumin MJ, Bergman NA, Holaday DA (1959) Carbon dioxide and oxygen blood levels with a carbon dioxide-controlled artificial respirator. Anesthesiology 20:313–320
3. Chapman FW, Newell JC, Roy RJ (1985) A feedback controller for ventilatory therapy. Ann Biomed Eng 13:359–372
4. Morozoff PE, Evans RW (1992) Closed-loop control of SaO_2 in the neonate. Biomed Instr Tech 26:117–123
5. Laubscher TP, Frutiger A, Fanconi S, Jutzi H, Brunner JX (1994) Automatic selection of tidal volume, respiratory frequency and minute ventilation in intubated ICU patients as startup procedure for closed-loop controlled ventilation. Int J Clin Monit Comput 11:19–30
6. Tong DA (1991) Weaning patients from mechanical ventilation: a knowledge-based system approach. Comput Methods Programs Biomed 35:267–78
7. Strickland JH jr, Hasson JH (1993) A computer-controlled ventilator weaning system. Chest 103:1220–1226
8. East TD, Morris AH, Wallace CJ, Clemmer TP et al (1992) A strategy for development of computerized critical care decision support systems. Int J Clin Monit Comput 8:263–269
9. Henderson S, Crapo RO, Wallace CJ, East TD et al (1992) Performance of computerized protocols for the management of arterial oxygenation in an intensive care unit. Int J Clin Monit Comput 8:271–280

10. East TD, Böhm SH, Wallace CJ, Clemmer TP et al (1992) A successful computerized protocol for clinical management of pressure control inverse ratio ventilation in ARDS patients. Chest 101:697–710
11. East TD, Tolle CR, Farrell RM, Brunner JX (1991) A non-linear closed-loop controller for oxygenation based on a clinically proven fifth-dimensional quality surface. Crit Care Med 19:S61

IV Control and Automation of Drug Delivery

a) Volatile Anesthetics

Adaptive Closed-Loop Control
of End-Tidal Concentrations of Volatile Agents

D.R. Westenskow

In inducing anesthesia with the volatile agents, the goal is to rapidly achieve the desired brain concentration without creating a dangerously high level in the arterial blood. One protocol uses high fresh-gas flows (5 l/min) and an initial inspired concentration of 3–4 MAC. When the end-tidal concentration reaches the desired level, the vaporizer setting is reduced to 120% of the desired level. After 5 min the vaporizer is set to the desired level and the fresh-gas flow reduced to 1 l/min. Automatic control of this process could be implemented in a very straightforward way. Automation would reduce the human variability and might avoid potential injury when a clinician is busy with other tasks and forgets to reduce the vaporizer setting at the appropriate time. This chapter will review the design of the automatic controller and present its clinical advantages.

Anesthesia can be induced most rapidly using a nonrebreathing system [1]. The controller delivers the volatile agent at the maximum allowable concentration, while observing the end-tidal concentration, breath-to-breath. Once the target end-tidal concentration is reached, the inspired concentration is reduced at a model-predicted rate. Typically, the desired end-tidal concentration is reached in 15–20 breaths. The one disadvantage of this system is that it uses high fresh-gas flows and large amounts of the volatile agent. The cost of the volatile agent may, however, be offset by a shorter stay in the operating room, because of the more rapid induction.

Closed-loop controllers have been developed to deliver agent to completely closed rebreathing circuits, thus using the minimum amount of gas and vapor. The inspired agent concentration is measured and an automatic controller adjusts the concentration of agent in the fresh-gas flow. To maintain a completely closed circuit, the fresh-gas flow rate must be limited; it may not exceed the patient's metabolic removal of gas from the rebreathing circuit (approximately 250 ml/min). A blower in the circuit significantly enhances mixing, improves the controller's response time, and renders the system independent of the patient's minute ventilation. Whether one uses a pole placement, fuzzy logic, classical PID, or adaptive control, the result is about the same. The desired inspired concentration is reached in 3.5 min [2].

Induction is more rapid when an automatic controller uses a high fresh-gas flow during induction and reverts to low fresh-gas flow when steady-state is reached. Fresh-gas flows begin at approximately 5 l/min and are reduced to 1 l/min once the desired agent concentration has been reached and maintained for several minutes. Using active control of fresh-gas flow and a classical PID controller for the volatile agent delivery, the desired oxygen concentration is reached in 7.7 min (0–90% response) [3]. The desired end-tidal concentration is reached in 3.6–5.6 min (depending on the size of the patient), 2.7–6.9 min (depending on cardiac output), or 3.5–5.8 min (depending on ventilation) [3]. When the process is controlled manually, the average clinician takes 10.6 ± 4.2 min to reach the desired end-tidal agent concentration [4]. The overshoot for the automatic controller is 9% over the target value, whereas anesthesiologists typically have an overshoot of 18% [4]. Regardless of the breathing circuit or the type of control, the time to reach the desired value ranges from 1.7 to 6 min [5, 7, 8].

The speed of induction is ultimately dependent on the rate at which agent is transferred from the arterial blood to the brain. Simulations, using an anesthetic uptake model, indicate that with a cardiac output of 10 l/min the brain rises to 50% of the desired level in 3 min, whereas with a cardiac output of 2.5 l/min, the brain reaches 50% of the desired concentration only after 10 min [9]. Even with very rapid control of end-tidal concentration, it is important to realize how cardiac output limits the rate of rise of the brain concentration.

To better control brain concentration, numerous investigators have controlled blood pressure, heart rate, or EEG [5]. Using isoflurane, the mean arterial pressure can be kept within 5 mmHg of the target value 89–94% of the time [10, 11]. These investigators found that the automatic controller performance was very similar to human performance. Blood pressure and heart rate are regulated by the sympathetic nervous system and rise with painful stimuli, making these controllers unreliable in some situations. The human operator must be careful to oversee their performance and quickly take action when not appropriate. In a very complex controller, Rehman et al. used heart rate, arterial pressure, respiratory rate, agent concentration, temperature, etc. as inputs to an artificial neural network [13]. They trained the network to predict the level of anesthesia and recommend the best inspired concentration. The network performed a nonlinear mapping and learned through examples to perform just as the anesthetist had performed. Although the relationship between clinical signs and anesthetic depth is not well defined, the network was able to find a relationship in the training data set. In simulated operation, using a patient model, Rehman et al. demonstrated the ability of a network to integrate data from a number of sources, as the clinician does, to assess depth of anesthesia.

Closed-loop control may become a valuable component of future anesthesia work stations, adding convenience, reliability, and safety. Under automatic control, the work station can mimic clinical practice, using high fresh-gas flows and high concentrations of the volatile anesthetic to induce anesthesia and then reducing the fresh-gas flow, once steady-state is reached. As in process control, aviation, etc., the human operator must always be present to oversee the controller's operation and to take quick action should the unexpected happen.

References

1. Tatnall ML, Morris P, West PG (1981) Controlled anaesthesia: an approach using patient characteristics identified during uptake. Br J Anaesth 53:1019–1025
2. Messer TM (1994) Control techniques for automated delivery of anesthesia: halothane system. Masters Thesis, University of Utah
3. Loughlin PJ (1988) Computer-assisted anesthesia: a control system to aid the anesthetist in efficiently administering oxygen and anesthetic gases. Masters Thesis, University of Utah
4. Smith NT, Quinn ML, Fukui Y, Fleming R, Coles JR (1984) Automatic control in anesthesia: a comparison in performance between the anesthetist and the machine. Anesth Analg 63:715–722
5. O'Hara DA, Bogen DK, Noordergraaf A (1992) The use of computers for controlling the delivery of anesthesia. Anesthesiology 77:563–518
6. Westenskow DR, Meline L, Pace NL (1987) Controlled hypotension with sodium nitroprusside: anesthesiologist versus computer. J Clin Monit 3:80–86
7. Fukui Y, Smith NT, Fleming RA (1982) Digital and sampled-data control of arterial blood pressure during halothane anesthesia. Anesth Analg 61:1010–1015
8. Zbinden AM, Frei R, Westenskow DR, Thomson DA (1986) Control of end-tidal halothane concentration. Br J Anaesth 58:563–571
9. Luttropp HH, Rydgren G, Tomasson R, Werner O (1991) A minimal-flow system for xenon anesthesia. Anesthesiology 75:896–902
10. Zwart A, Smith NT, Beneken JEW (1972) Multiple model approach to uptake and distribution of halothane: the use of an analog computer. Comput Biomed Res 5:228–238
11. Millard RK, Monk CP, Prys-Roberts C (1988) Self-tuning control of hypotension during ENT surgery using a volatile anaesthetic IEE Proc 135D:95–105
12. Monk CR, Millard RK, Hutton P, Prys-Roberts C (1989) Automatic arterial pressure regulation using isoflurane: comparison with manual control. Br J Anaesth 63:22–30
13. Rehman HU, Linkens DA, Asbury AJ (1993) Neural networks and nonlinear regression modeling and control of depth of anaesthesia for spontaneously breathing and ventilated patient. Comput Methods Programs Biomed 40:227–247

Fuzzy Control of Arterial Blood Pressure by Volatile Anesthetics

A.M. Zbinden, M. Derighetti, S. Petersen, and P. Feigenwinter

While feedback control has found wide application in many areas of modern civilization (such as the regulation of the speed of rapid trains, cars, and cameras), medicine is still – with a few exceptions – exempt. For many controlled parameters during anesthesia automatic feedback control can be applied because the input and output values are well defined and can be easily measured. Anesthetists have to perform many tasks simultaneously; if they can be released from some of the repetitive tasks they can devote more attention to the patient. Automatic feedback systems can help not only to save manpower but also potentially expensive anesthetic gases by minimizing fresh-gas flow. Feedback systems can be used for many tasks, such as:

- Adjusting *tidal volume and frequency* depending on the measured expired CO_2 concentration and/or the mean airway pressure (or other parameters used to estimate optimization of ventilation)
- Adjusting the *fresh-gas concentration of oxygen nitrous oxide, and/or volatile anesthetics*, so that the desired inspired and/or end-tidal concentration is obtained
- Adjusting the *inspired and/or end-tidal concentration of volatile anesthetics*, so that a desired mean arterial blood pressure is obtained
- *Minimizing fresh-gas flow* of oxygen and nitrous oxide, so that costs for anesthetic gases are reduced while at the same time the ability to adjust rapidly the different gas concentrations is maintained

The goal would be to create an anesthesia system which, after having been connected to the patient, automatically adjusts gas concentrations and ventilation, while at the same time minimizing gas consumption. Feedback systems can be used whenever input signals are well defined and can be measured easily without artifacts. Long delay times are the enemy of any control system. Characteristics of good control systems are rapid reactions, the absence of over- or undershooting, as well as of oscillations, a well-defined and – if possible – simple structure, and the absence of software and hardware errors. A well-defined structure is a must if the control system is to be approved by a licensing institution.

Several feedback-control strategies exist: proportional-integral-derivative (PID) controllers [1], adaptive controllers [2], and state estimation controllers, which update initial values using least-squares online estimation [3]. The classical PID approach can be used whenever the "between" and "within" individual variability remains small. Control can be improved if a good mathematical model of the process is available. As in many biomedical settings, the great variance of the plant[1] has lead to oscillation of the controller; the investigation of self-adaptive control strategies, and later of self-organizing controllers, was needed. Although self-adaptive controllers have been successful, considerable work was required to select the right design parameters. The pharmacokinetic and -dynamic properties of inhaled anesthetics are nonlinear [4], time varying [5], and difficult to model. If the effects of surgery, the anesthesia breathing system, and concomitantly used intravenous anesthetics also have to be considered, modeling becomes very difficult. This is a typical setting where fuzzy logic control can be applied. Fuzzy logic was introduced in the 1960s and is now very popular in many areas [6]. It uses linguistic rules which describe fuzzy sets, the members of which are not crisp (binary), but can range from 0 to 1.

The feedback control used in our institution has been described in part previously [7]. The development of a fuzzy controller can be divided into five steps, as shown, using control of mean arterial blood pressure (MAP) with isoflurane as an example.

Step 1 brings together the knowledge and skill of users and engineers in order to define rules based on the requirements of the user; i.e., if blood pressure is high then give a high concentration of isoflurane.

In *step 2* the input data are fuzzified. For each set a membership function is defined. Assume a measured MAP of 85, the set MAP being 80. The error thus is (80–85)/80 = −0.0625. Thus the negative medium rule will become 100% active and the negative small rule will become some 20% active (see Fig. 1).

Step 3 uses if-then-else rules to connect input rules to output rules, e.g., if the error in MAP is large negative, then use a very large, positive inspired isoflurane concentration.

In *step 4*, using the various input data a single output variable is defined; this means that the input data are defuzzified.

Step 5 is probably the most difficult. It consists of the optimization of the fuzzy controller. As no mathematical tool exists for this stage, a great deal of the work is based on the subjective feeling and the skill of both the engineer and the physician. In order to reduce the number of experiments, the use of computer simulation is recommended. Plotting the frequency of the occurrence of the rules is a good method to detect which rules are important and which can be deleted without affecting the function of the controller. The rules then have to be improved quantitatively using data obtained from patients.

Using isoflurane to control MAP can be questioned, as the end-tidal isoflurane concentration is probably not directly related to the blood pressure increase caused by surgical stimulation [8]. On the other hand, it is common practice to

---

[1] *A plant*, in the language of the engineer, is not a flower. It is that miraculous thing that occurs between input and output; in our setting, it describes what the anesthesia circuit and the human body are doing to the input signal (e.g., the fresh-gas isoflurane concentration).

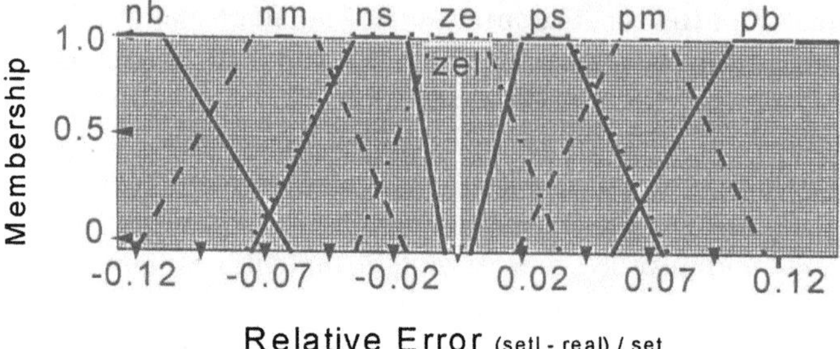

Fig. 1. Fuzzy logic membership functions relating the relative error to one or several values: *nb*, negative big; *nm*, negative medium; *ns*, negative small; *ze*, zero; *zel*, zero large; *ps*, positive small; *pm*, positive medium; *pb*, positive big

adjust isoflurane concentration using MAP, since other signs such as pupil size are no longer applicable during modern anesthesia. Isoflurane has a rapid and well-defined effect on blood pressure, and the inspired and/or end-tidal isoflurane concentration can be easily measured. However, when MAP is used to control isoflurane concentration, abrupt changes in surgical stimulation such as skin incision cannot be anticipated by an automatic control system but can be anticipated by the anesthesiologist. Furthermore, isoflurane is not able to suppress the increase of blood pressure caused by surgical stimulation, but the prestimulation MAP can be decreased [8].

The concept of the controller used in the future may be based on a cascade design with an inner loop that controls the inspired isoflurane concentration, therefore accounting mainly for the effects of the anesthesia breathing system, and an outer loop that controls MAP by setting the inspired isoflurane concentration, thus accounting mainly for patient effects. The aim of the construction of the inner loop was to reduce both the time response and gas consumption. The advantage of this system is that if the outer loop breaks down, e.g., due to measurement errors, the control system can switch to the inner loop and maintain a certain inspired concentration. Furthermore, the inner loop may be equipped with a system which minimizes the fresh-gas flows so that costly anesthetic gases are not wasted, but the ability to change concentration rapidly is maintained. Figure 2 shows an example of the response to a step change of the isoflurane concentration of the inner loop. Figure 3 shows the changes of fresh-gas flows adjusted by the controller in order to obtain a rapid adjustment of the inspired gas concentrations.

Safety is probably one of the major features of such a control system. It has to be guaranteed that adequate control is maintained, even when the input signal is disturbed (e.g., by a clotted arterial cannulation, motion artifacts, or calibration errors). This can be achieved by using a redundant measuring system (the signal for the feedback system originates from a system which is independent from the system used to display the measured values to the anesthesiologist) and by using a supervisor system. The latter incorporates a model which simulates the anesthesia breathing system and the human body with the uptake and the pharmacodynamic effects of the inhaled anesthetic. The supervisor system

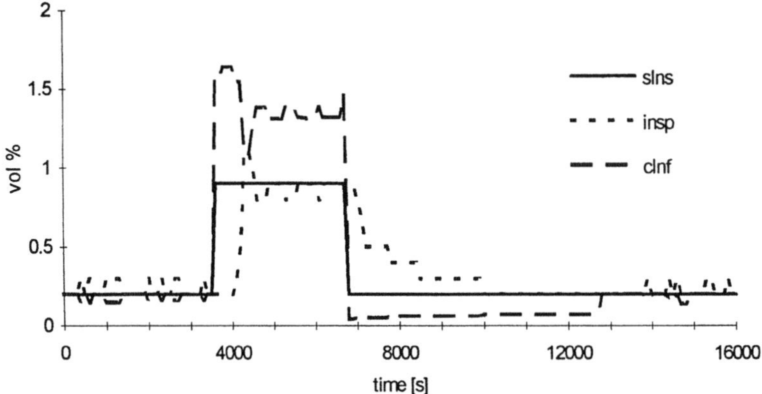

Fig. 2. Step response of the inspired isoflurane concentration during surgery. *sIns*, Set inspired isoflurane concentration; *insp*, measured inspired isoflurane concentration; *clnf*, fresh-gas isoflurane concentration

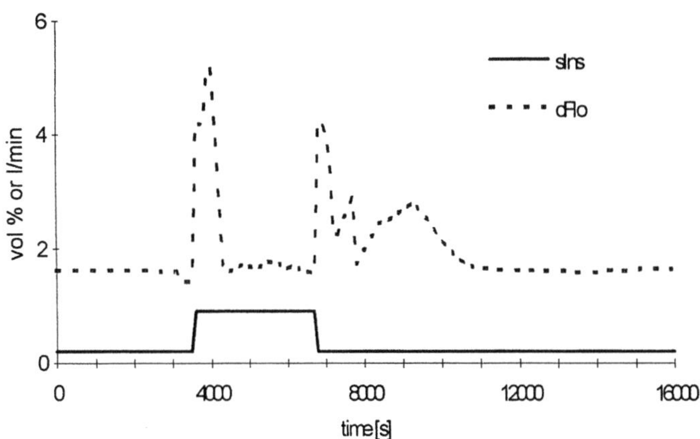

Fig. 3. Step response of the inspired isoflurane concentration during surgery. *sIns*, Set inspired isoflurane concentration; *cFlo*, fresh-gas flow set by the controller. A change in *sins* results in a temporary increase of *cFlo*

displays an alarm message as soon as one of the input parameters substantially differs from the corresponding parameter calculated by the supervisor model.

There is still a long way to go before feedback systems are introduced onto the market. The first feedback system will probably be a system which adjusts the fresh-gas concentration so that the desired inspired concentration of oxygen, nitrous oxide, and isoflurane is achieved while at the same time fresh-gas consumption is minimized. In a later stage, the inspired concentration may be automatically adjusted so that a desired end-tidal concentration is achieved. Both above-mentioned systems depend not only on the introduction of control algorithms, but also on the availability of the corresponding electronically controlled actuators (flowmeters, vaporizers). Whether automatic control systems will finally be introduced into clinical routine depends not only on technological progress, but also on acceptance by the users and the possibility of relieving the anesthesiologists so that they can concentrate more on the patients themselves.

References

1. Sheppard LC (1980) Computer control of the infusion of vasoactive drugs. Ann Biomed Eng 8:431–444
2. Vishnoi R, Roy FJ (1991) Adaptive control of closed circuit anesthesia. IEEE Trans Biomed Eng 38:39–46
3. Rametti LB, Bradlow HS, Uys PC (1985) On-line parameter estimation and control of d-tubocurarine induced muscle relaxation. Med Biol Eng Comput 23:556–564
4. Ashman MN, Blesser WB, Epstein RM (1970) A nonlinear model for the uptake and distribution of halothane in man. Anesthesiology 33:419–429
5. Petersen S, Zbinden AM, Fischer M, Thomson DA (1993) Isoflurane MAC decreases during anesthesia and surgery. Anesthesiology 79:959–965
6. Zadeh LA (1965) Fuzzysets. Information Control 8:338–352
7. Meier R, Nieuwland J, Zbinden AM, Hacisalihzade SS (1992) Fuzzy logic control of blood pressure during anesthesia. IEEE Control Systems Magazine 12:12–17
8. Zbinden AM, Petersen-Felix S, Thomson DA (1994) Defining anesthetic depth using multiple noxious stimuli during isoflurane/oxygen anesthesia. Part 2. Hemodynamic responses. Anesthesiology 80:261–267

Model-Based Adaptive Control of Volatile Anesthetics by Quantitative EEG

H. Schwilden and J. Schüttler

Automatic feedback control of the delivery of volatile anesthetic agents has been realized in the past using inspired concentrations as well as expired concentrations (see D.R. Westenskow, this volume, pp 155–157) as feedback signal. These approaches used a proportional-integral-derivative (PID) controller for feedback control of the volatile anesthetic agents. This paper deals with a model-based adaptive feedback control system of the delivery of volatile anesthetics using the EEG as the pharmacodynamic response variable to be controlled. Specifically, we used the median EEG frequency.

Theoretical Considerations

Figure 1 depicts the block schematics of a model-based feedback control system. The input to the system is the vaporizer setting; the output of the system is the median EEG frequency as measured from the scalp of the patient. The task of the feedback system is to dial the vaporizer setting such that the measured output is within the desired range. The core of the feedback system is a model of the patient with respect to the relationship between drug dosing and drug effect.

Such a model can be used in two directions. In the forward direction it can give a prediction of the measured output. In the backward direction it can be used to determine the necessary input to achieve and maintain a certain level of output.

Given such a model, the system incorporates three values for the effect. Let E_m denote the effect which is actually measured, E_p the effect which is predicted by the model, and E_s the chosen set point. Ideally, all three values coincide

$$E_m = E_s = E_p \tag{1}$$

De facto, these three values will differ, allowing the construction of two differences, for instance $E_m - E_p$ and $E_m - E_s$. A non-zero difference $E_m - E_p$ means that the measured effect is different from the predicted effect indicating that the model does not precisely describe the actual patient. The difference $E_m - E_s$ means that the measured effect is not at the set point. These two differences can be used in the following way: The difference between E_m and E_p is used to adapt the model to the patient. That is to say, the parameter values are modified such that the model prediction will coincide with the measured value. On the basis of the updated

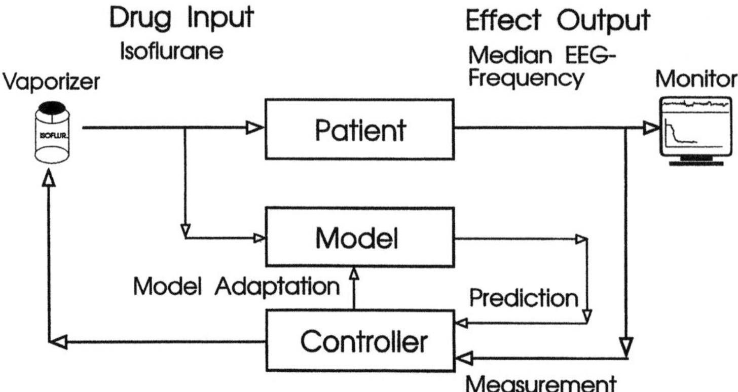

Fig. 1. Model-based adaptive feedback control system

model, a new dosing scheme is calculated which should bring the measured output
to the set point and maintain it.

The Integrated Pharmacokinetic-Pharmacodynamic Model

The classic dose-response relationship (in vivo) relates a given dose of a compound to the effect at a certain moment in time. Static concentration response relationships are generated, in general, with isolated organs or tissues; their response is studied in a bath of defined drug concentration. Pharmacokinetic-pharmacodynamic modeling aims at integrating and generalizing the dose-response and concentration-response relationship by modeling the time-varying effect as a function of the time-varying drug input. From this point of view, one may consider pharmacokinetics a functional K, mapping the time course of drug delivery $I(t)$ to the time course of drug concentration $c(t)$, and pharmacodynamics may be considered a functional D, mapping the time course of drug concentration $c(t)$ to the time course of drug effect $E(t)$:

$$c(t) = K[I(t')]$$
$$E(t) = D[c(t')] \tag{2}$$

For volatile anesthetic agents one has to discuss the meaning of the drug delivery function $I(t)$. For intravenous anesthetic agents drug delivery is the amount of drug given to the systemic circulation via the intravenous route per unit time. For the volatile anesthetic agents one may consider three different definitions depending on the purpose they are used for. From the point of view of drug consumption, the drug-delivery function $I(t)$ may be defined as fresh-gas flow times vaporizer setting (flow $\times$ c_{vap}); from the point of view of the patient's exposure to the vapor, one may define the drug-delivery function $I(t)$ as the product of the inspired concentration c_{insp} times total minute ventilation $\dot{V}_T$. A third aspect could be to consider the amount of volatile agent that reaches the systemic circulation per unit time. This rate is given approximately by

$$I(t) = (c_{et} - c_{insp}) \times \dot{V}_A \tag{3}$$

whereby $\dot{V}_A$ denotes alveolar ventilation and c_{et} the end-tidal concentration of the volatile agent. As the problem of the feedback system is to dial the appropriate vaporizer concentration or fresh-gas concentration c_{vap} which leads to the desired effect, we define drug delivery for our purposes as $I(t) = $ flow $\times c_{vap}$. Given c_{vap}, one has to establish the chain of the following relations: $c_{vap} - c_{insp}$, $c_{insp} - c_{et}$, $c_{et} - c_{biophase}$, $c_{biophase} - $ effect.

The relation between vaporizer setting and inspiratory concentration is, in general, a complex one which depends on the geometry and technical realization of the anesthesia machine as well as on the fresh-gas flow, minute ventilation, and end-tidal concentration. At large fresh-gas flows one may, however, choose the approximation

$$c_{insp}(t) = \int dt' \exp(-\text{flow}(t - t')/V_c)c_{vap}(t') \tag{4}$$

whereby V_c denotes the virtual volume of distribution of the volatile agent for the circle system. The relation between inspiratory and expiratory concentration can be written as a convolution integral

$$c_{et}(t) = \int dt' G(t - t')c_{insp}(t') \tag{5}$$

whereby the function $G(t)$ describes the disposition of the volatile agent in the body.

The function $G(t)$ can be estimated by two entirely different approaches. One may construct $G(t)$ from an explicit model of the tissue composition of the body (Fig. 2). Given the tissue/gas partition coefficients and the volumes and perfusions of the diverse tissues, $G(t)$ can be calculated explicitly, under the assumption that equilibration between blood and tissue occurs within the transit time through the tissue [1]. Depending on the number of tissues and other volumes of distribution to be considered, $G(t)$ might depend on too many exponential terms

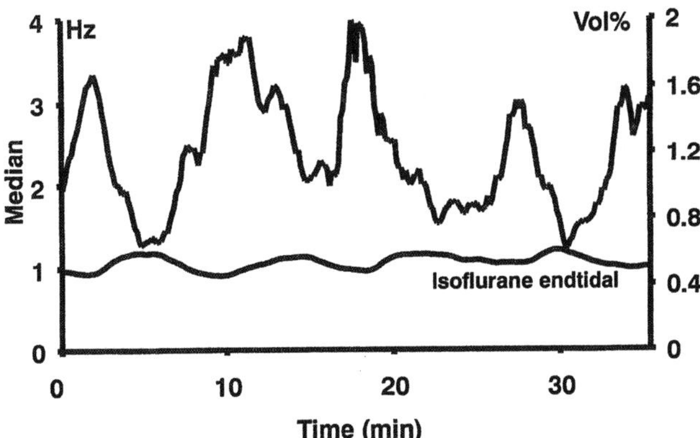

Fig. 2. Concentration response and hysteresis

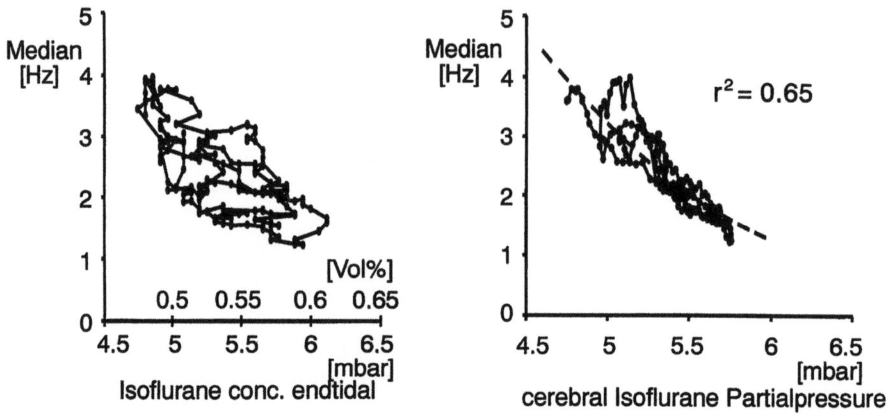

Fig. 3. Determination of hysteresis and half-maximum effect

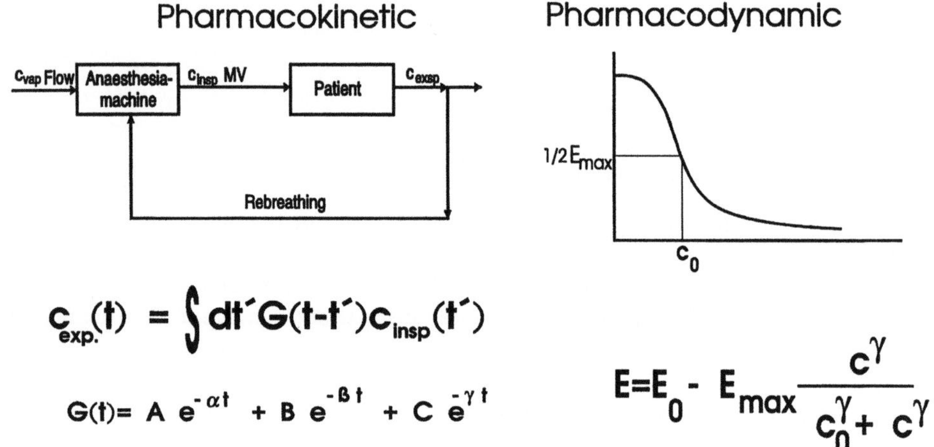

$$c_{exp.}(t) = \int dt'\, G(t-t')\, c_{insp}(t')$$

$$G(t) = A\, e^{-\alpha t} + B\, e^{-\beta t} + C\, e^{-\gamma t}$$

$$E = E_0 - E_{max}\frac{c^\gamma}{c_0^\gamma + c^\gamma}$$

Fig. 4. Pharmacokinetic-pharmacodynamic model used for feedback control

to be easily suited for numerical analysis. The other approach is to fit the function G(t) to measured inspired and expired concentration. This approach will lead, in general, to no more than three to four exponential terms [2]. The last step in developing the entire pharmacokinetic-pharmacodynamic model is to establish the relationship between end-tidal concentrations and the effect via biophase concentrations. To do so, we measured simultaneously end-tidal concentrations and median EEG frequency (Fig. 2). Plotting median EEG frequency against isoflurane concentrations results in hysteresis loops (Fig. 3, left); minimization of the hysteresis loop (Fig. 3, right) yields the desired half-life of distribution to the biophase. For isoflurane we found a typical half-life between 90 and 120 s. Figure 4 depicts the pharmacokinetic-pharmacodynamic model used for the feedback control.

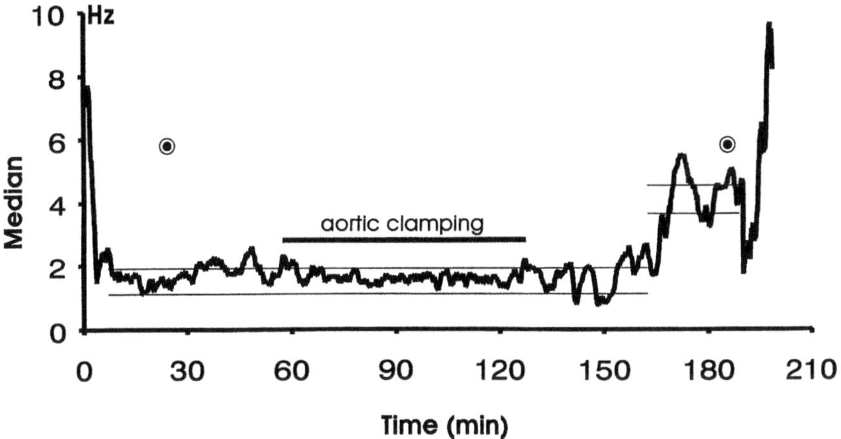

Fig. 5. Closed-loop feedback control of isoflurance delivered during surgery for infrarenal aortic aneurysm in a 68-year-old man

Specifically, the feedback system works as follows [3]: The EEG is recorded via a Siemens EEG monitor. One lead is segmented into epochs of 8.2 s length and digitized at a rate of 125 Hz. The power spectrum is calculated between 0.5 and 30 Hz, and median EEG frequency is determined. Initial vaporizer setting is based on the model and the set point. If, subsequently, median EEG frequency differs from the set point, the model is adapted and a new vaporizer setting is calculated. The vaporizer may be set automatically by a specially designed piece of hardware which moves the hand screw of the vaporizer, or it may be set manually, according to the advice of the feedback program.

Figure 5 depicts an example of the time course of median EEG frequency during a surgical procedure (infrarenal aortic aneurysm) while delivering the volatile agent by the feedback system. The relatively stable time course of median EEG frequency has to be opposed to rapidly changing inspired and expired concentration of the volatile agent, which is depicted in Fig. 6. Especially around the phase of aortic clamping, one recognizes these large varying concentrations, which are damped to a rather constant concentration in the period following. Most likely, the oscillating behavior reflects the instable hemodynamic situation which is accompanied and induced by the aortic clamping.

The Feedback System as a Research Tool

It has been shown that the interaction between nitrous oxide and volatile agents such as halothane, enflurane, or isoflurane is additive, in the sense that the combination of two MAC fractions of nitrous oxide and the volatile agent leading to 1.0 MAC also suppresses movement in response to skin incision in 50% of patients [4–6]. The additivity of MAC supports the "unitary theory of narcosis," which

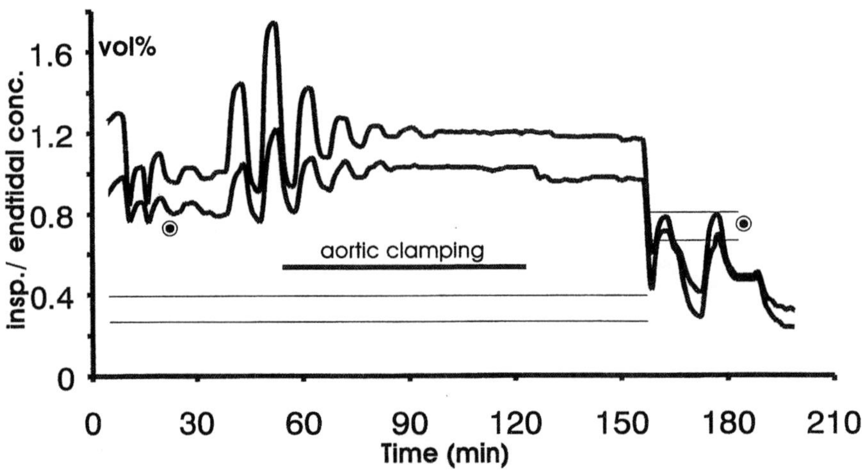

Fig. 6. Same situation as in Fig. 5; rapid change in inspired and expired concentration of isoflurane

asserts that all anesthetics act in the same way. This theory requires an identity of action at the molecular level [7].

Recent studies by Cole et al. [8, 9] are claimed to have shown a nonlinear contribution to the interaction of nitrous oxide with halothane, enflurane, and isoflurane in rats. Chortkoff et al. examined the ED_{50} for suppression of learning and the ability to respond appropriately to verbal command (MAC-awake) using a combination of isoflurane and 40% nitrous oxide. The MAC-awake and the ED_{50} for suppression of learning were higher than their values predicted by additivity [10]. A study by Yli-Hankala et al. showed that the addition of nitrous oxide to isoflurane decreases the frequency and duration of isoflurane-induced burst suppressions in the EEG, indicating a nonadditive interaction [11].

The type and degree of interaction between two anesthetics depend also on the clinical end point used. Deady et al. [12] demonstrated that the ratio of anesthetic concentration to maintain upright position in response to tail-clamp stimulus and the ratio of anesthetic concentration to maintain upright position in response to heat applied to the tail differs for the anesthetics nitrous oxide, isoflurane, enflurane, and halothane in mice. Their findings do not support a unitary mechanism of anesthetic action. Instead, righting reflex and response to tail-clamp test or heat test seem to be depressed by different mechanisms.

The aim of our study was to investigate the potency of nitrous oxide to substitute isoflurane at a median EEG frequency between 2 and 3 Hz during surgery.

Methods

After the study protocol had been approved by the local Ethics Committee, written informed consent was obtained from 25 female patients, ASA I or II, aged 39 ± 8 years, scheduled for gynecological laparotomies. We did not include patients with apparent neurological deficit, hypo- or hyperthyroidism, or pregnancy, or patients who had received drugs affecting central neurotransmitter release. Patients were premedicated with oral midazolam 7.5 mg 2 h prior to surgery. Anesthesia was induced with 0.5 mg alfentanil and 3 mg/kg thiopental. Vecuronium was administered for neuromuscular block, and no anticholinergic agent was used. Once the trachea had been intubated, anesthesia was maintained with isoflurane and nitrous oxide. In addition to nitrous oxide, patients were ventilated with O_2 and air. End-tidal pCO_2 was monitored and kept constant at 35 mmHg. Blood pressure and heart frequency were measured noninvasively with a Dinamap Vital Daten Monitor (Criticon INC., Tampa, FL) at intervals of 3 min. Esophageal temperature was registered.

One EEG lead in the F_3 and P_3 position (international 10–20 system) (Sirecust 404, Siemens, Germany) was used for online signal analysis. The raw signal was filtered between 0.5 and 32 Hz and divided into epochs of 8.192 s duration, which were digitized at a rate of 125 Hz. The median EEG frequency (50% quantile of the power spectrum) and the percentage of activity in the frequency bands 0.5–2, 2–5, 5–8, 8–13, and 13–32 Hz were calculated. A moving average over seven epochs was used for data smoothing. Isoflurane vaporizer settings were chosen so that the median EEG frequency was held between 2 and 3 Hz. End-tidal isoflurane concentrations were measured by a Normac anesthetic gas analyzer (Datex, Kopenhagen, Denmark). For each patient, the analyzer was calibrated without any anesthetic and with a standard concentration of volatile anesthetic. Nitrous oxide was administered in randomized concentrations of 0, 20, 40, 60, and 75 vol%; each concentration was given to ten patients. After induction of anesthesia, a 60-min waiting period allowed the effects of thiopental and alfentanil to disappear. Required isoflurane concentration was defined as the mean end-tidal isoflurane concentration over a period of 15 min. These periods were allocated during surgical stimulation between opening and closure of the peritoneum. A period of 30 min for equilibration of nitrous oxide and isoflurane was allowed after each nitrous oxide change and prior to the next measurement period.

The hypothesis of additivity between the two anesthetic agents was tested with the method of isoboles. For each chosen concentration of nitrous oxide we measured the concentration of isoflurane necessary to maintain the median EEG frequency between 2 and 3 Hz. Additivity is present if all pairs of concentrations of both agents ($C_{isoflurane}$, $C_{nitrous\ oxide}$) which lead to the same effect obey the equation

$$\alpha \times C_{isoflurane} + \beta \times C_{nitrous\ oxide} = 1 \text{ with suitable coefficients}$$
$$\alpha > 0 \text{ and } \beta > 0. \tag{6}$$

Thus additive interaction is present if data points lie on a straight line. Deviations from linearity indicate a nonadditive interaction.

Differences in age, temperature, and median EEG frequency in the different nitrous oxide concentration groups were tested with analysis of variance. We used a regression analysis to quantify the nature and strength of the relationship between chosen nitrous oxide concentrations and end-tidal isoflurane concentrations necessary to keep median EEG frequency between 2 and 3 Hz, and the relationship between blood pressure, heart rate, and nitrous oxide concentrations. Statistical significance was assumed at probability levels ≤ 0.05.

Results

Age, temperature, and median EEG frequency did not differ between the various nitrous oxide concentration groups (Table 1). Figure 7 depicts the isobole of required end-tidal isoflurane concentrations to keep the median EEG frequency between 2 and 3 Hz versus the chosen nitrous oxide concentrations. Regression analysis was performed by fitting linear and quadratic models relating isoflurane concentrations to independently chosen nitrous oxide concentrations. Lowest

Table 1. Age, temperature, median EEG frequency, required end-tidal isoflurane concentrations, and total anesthetic requirement at different nitrous oxide concentrations

Nitrous oxide (vol%)	Age (years)	Temp. (°C)	Median EEG frequency (Hz)	Required end-tidal isoflurane (vol%)	Total anesthetic requirement (MAC)
0	38.4 ± 8.0	35.7 ± 0.6	2.51 ± 0.12	1.06 ± 0.24	0.92 ± 0.21
20	40.9 ± 9.3	35.7 ± 0.6	2.47 ± 0.08	1.04 ± 0.25	1.09 ± 0.22
40	37.3 ± 6.4	35.9 ± 0.5	2.45 ± 0.06	0.87 ± 0.27	1.14 ± 0.23
60	38.0 ± 9.4	35.6 ± 0.7	2.48 ± 0.10	0.77 ± 0.15	1.24 ± 0.13
75	38.7 ± 9.7	35.7 ± 0.5	2.46 ± 0.07	0.79 ± 0.23	1.41 ± 0.20

Data are mean ± SD.

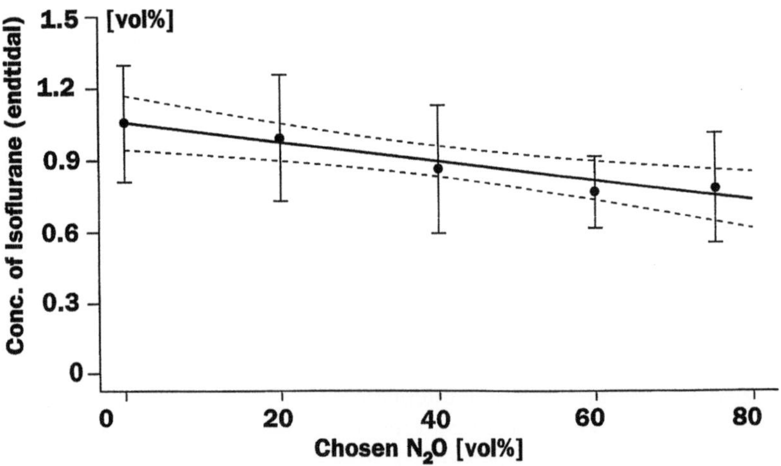

Fig. 7. End-tidal concentrations of isoflurane required to maintain median EEG frequency between 2 and 3 Hz, dependent on nitrous oxide concentrations

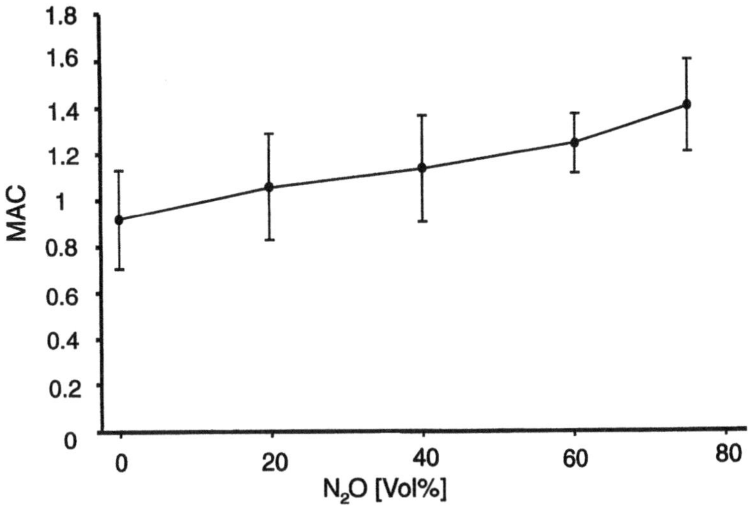

Fig. 8. Total minimum alveolar concentrations (*MAC*) of isoflurane and nitrous oxide required to maintain median EEG frequency at 2–3 Hz

standard error of estimation was found for a linear model. The line of regression was calculated as:

$$C_{\text{isoflurane}} = 1.05 \text{ vol\%} - 0.0041 \times C_{\text{nitrous oxide}} \tag{7}$$

The probability level for dependence of the required isoflurane concentration on nitrous oxide concentration (slope $\neq 0$) is 0.015. The correlation coefficient is -0.93, R-squared is 89.6%, and standard error of estimation is 0.05.

If the total anesthetic requirement is expressed as the sum of isoflurane and nitrous oxide MAC fractions (assuming 1.0 MAC of isoflurane to be 1.15 vol.% and 1.0 MAC of nitrous oxide to be 1.04 atm absolute), there is a significant increase in the total anesthetic MAC multiples with increasing nitrous oxide concentrations (Fig. 8).

Table 2. Hemodynamic parameters and EEG frequency bands for different nitrous oxide concentrations

Nitrous oxide (vol%)	BP$_{sys}$ (mmHg)	BP$_{dia}$ (mmHg)	HR (min⁻¹)	delta 1 0.5–2 Hz (%)	delta 2 2–5 Hz (%)	theta 5–8 Hz (%)	alpha 8–13 Hz (%)	beta 13–32 Hz (%)
0	112 ± 4	66 ± 8	80 ± 15	47.1 ± 2.1	14.8 ± 2.7	13.7 ± 3.6	8.6 ± 4.7	1.9 ± 0.7
20	113 ± 14	69 ± 13	80 ± 11	46.9 ± 2.7	15.6 ± 3.4	13.0 ± 2.5	7.9 ± 4.3	2.2 ± 0.9
40	112 ± 15	73 ± 15	72 ± 8	46.8 ± 3.9	15.1 ± 4.2	12.0 ± 3.7	9.4 ± 4.7	3.0 ± 1.7
60	112 ± 11	69 ± 11	77 ± 12	46.4 ± 3.1	16.8 ± 3.4	11.4 ± 3.8	6.8 ± 3.1	3.2 ± 1.0
75	114 ± 15	71 ± 13	76 ± 15	46.6 ± 2.5	18.3 ± 3.7	10.8 ± 5.0	4.8 ± 2.1	3.1 ± 1.6

Data are mean ± SD.
BP$_{sys}$, Systolic blood pressure; *BP$_{dia}$*, diastolic blood pressure; *HR*, heart rate.

No significant difference in systolic blood pressure, diastolic blood pressure, heart rate, or the percentage of activity in the EEG frequency bands between the various nitrous oxide concentration groups was observed (Table 2).

Discussion

This study shows that in a dose range of 0–75 vol% nitrous oxide decreases linearly the isoflurane requirement to maintain median EEG frequency between 2 and 3 Hz during surgery. This is compatible with an additive type of interaction between nitrous oxide and isoflurane on median EEG frequency.

Cole et al. reported deviations from linearity of the interaction between nitrous oxide and halothane, enflurane, or isoflurane on MAC in rats [8, 9]. The observed deviations, however, were judged as rather small, so that Eger continued to consider this interaction to be additive [13]. Additivity was also verified for the interaction of nitrous oxide and isoflurane on MAC in children [14].

The potency of nitrous oxide to decrease the concentration of isoflurane necessary to keep median EEG frequency between 2 and 3 Hz is lower than the potency of nitrous oxide to decrease the concentration of isoflurane necessary to suppress movement in response to skin incision in 50% of patients (MAC). Using Eq. (7), we can estimate that every 10% addition of nitrous oxide decreases the isoflurane requirement as defined by the EEG criterion by approximately 0.04 vol%, while, in terms of MAC, each 10% addition of nitrous oxide decreases the isoflurane requirement by approximately 0.11 vol% (assuming additive interaction and MAC isoflurane, 1.15 vol% [6], and MAC nitrous oxide, 1.04 atm absolute [15]).

Other recent studies can be used to estimate the interaction of isoflurane and nitrous oxide when the level of clinical judgement or memory functions are considered (Fig. 8). Eger et al. compared isoflurane anesthesia with and without 60% nitrous oxide for several kinds of surgical procedures [16]. Without nitrous oxide, an average end-tidal concentration of 0.85 vol% isoflurane was determined to be necessary by the attending anesthesiologist, while 60% nitrous oxide allowed a reduction of isoflurane to 0.64 vol%. Assuming a linear relationship, every 10% of nitrous oxide reduces the isoflurane requirement by 0.035 vol%. Eger et al. found lower levels of isoflurane than in our study. This could be explained by the co-administration of 0.23 mg fentanyl, which was not used in our study. In another study, Dwyer et al. determined the dose of isoflurane and nitrous oxide that suppressed memory by 50% (ED_{50}) [17]. The ED_{50} was 0.2 MAC for isoflurane and 0.5 MAC for nitrous oxide. Assuming linear dependence, every 10% of nitrous oxide decreases the isoflurane requirement by 0.045 vol%.

The differences in the potency of nitrous oxide to substitute isoflurane confirm the results of previous studies: the relative potencies of inhaled anesthetic agents depend upon the end point measured [12, 18, 19]. These studies do not support the hypothesis that both anesthetics act in the same way. One possible explanation is that these anesthetics act at different anatomic sides. On the one hand, the EEG is known to represent the electrical activity of cortical structures.

On the other hand, more recent studies suggest that MAC is a test of anesthetic potency that evaluates depression of a spinal reflex. Rampil et al. demonstrated that, with regard to MAC, the anesthetic potency of isoflurane is independent of forebrain structures of the rat [20]. They concluded that surgical unresponsiveness appears to be supported, and may be determined, by subcortical structures. In a further study, Rampil demonstrated that acute spinal transection at T_1 in rats does not change MAC [21]. Antigonini and Schwartz measured MAC in goats and found a large increase in isoflurane requirement (from 1.2 vol% up to 2.9 vol%) when the brain was preferentially anesthetized [22]. They concluded that subcortical structures modulate movement in response to painful stimuli during general anesthesia.

Quantitative EEG measurement during anesthesia with isoflurane and nitrous oxide at 1.3 and 1.5 MAC showed dose-related dependence [23], but comparison of EEG and movement response to noxious stimulation showed no correlation [24]. One conclusion might be that EEG effects and movement response to noxious stimulation are to be regarded as components of anesthesia which results from separate pharmacological actions.

The degree of interaction between nitrous oxide and isoflurane, as measured by the slope of the isoboles in the study of Eger et al. [16] and in our study, was approximately equal. This leads to the conclusion that the EEG median frequency reflects better what an attending anesthesiologist considers clinically appropriate anesthesia than does the addition of MAC fractions of both agents.

In spite of its analgesic properties [25], nitrous oxide is known to have only weak anesthetic potency. Due to its high MAC value, it cannot be used effectively as a sole anesthetic at normal atmospheric pressure. This study of its interaction with isoflurane on the EEG indicates that the potency of nitrous oxide to substitute isoflurane is much lower than might be expected from its MAC value. If 60% nitrous oxide reduces the required isoflurane concentration by only 0.25 vol%, it may be questioned whether nitrous oxide is at all an essential anesthetic component of inhalation anesthesia.

In conclusion, this paper has shown an additive interaction of isoflurane and nitrous oxide on median EEG frequency. The degree of interaction for this end point is weaker than that on the MAC basis, but it seems to reflect more appropriately the clinical handling of both drugs.

References

1. Zuntz N (1897) Zur Pathogenese und Therapie der durch rasche Luftdruckänderungen erzeugten Krankheiten. Fortschr Med 15:632
2. Schwilden H, Stoeckel H, Schüttler J, Lauven PM (1982) Pharmacokinetic data of fentanyl, midazolam and enflurane as obtained by a new method for arbitrary schemes of administration. In: Prys-Roberts C, Vickers MD (eds) Cardiovascular measurement in anaesthesiology. Springer, Berlin Heidelberg New York, pp 22–29
3. Stoeckel H, Schwilden H (1986) Methoden der automatischen Feedback-Regelung für die Narkose. Konzepte und klinische Anwendung. Anaesth Intensivther Notfallmed 21:60–67

4. Saidman LJ, Eger EI (1964) Effect of nitrous oxide and of narcotic premedication on the alveolar concentration of halothane required for anesthesia. Anesthesiology 25:302–306

5. Torri G, Damia G, Fabiani ML (1974) Effect of nitrous oxide on the anesthetic requirement of enflurane. Br J Anaesth 46:468–472

6. Stevens WC, Dolan WM, Gibbons RT, White A, Eger EI, Miller RD, De Jong RH, Elashoff RM (1975) Minimum alveolar concentrations (MAC) of isoflurane with and without nitrous oxide in patients of various ages. Anesthesiology 42:197–200

7. DiFazio CA, Brown RE, Ball CG, Heckel CG, Kennedy SS (1972) Additive effects of anesthetics and theories of anesthesia. Anesthesiology 36:57–63

8. Cole DJ, Kalichman MW, Shapiro HM (1989) The nonlinear contribution of nitrous oxide at sub-MAC concentrations to enflurane MAC in rats. Anesth Analg 68:556–562

9. Cole DJ, Kalichman MW, Shapiro HM, Drummond JC (1990) The nonlinear potency of sub-MAC concentrations of nitrous oxide in decreasing the anesthetic requirement of enflurane, halothane, and isoflurane in rats. Anesthesiology 73:93–99

10. Chortkoff BS, Bennet HL, Eger EI (1993) Does nitrous oxide antagonize isoflurane-induced suppression of learning? Anesthesiology 79:724–732

11. Yli-Hankala A, Lindgren L, Porkkala T, Jäntti V (1993) Nitrous oxide-mediated activation of the EEG during isoflurane anaesthesia in patients. Br J Anaesth 70:54–57

12. Deady JE, Koblin DD, Eger EI, Heavner JE, D'Aoust B (1981) Anesthetic potencies and the unitary theory of narcosis. Anesth Analg 60:380–384

13. Eger EI (1989) Does 1 + 1 = 2? (Editorial) Anesth Analg 68:551–552

14. Murray DJ, Metha WP, Forbes RB (1991) The additive contribution of nitrous oxide to isoflurane MAC in infants and children. Anesthesiology 75:186–190

15. Hornbein TF, Eger EI, Winter PM, Smith G, Wetstone D, Smith KH (1982) The minimum alveolar concentration of nitrous oxide in man. Anesth Analg 61:553–556

16. Eger EI, Lampe GH, Wauk LZ, Whitendale P, Cahalan MK (1990) Clinical pharmacology of nitrous oxide: an argument for its continued use. Anesth Analg 71:575–585

17. Dwyer R, Bennett HL, Eger EI, Heilbron D (1992) Effects of isoflurane and nitrous oxide in subanesthetic concentrations on memory and responsiveness in volunteers. Anesthesiology 77:888–898

18. Shim CY, Andersen NB (1992) Minimal alveolar concentration (MAC) and dose-response curves in anesthesia. Anesthesiology 36:146–151

19. Kissin I (1993) General anesthetic action: an obsolete notion? Anesth Analg 76:215–218

20. Rampil IJ, Mason P, Singh H (1993) Anesthetic potency (MAC) is independent of forebrain structures in the rat. Anesthesiology 78:707–712

21. Rampil IJ (1993) Is MAC testing a spinal reflex? Anesthesiology 79:A422 (abstract)

22. Antigonini JF, Schwartz K (1993) Exaggerated anesthetic requirements in the preferentially anesthetized brain. Anesthesiology 79:1244–1249

23. Schwilden H, Stoeckel H (1987) Quantitative EEG analysis during anaesthesia with isoflurane in nitrous oxide at 1.3 and 1.5 MAC. Br J Anaesth 59:738–745

24. Rampil IJ, Laster MJ (1992) No correlation between quantitative electroencephalographic measurement and movement response to noxious stimuli during isoflurane anesthesia in rats. Anesthesiology 77:920–925

25. Komatsu T, Shingu K, Tomemori M, Urabe N, Mori K (1981) Nitrous oxide activates the supraspinal pain inhibition system. Acta Anaesth Scand 25:519–522

IV Control and Automation of Drug Delivery

b) Intravenous Anesthetics

The Target of Control: Plasma Concentrations or Drug Effect

P.S.A. GLASS

Introduction

The objective of any drug-administration scheme is to obtain a desired effect. The therapeutic process consists of administering a drug to the patient to provide the desired effect. As a result of the disposition of the drug within the patient, the administered dose will result in a plasma concentration of the drug. This concentration will then determine the effect of the drug (Fig. 1). This drug effect is observed or monitored by the physician, and the drug dosage is then adjusted to achieve the desired therapeutic goal.

Automated Closed-Loop Drug Delivery

The above is a brief description of a manual, physician-based, closed-loop system. From this, it is obvious that the target of control is always the effect. Such a manual, physician, closed-loop system, although obtaining the desired effect, will continuously oscillate around this effect, unless (a) drug disposition is accounted for in the dosing scheme and (b) the effect can be precisely monitored so as to continuously adjust drug dose to clinical effect. Recent developments in pharmacokinetics and technology have enabled the development of automated drug-delivery systems; these enable the physician to target either a desired drug concentration or, where there is a measurable feedback system, a desired effect.

These automated systems are described in the chapter on drug-delivery systems. Automated closed-loop drug delivery is able to precisely obtain and maintain the targeted effect. Such systems, however, are dependent on a monitor that can qualitatively and quantitatively measure the effect that is under control. Thus, automated closed-loop drug delivery is readily available for the control of, e.g., blood pressure or neuromuscular blockade.

For drugs used to provide the anesthetic state, a precise measure of depth of anesthesia is not yet available. The EEG and its derivatives, auditory evoked potentials and hemodynamics, have been proposed as measures of anesthetic depth [1–5]. Unfortunately, none of these measures have been proven to provide quantitative measures of anesthetic depth, nor are they robust across all anesthetic drugs and techniques [5]. In addition, it appears that motor responses to stimulation during anesthesia are controlled at a subcortical level, thus implying that

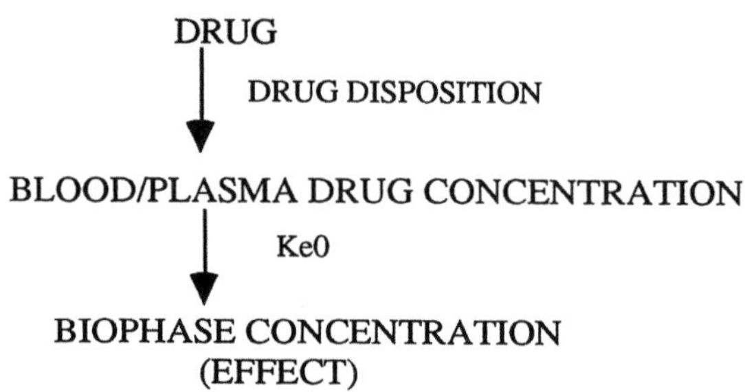

Fig. 1. The pharmacokinetic process that determines the effect of drug dose

cortical measures may be inappropriate as measures of anesthetic depth [6]. Even though the above arguments would imply that the measures mentioned could not be used to control the depth of anesthesia, both auditory evoked potentials and median EEG frequency [4, 7] have been used successfully in automated closed-loop delivery systems to provide anesthesia to a limited number of patients undergoing surgery. However, it cannot be assumed, based on our present knowledge of the EEG and auditory evoked potentials, that such systems can stand up to the rigors of clinical practice.

Target Concentration Drug Delivery

If we are unable to measure the desired effect with a quantitative monitor, our next best choice is to target drug concentration, as it is assumed that blood-drug concentration is related to the resultant effect. By utilizing pharmacokinetic parameters, it is possible to design dosing regimens to provide target plasma/blood concentrations [8]. Manual infusion schemes using the classic approach of Wagner [9] have been described for many of the intravenous anesthetics [8]. As described in the chapter on drug-delivery systems, pharmacokinetic model-driven infusion systems are capable of administering drug to a target plasma concentration and adjusting this target plasma concentration as required.

Such systems that target the plasma concentration have proven to be effective in providing anesthesia [9]. The plasma, however, is not the site of drug effect. The site of drug effect is termed the biophase and, for anesthetics, resides within the central nervous system. It is well known that when a drug is administered intravenously, although its plasma drug concentration will peak almost instantaneously, the peak drug effect will be somewhat delayed. This delay is due the transfer of drug from plasma into the biophase. The biophase can be thought of as simply another compartment with which the plasma equilibrates. It is the concentration in this biophase compartment that truly determines the effect of the drug. In human beings it is obviously impossible to measure the concentration within the biophase, but it is possible to determine the rate of equilibration between the plasma concentration and drug effect. This is achieved by administering a dose of the drug and then measuring both plasma drug concentration and

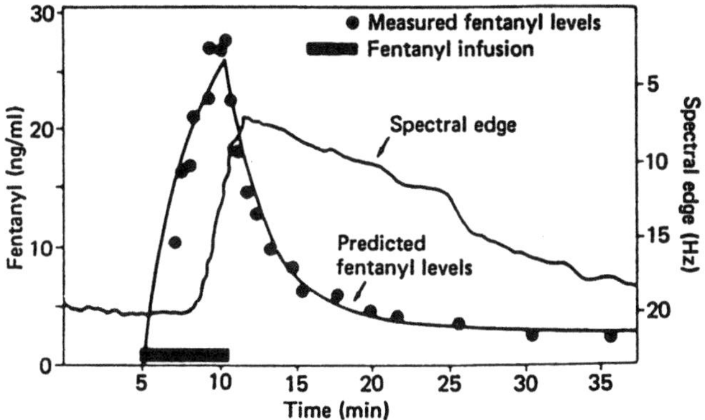

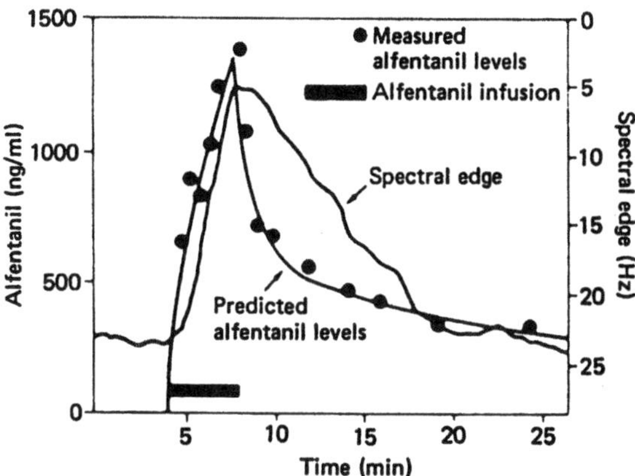

Fig. 2. Simultaneous measurement of drug concentration (alfentanil and fentanyl) and the bispectral edge of the EEG (a measure of drug effect). Note the differences in the relationship between onset and offset of drug concentration to drug effect between fentanyl and alfentanil. This demonstrates their differences in the equilibration between plasma and their biophase. (From [2] with permission)

drug effect [2] (Fig. 2). It will be observed (Fig. 3) that if drug concentration is then plotted against drug effect, a hysteresis loop results. This hysteresis loop occurs as a result of the equilibration time between the plasma and the biophase. The intercompartmental rate constant that determines the rate of equilibration between the plasma and the apparent effect compartment concentration is that value that causes the hysteresis loop to collapse so that the plasma concentration relates linearly to drug effect [10]. This rate constant is termed the ke0. The larger the ke0, the more rapid the rate of equilibration between the plasma and the biophase. Utilizing the ke0 value, it is possible to program automated drug-delivery systems to target an effect compartment concentration rather than a plasma drug concentration [11, 12]. The $T1/2$ ke0 (0.693/ke0) represents the half-life for equilibration between the plasma drug concentration and the biophase.

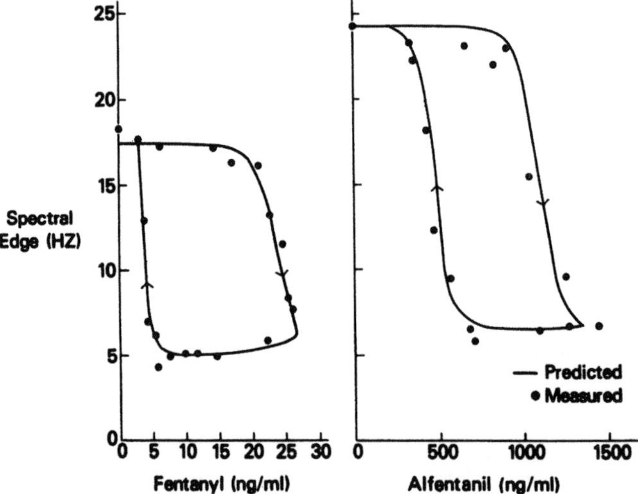

Fig. 3. The hysteresis loop that results from a plot of the plasma concentration and the measured effect (bispectral edge of the EEG) following a rapid infusion of alfentanil or fentanyl. (From [2] with permission)

Table 1. Time to peak effect, and $t_{1/2}$ keo

Drug	Time to peak effect (min)	$T_{1/2}$ keo (min)
Fentanyl	3.6	4.7
Alfentanil	1.4	0.9
Sufentanil	5.6	3
Propofol	2.2	2.4
Thiopental	1.7	1.5
Midazolam	2.8	4
Etomidate	2	1.5

Table 1 lists the $T1/2$ ke0 and time to peak effect of most of the commonly used intravenous anesthetics.

Drugs with a small ke0 value (i.e., a long equilibration time) will have marked differences between the target drug plasma concentration and the resultant biophase concentration (and therefore effect), as these are titrated during the course of an anesthetic. For drugs with a large ke0 value, drug equilibrates rapidly with the biophase, and there are only small differences between the target plasma concentration and the resultant biophase concentration. Thus, the advantage of targeting the effect site of drug concentration rather than the plasma drug concentration becomes more obvious with drugs that have slow equilibration times.

An appreciation of ke0 value is important for even simple dosing strategies if one wishes to achieve a desired effect rapidly. First, when utilizing a manual

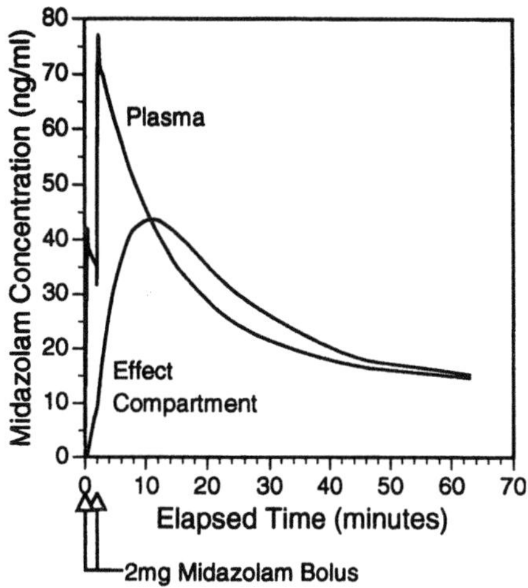

Fig. 4. The simulated plasma concentration and biophase concentration following two 1-mg doses of midazolam spaced only 1 min apart. Note how the biophase concentration continues to rise, so that the peak effect of the first dose is not observed prior to the administration of the second dose

infusion scheme to obtain the desired effect with the initial loading dose, it is best to determine the loading dose on the volume of distribution that incorporates the biophase and not on the initial volume of distribution, as described by most classic texts [13]. For example, when aiming to provide a plasma concentration of 1 ng/ml with fentanyl, simply giving the loading dose based on the initial volume of distribution (e.g., 1 μg/kg followed by 1 μg/kg/h) would result in an effect of 1 ng/ml only at 20 min. If the loading dose is calculated by utilizing the volume of distribution incorporating the biophase, e.g., 3 μg/kg, although the measured plasma concentration will far exceed the desired 1 ng/ml, the actual effect concentration of 1 ng/ml will be achieved almost immediately.

Second, the ke0 also determines the time to peak drug effect following a bolus dose. It is important to be aware of when the peak effect occurs, so that intermittent doses are appropriately spaced. A typical example of this is in the titration of diazepam and midazolam. The time to peak drug effect for diazepam is more rapid than that of midazolam. Thus, the peak effect observed for midazolam occurs later than that for diazepam. Clinicians who were familiar with diazepam when they first changed to midazolam tended to space the midazolam doses based on their previous experience with diazepam. Thus, it was possible for an overdose to be administered, as the second dose of midazolam was given prior to its peak effect being observed (Fig. 4). Finally, the ke0 value will determine the optimal infusion rate of the initial loading dose to prevent an overshoot in the biophase concentration. For drugs with a narrow therapeutic margin, overshoot in the effect compartment results in undesirable side effects. A typical example of this is propofol, which, if given at the optimal infusion rate, will result in a lower total dose of drug being given and fewer hemodynamic perturbations [14].

The ke0 values have thus far been determined using the EEG as a continuous measure of effect. As stated above, the EEG may not necessarily reflect for all drugs a measure of anesthesia. It is also impossible to actually measure (at least in human beings) the concentration of drug in the biophase. Thus, although the concept of using of the ke0 to provide an appropriate effect compartment concentration is correct, it is important that we test these values to ensure that they truly reflect the equilibration rate between plasma concentration and actual observed anesthetic effect. Recently, several studies have supported the published values for the ke0 of both thiopental and propofol. In the first study, Avram et al. [15] investigated the relationship between the variability in the dose of thiopental required for loss of consciousness and population pnarmacokinetics. In an editorial that accompanied their paper, Jacobs and Reves [16] were able to demonstrate that if the Ke0 value for thiopental was incorporated into the model, the dose determined to provide loss of consciousness in 50% of patients resulted in a thiopental effect compartment concentration that was consistent with the previously demonstrated concentration, which resulted in loss of consciousness in 50% of patients. Thus, the incorporation of the ke0 value into the model exactly described the expected relationship between dose and loss of consciousness. A second study by the same group investigated the relationship between infusion rate and dose for loss of consciousness [17]. As discussed above, because of equilibration with the effect compartment, the dose for loss of consciousness would be expected to vary according to the infusion rate administered. When previously published ke0 values were incorporated into a simulation model, the dose predicted to achieve loss of consciousness for each infusion rate was exactly equal to the dose that was required for their patients to achieve loss of consciousness, thus confirming that the ke0 value used in the model was correct. In an unreported study by our group, we divided patients into two groups. One group was administered propofol using CACI (our automated drug-delivery device) to target an *effect* compartment concentration of 5.4 μg/ml. This is the plasma concentration that will result in hypnosis in 95% of patients [18]. The other group was administered propofol to a target *plasma* concentration of 5.4 μg/ml. The ke0 value that was used in CACI was taken from the literature [19]. The time to loss of consciousness was then observed. It was significantly longer in the patients in whom propofol was administered to a target plasma concentration. In addition, in both groups loss of consciousness occurred when the effect compartment concentration reached 5.4 μg/ml. Thus, it would appear that even though the ke0 value is based on the EEG, it does represent the rate of equilibration of drug between the plasma and the biophase.

Conclusion

It is clearly optimal to target the measured effect via an automated closed-loop delivery system. Where there is no monitor of the desired effect available, it is possible to administer drug to a target effect compartment concentration rather than to the plasma concentration. It must be remembered that the anesthetic state is dependent not only on the concentration of drug within the biophase, but also on the patient's individual response to that drug concentration, as well as on the intensity of the surgical stimulus. In addition, like any other pharmacokinetic parameter, the value of ke0 varies from patient to patient. Thus, although present studies confirm the accuracy of the ke0 value, this simply represents the average for the population. In addition, an adequate anesthetic state can rarely be provided by a single drug, and the interaction between anesthetics in providing anesthesia is complex [20]. The net result is that it is incorrect to target an effect compartment concentration and assume that the desired effect will be obtained. More importantly, when one is targeting a plasma or effect concentration, a delivery system that is able to titrate the target drug concentration is needed so that the desired effect of adequate anesthesia is always obtained.

References

1. Schwilden H, Stoeckel H, Schuttler J (1989) Closed-loop feedback control of propofol anaesthesia by quantitative EEG analysis in humans. Br J Anaesth 62:290–296
2. Scott JC, Ponganis KV, Stanski DR (1985) Quantitation of narcotic effect: the comparative pharmacodynamics of fentanyl and alfentanil. Anesthesiology 62:234–241
3. Vernon J, Bowles S, Sebel PS, Chamoun MS (1992) EEG bispectrum predicts movement on skin incision during isoflurane or propofol anesthesia. Anesthesiology 77:A502
4. Kenny GNC, Davies FW, Mantzardis H, Fisher AC (1992) Closed-loop control of anesthesia. Anesthesiology 77:A328
5. Stanski DR (1994) Monitoring depth of anesthesia. Intravenous drug delivery systems. In: Miller RD (ed) Anesthesia, 4th edn. Churchill Livingstone, New York, pp 1127–1160
6. Rampil IJ, Mason P, Singh H (1993) Anesthetic potency (MAC) is independent of forebrain structures in the rat. Anesthesiology 78:707–712
7. Schwilden H, Stoeckel H (1990) Effective therapeutic infusions produced by closed-loop feedback control of methohexital administration during total intravenous anesthesia with fentanyl. Anesthesiology 73:225–229
8. Glass PSA, Shafer SL, Jacobs JR, Reves JG (1994) Intravenous drug delivery systems. In: Miller RD (ed) Anesthesia, 4th edn. Churchill Livingstone, New York, pp 389–416
9. Wagner JG (1974) A safe method for rapidly achieving plasma concentration plateaus. Clin Pharmacol Ther 16:691–700
10. Sheiner LB, Stanski DR, Vozeh S et al (1979) Simultaneous modelling of pharmacokinetics and pharmacodynamics; application to d-tubocurarine. Clin Pharmacol Ther 25:358–371
11. Shafer SL, Gregg K (1992) Algorithms to rapidly achieve and maintain stable drug concentrations at the site of drug effect with a computer-controlled infusion pump. J Pharmacokinet Biopharm 20:147–169
12. Jacobs JR, Williams EA (1993) Algorithm to control "effect compartment" drug concentrations in pharmacokinetic model-driven drug delivery. IEEE Trans Biomed Eng 40:993–999
13. Shafer SL, Varvel JR (1991) Pharmacokinetics, pharmacodynamics, and rational opioid selection. Anesthesiology 74:53–63
14. Peacock JE, Lewis RP, Reilly CS, Nimmo WS (1990) Effects of different rates of infusion for induction of anaesthesia in elderly patients. Br J Anaesth 65:346–352
15. Avram MJ, Sanghvi R, Henthorn TK, Krejcie TC, Shanks CA, Fragen RJ, Howard KA (1993) Determinants of thiopentone induction dose requirements. Anesth Analg 76:10–17
16. Jacobs JR, Reves JG (1993) Effect site equilibration time is a determinant of induction dose requirement. Anesth Analg 76:1–6

17. Gentry WB, Krejcie TC, Henthorn TK, Shanks CA, Howard KA, Gupta DK, Avram MJ (1994) Effect of infusion rate on thiopental dose-response relationships: assessment of a pharmacokinetic-pharmacodynamic model. Anesthesiology 81:361–324
18. Smith C, McEwan AI, Jhaveri R et al (1994) Reduction of propofol Cp50 by fentanyl. Anesthesiology (in press)
19. Dyck JB, Varvel J, Hung O, Shafer SL (1991) The pharmacokinetics of propofol versus age. Can J Anaesth 38:A129
20. McEwan AI, Smith C, Dyar O, Goodman D, Glass PSA (1993) Isoflurane MAC reduction by fentanyl. Anesthesiology 78:864–869

Open-Loop Control Systems and Their Performance for Intravenous Anaesthetics

J.W. Sear

Introduction

Anaesthetists often provide anaesthesia by continuous infusion of intravenous drugs, using open-loop control systems. Such systems include syringe pumps and volumetric pumps.

There are a number of different approaches that the anaesthetist can use to achieve a given target site concentration [be it the blood or effector site (biophase)]. If the drug is administered as a zero-order infusion, it will take three to five times the elimination half-life to reach stable concentrations. The time can be reduced when a loading dose of the drug is given "up front," either as a single intravenous injection or as a fast-rate infusion. For each of these techniques, the maintenance rate will be the resultant of the target concentration times the drug's systemic clearance.

Despite knowledge of a drug's kinetics, the anaesthetist is well aware that variability exists within any studied population, such that there are differences between the predicted and measured target concentrations. Some of the factors affecting drug disposition have been discussed elsewhere by Wood [30, 31] and Sear [16, 17]

In this chapter, evaluation of the predictive accuracy of two different manually controlled infusion regimens has been made in anaesthetised surgical patients. Predicted concentrations (modelled from published kinetic data sets) have been compared with the actually achieved concentrations of etomidate and propofol. From these differences, the bias, inaccuracy and dispersion of the data have been calculated as the median performance error (MDPE), median absolute performance error (MADPE) and dispersion (95% confidence limits).

Methods

Thirty-seven patients (ten male) undergoing either spinal surgery or abdominal or major body-surface surgery were recruited to two separate studies, both of which have been reported in preliminary communications elsewhere [19, 20]. All patients were ASA status 1 or 2 and were receiving no significant intercurrent medication. Each patient consented to one or the other of the studies, which had been approved by the local hospital ethics committees.

Evaluation of a Double Infusion Regimen for the Maintenance of Anaesthesia by a Continuous Infusion of Etomidate

Twelve patients (seven male) were premedicated with 10 mg diazepam and 10 mg metoclopramide orally, given 1 h prior to induction. Anaesthesia was induced with a fast-rate etomidate infusion (100 μg/kg/min) maintained over 10 min, the infusion then being decreased to a maintenance rate of 10 μg/kg/min. Neuromuscular blockade was achieved with alcuronium, and following endotracheal intubation, ventilation was continued with 67% nitrous oxide in oxygen ($n = 6$, group I), or oxygen-enriched air ($n = 6$, group II). Additional analgesia was provided by fentanyl. An initial bolus dose was given prior to induction, followed by supplements when clinically indicated. The total dose received by the two groups was similar; group I 447 μg (SD 237), group II 681 μg (88).

For pharmacokinetic sampling, venous blood samples (10 ml) were collected before and during the infusion of etomidate at the following time intervals: 5, 10, 15, 30, 60, 90, and 120 min and then every half hour to the end of surgery. After centrifugation, plasma was stored at -20°C until plasma etomidate concentrations were measured by GLC using an alkaline flame ionisation detector [20].

Evaluation of a Stepped Infusion Regimen for the Maintenance of Anaesthesia by a Continuous Infusion of Propofol

Twenty-five patients (three male, ASA I or II, aged 16–60 years and weighing 50–90 kg) were studied whilst undergoing major body surface or abdominal surgery. After premedication with 20 mg temazepam given orally 1 h before surgery, sleep was induced with propofol, the trachea was intubated following vecuronium 0.1 mg/kg, and anaesthesia was then maintained with an infusion of propofol to supplement nitrous oxide. Additional analgesia was provided by a single bolus of 10 mg morphine i.v. prior to the start of surgery.

During surgery, clinically inadequate anaesthesia (systolic blood pressure >15% above awake value; heart rate >90 beats per minute; movement in response to the initial incision; autonomic responses – sweating, tears, reacting pupils), was treated by supplementing the propofol infusion with isoflurane (0.5–1.0%). Inadequate neuromuscular blockade (as assessed by hiccoughing or evidence of unsatisfactory surgical conditions) was treated by increments of vecuronium (1–2 mg). At the end of surgery, the infusions of propofol and nitrous oxide were discontinued and residual neuromuscular blockade was reversed with neostigmine and glycopyrrolate.

Patients received an infusion of propofol based on body weight. An induction dose of 1 mg/kg was followed by an infusion of 10 mg/kg/h for 10 min, 8 mg/kg/h for the next 10 min and 6 mg/kg/h thereafter. This regimen [12] was designed on the basis of the kinetic parameters reported by Tackley et al. [24].

For pharmacokinetic sampling, venous blood samples for propofol concentrations were taken at incision, at 35, 40 and 45 min after the start of the propofol infusion, at the end of the infusion, and at recovery (eyes open to command). Additional samples were taken at times of clinically inadequate anaesthesia.

Whole blood propofol concentrations were measured by HPLC according to Plummer [9]. The interassay CV for paired samples was between 4.6 and 8.8% over the concentration range $1-6\,\mu g/ml$, and the limit of detection was $10\,ng/ml$.

In all patients, the electrocardiogram, heart rate and blood pressure were monitored continuously throughout surgery.

Data Analysis

For both studies, computer simulation of the actual etomidate and propofol dose regimen used in each patient (in µg/kg/min or mg/kg and mg/kg/h) provided information on the predicted plasma etomidate or blood propofol concentrations at those times when actual concentrations were measured. Simulations were conducted with pharmacokinetic input parameters described by Schüttler et al. [13] and Tackley et al. [24]. As these two publications describe a number of different subsets of rate constants, the actual values used in the present study are shown in Table 1.

The accuracy with which the infusion regimen achieved the predicted drug concentration, derived by computer simulation, was assessed by calculation of performance errors. For a given estimate of blood concentration, the performance error (PE) was calculated as:

$$PE = (C_M - C_P)/C_P \times 100\%$$

where C_M is the measured blood concentration of propofol, and C_P the predicted concentration according to the kinetic model used [23, 27]. The individual errors of all samples were then summated; the bias (systemic error above or below the predicted concentration, %) was calculated as the median PE (MDPE) and inaccu-

Table 1. Pharmacokinetic parameters for etomidate and propofol according to Schüttler et al. [13] and Tackley et al. [24]

Parameter	Schüttler et al.	Tackley et al.
V_1	$21.0\,l$	$24.32\,l$
K_{10}	$0.079\,min^{-1}$	$0.0827\,min^{-1}$
K_{12}	$0.164\,min^{-1}$	$0.1050\,min^{-1}$
K_{21}	$0.035\,min^{-1}$	$0.0640\,min^{-1}$
K_{13}		$0.0220\,min^{-1}$
K_{31}		$0.0034\,min^{-1}$
Cl	$1.657\,l/min$	$2.011\,l/min$

V_1, Initial volume of distribution; Cl, systemic clearance; K_{10}, K_{12}, K_{21}, K_{13}, K_{31}, microconstants describing a two- or three-compartment mammillary model.

racy (size of the typical miss) as the median absolute performance error (MADPE). If the 95% confidence intervals of the population median PE included zero, it was concluded that no significant bias existed.

Statistics

Data are shown as medians (and 95% confidence limits) except where otherwise stated. Performance errors (PE) and absolute performance errors (APE) were compared using the Mann-Whitney U test between treatment regimens for the etomidate patients and the Wilcoxon Matched-Pairs Signed-Rank test for the effects of time. Drug concentrations are quoted or shown in Fig. 1 as mean (SD).

Results

Anaesthesia and surgery were uneventful in all patients; the duration of anaesthesia ranged between 85 and 151 min for the etomidate patients and between 43 and 110 min for patients receiving propofol.

Etomidate by Infusion

Figure 1 shows plasma concentrations of etomidate in the two groups of patients. In the group receiving nitrous oxide (group I), plasma concentrations were consistently higher than in the patients receiving oxygen-enriched air (group II). The mean plasma etomidate concentration during the maintenance infusion phase

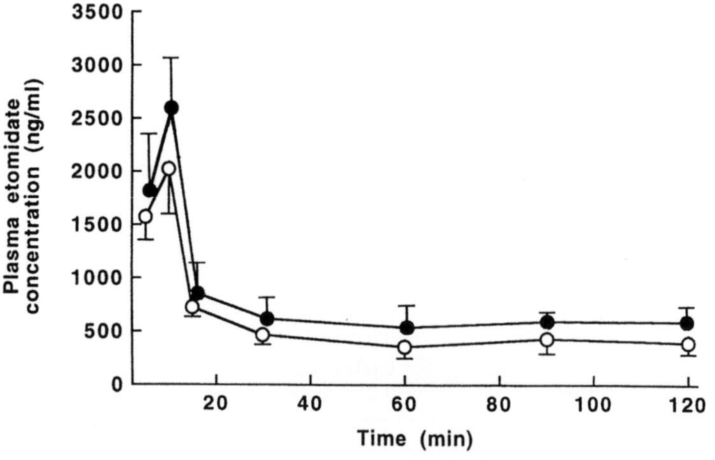

Fig. 1. Plasma etomidate concentrations (ng/ml) during the infusion phase. Data are shown as the mean (SD). *Closed circles*, Group I (receiving 67% nitrous oxide in oxygen); *open circles*, group II (receiving oxygen-enriched air)

(calculated as the average of values obtained from 60 min to the end of the infusion) was 501 ng/ml (SD 135) for group I and 367 ng/ml (SD 110) for group II. Similarly, the AUC (time 0 to end of infusion) was greater for group I than for group II [85.3 μg·min/ml (SD 7.9) vs. 64.7 μg·min/ml (4.4); $p < 0.05$].

Comparison of measured and predicted etomidate concentrations showed individual patient values of the PE ranging between -43.9% and 146.4% in group I and between -48.1% and 129.9% in group II. The overall median PEs of the two groups were 41.0% (95% CI: 18.1–73.2) and 7.9% (-4.8–36.0), and the overall median APE 42.1% (31.5–73.2) and 32.8% (18.2–44.6), respectively.

During the fast infusion phase, the median PE was 44.7% (5.1–84.4) for group II and 79.2% (21.2–128.6) for group I; these values were both significantly different from zero. For the remainder of the infusion period, the median PE was -0.3% (-13.1–23.8) for group II and 29.5% (0.5–61.7) for group I, only the latter being significantly different from zero.

Propofol by Infusion

The 25 patients provided 120 samples of intraoperative data. The apparent steady-state propofol concentration (calculated as the mean of concentration values between 35 and 45 min) was 3.42 μg/ml (SD 0.69). Predicted propofol concentrations were compared with the measured values (Fig. 2). The median PE was 16.1% (12.4–

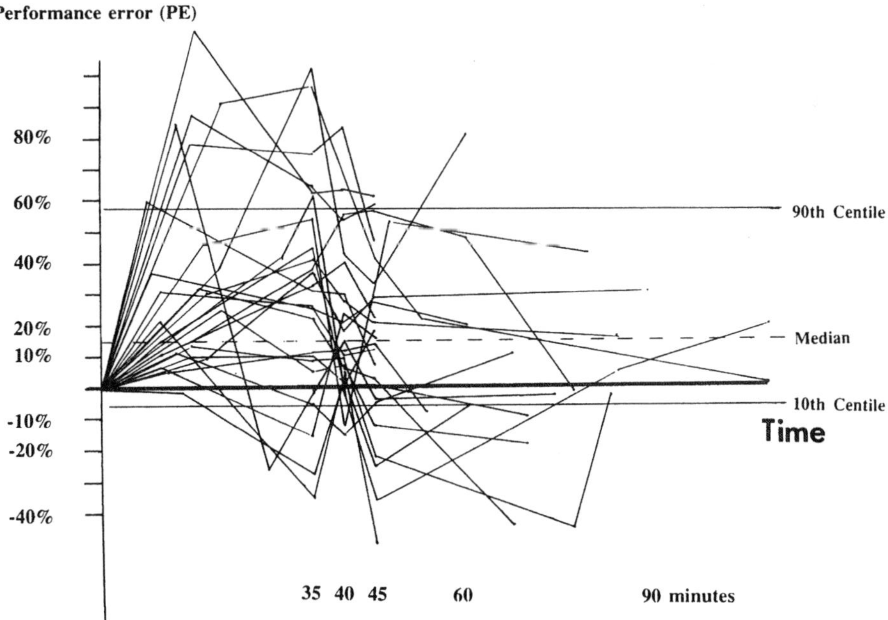

Fig. 2. Individual performance errors for the 25 patients receiving propofol by infusion to supplement 67% nitrous oxide in oxygen. The dispersion of the data is shown by the 10th and 90th centile lines

21.8) and the MADPE 21.5% (16.3–26.8). For both estimates the results were significantly different from zero ($p < 0.01$).

As in the etomidate infusion group, the magnitude of the individual median PEs varied with the duration of the infusion. The median value of the individual sample performance errors was 26.9% (12.4–42.8%) during the first 30 min of infusion, 16.8% (10.4–26.8%) during 35–45 min of infusion, and 3.0% (−5.9–20.3%) for samples taken after more than 60 min infusion (the median values in the first two time periods being significantly different from zero; $p < 0.01$).

Discussion

This paper has described an evaluation of two manually controlled infusion regimens for administration of etomidate and propofol to supplement nitrous oxide or oxygen-enriched air anaesthesia in patients undergoing abdominal, major body surface or spinal surgery. The cardiovascular responses to the initial surgical incision and subsequent surgery were minimal in both studies and were similar to those seen in patients of comparable age and ASA status receiving volatile or opioid supplementation to nitrous oxide anaesthesia [10, 21] or hypnotic infusion-nitrous oxide for maintenance of anaesthesia [18].

The infusion regimen described by Schüttler et al. [13] for etomidate was based on a two-phase infusion strategy as reported by Wagner [29] and was aimed at achieving stable drug concentrations. There was a significant effect of nitrous oxide on the disposition of etomidate; the plateau concentration (60 min to end of infusion) was greater in the nitrous oxide group, as was the AUC (time zero to the end of infusion). In evaluating the predictability of the regimen to achieve a target concentration of around 500 μg/ml, the overall median PE was 41.0% for the nitrous oxide group and 7.9% for those patients receiving oxygen-enriched air.

The infusion regimen described by Roberts et al. [12] for a constant propofol concentration was calculated as a manual approximation to a complex infusion scheme based on Vaughan and Tucker [28], with a target concentration of between 2.5 and 3.0 μg/ml. After the initial bolus dose and two fast-infusion phases, we measured individual blood propofol concentrations during the maintenance infusion phase (6 mg/kg/h). These ranged between 1.63 and 5.55 μg/ml when the infusion rate was administered on a per kg body wt. basis, and represents a threefold variability. This reflects both kinetic variability and the influences of abdominal surgery on liver blood flow, and hence propofol clearance [2, 3].

Several other studies have looked at the predictability of infusion regimens in terms of measured and predicted blood or plasma propofol concentrations. For example, Schüttler et al. [15] found the measured-to-predicted ratio for propofol to be 0.88 when comparing 508 samples collected from 20 patients receiving alfentanil–oxygen-enriched air–propofol anaesthesia. For a predicted propofol concentration of 2.5 μg/ml, measured concentrations varied between 1 and 3.5 μg/ml. Marsh et al. [8] described a computer-driven infusion system for children based on the infusion kinetics of Gepts et al. [4]. This produced a median PE of

−18.5% (due partly to the larger volume of distribution of propofol in the paediatric patient) and a median APE of 25.4%. Using a computer-driven infusion pump based on the pharmacokinetic model of Gepts et al. [4], Glass et al. [5] found a mean PE of 5% and a median APE of 29% for propofol given to adult patients.

For both our infusion regimens, there was a time dependency in the performance errors, with significantly greater errors during the initial infusion phases. Several possible aetiological factors may be identified:

- Assay errors
- Sampling site differences (sampling venous blood rather than arterial blood, with the resulting inadequate delineation of the initial volume of drug distribution)
- Influence of anxiety prior to surgery on drug disposition (in the case of the etomidate model, the kinetic parameters were defined in volunteers)
- Effect of the concurrent surgery
- Kinetic interaction of hypnotic drug and fentanyl or nitrous oxide

This latter aspect has been studied by Schüttler and colleagues [14], who found a significant reduction in etomidate clearance and volume of distribution when etomidate was given in the presence of a steady-state fentanyl concentration of 10 ng/ml. In both groups I and II of the etomidate patients reported in this paper, clearance estimates were similar to those reported by other authors. This study shows that addition of 67% nitrous oxide alters the disposition of etomidate, with a greater median PE in group I. This may be the result of a dose-dependent reduction in cardiac output [7, 26].

Smaller estimates of both performance indices could be achieved by examining *fewer* patients with *more* samples per patient. The observed magnitude of the present estimates reflect closely interindividual kinetic variability (±30%) in surgical patients. Similar values for MDPE and MADPE have been demonstrated for other kinetically based infusion regimens. Raemer et al. [11] measured a MDAPE of 52–55% for alfentanil, and Glass et al. [6] showed the MDPE to be −4% and MADPE 21% using a computer-assisted fentanyl infusion system. These data are similar to MDAPEs between 13 and 59% for fentanyl, as reported by Shafer and colleagues [22].

More recently, Buhrer et al. [1] have reported population MDPE and MDAPE estimates of 5% and 16%, respectively, for thiopentone by infusion to volunteers, and Theil et al. [25] median PE and APE estimates of −14% and 28%, respectively, for fentanyl, and 9% and 25% for midazolam during computer-assisted continuous infusions for cardiac surgery.

From calculation of these performance errors, we can revise the kinetic model that describes drug behaviour during continuous infusion, so that the anaesthetist, unable to measure the blood or biophase concentration in real time, has a better input model in terms of the drug infusion regimen. However, significant improvement of the predictive accuracy of kinetically designed open-loop infusion models may require the use of either individualised population kinetic data sets or Bayesian forecasting.

References

1. Buhrer M, Maitre PO, Hung OR, Ebling WF, Shafer SL, Stanski DR (1992) Thiopental pharmacodynamics. I. Defining the pseudo-steady-state concentration–EEG effect relationship. Anesthesiology 77:226–236
2. Cowan RE, Jackson BT, Grainger SL, Thompson RPH (1991) Effects of anesthetic agents and abdominal surgery on liver blood flow. Hepatology 14:1161–1166
3. Gelman SI (1976) Disturbances of hepatic blood flow during anesthesia and surgery. Arch Surg 111:881–883
4. Gepts E, Camu F, Cockshott ID, Douglas EJ (1987) Disposition of propofol administered as constant rate intravenous infusions in humans. Anesth Analg 66:1256–1263
5. Glass PS, Goodman DK, Ginsberg B, Reves JG, Jacobs JR (1989) Accuracy of pharmacokinetic model-driven infusion of propofol. Anesthesiology 71:A277 (abstract)
6. Glass PSA, Jacobs JR, Smith LR, Ginsberg B, Quill TJ, Bai SA, Reves JG (1990) Pharmacokinetic model-driven infusion of fentanyl: assessment of accuracy. Anesthesiology 73:1082–1090
7. McDermott RW, Stanley TH (1974) The cardiovascular effects of low concentrations of nitrous oxide during morphine anesthesia. Anesthesiology 41:89–91
8. Marsh B, White M, Morton N, Kenny GNC (1991) Pharmacokinetic model-driven infusion of propofol in children. Br J Anaesth 67:41–48
9. Plummer GF (1987) An improved method for the determination of propofol (ICI 35868) in blood. J Chromatogr Biomed Appl 421:171–176
10. Prys-Roberts C (1982) Cardiovascular effects of continuous intravenous anaesthesia compared with those of inhalational anaesthesia. Acta Anaesth Scand 26 [Suppl 75]:10–17
11. Raemer DB, Buschman A, Varvel JR, Philip BK, Johnson MD, Stein DA, Shafer SL (1990) The prospective use of population pharmacokinetics in a computer-driven infusion system for alfentanil. Anesthesiology 73:66–72
12. Roberts FL, Dixon J, Lewis GTR, Tackley RM, Prys-Roberts C (1988) Induction and maintenance of propofol anaesthesia. A manual infusion scheme. Anaesthesia 43 [Suppl]:14–17
13. Schüttler J, Wilms M, Lauven PM, Stoeckel H, König A (1980) Pharmakokinetische Untersuchungen über Etomidat beim Menschen. Anaesthesist 29:658–661
14. Schüttler J, Wilms M, Stoeckel H, Schwilden H, Lauven PM (1983) Pharmacokinetic interaction of etomidate and fentanyl. Anesthesiology 59:A247 (abstract)
15. Schüttler J, Kloos S, Schwilden H, Stoeckel H (1988) Total intravenous anaesthesia with propofol and alfentanil by computer-assisted infusion. Anaesthesia 43[Suppl 2]:2–7
16. Sear JW (1987) Toxicity of i.v. anaesthetics. Br J Anaesth 59:24–45
17. Sear JW (1987) Variability in drug disposition. In: Bergmann H, Steinbereithner K (eds) Seventh European Congress of Anaesthesiology, Proceedings III (workshops 1–8; WFSA Forum). Beitr Anaesthesiol Intensivmed 21:165–174
18. Sear JW (1989) Intravenous anaesthetics. Ballieres Clin Anaesthesiol 3:217–242
19. Sear JW (1991) Should propofol infusion rate be related to body weight? In: Prys-Roberts C (ed) Focus on infusion: intravenous anaesthesia. Current Medical Literature, London, pp 100–101
20. Sear JW, Walters FJM, Wilkins DG, Willatts SM (1984) Etomidate by infusion for neuroanaesthesia. Kinetic and dynamic interactions with nitrous oxide. Anaesthesia 39:12–18
21. Sear JW, Shaw A, Wolf A, Kay NH (1988) Infusions of propofol to supplement nitrous oxide-oxygen for the maintenance of anaesthesia. A comparison with halothane. Anaesthesia 43[Suppl]:18–22

22. Shafer SL, Varvel JR, Aziz N, Scott JC (1990) Pharmacokinetics of fentanyl administered by computer-controlled infusion pump. Anesthesiology 73:1091–1102
23. Sheiner LB, Beal SL (1981) Some suggestions for measuring predictive performance. J Pharmacokinet Biopharm 9:503–512
24. Tackley RM, Lewis GTR, Prys-Roberts C, Boaden RW, Dixon J, Harvey JT (1989) Computer-controlled infusion of propofol. Br J Anaesth 62:46–53
25. Theil DR, Stanley TE, White WD, Goodman DK, Glass PSA, Bai SA, Jacobs JR, Reves JG (1993) Midazolam and fentanyl continuous infusion anesthesia for cardiac surgery; a comparison of computer-assisted versus manual infusion systems. J Cardiothorac Vasc Anesth 7:300–306
26. Thomson IA, Hughes RL, Fitch W, Campbell D (1982) Effects of nitrous oxide on liver haemodynamics and oxygen consumption in the greyhound. Anaesthesia 37:548–553
27. Varvel JR, Donoho DL, Shafer SL (1992) Measuring the predictive performance of computer-controlled infusion pumps. J Pharmacokinet Biopharm 20:63–94
28. Vaughan DP, Tucker GT (1975) General theory for rapidly establishing steady-state drug concentrations using two consecutive constant rate infusions. Eur J Clin Pharmacol 9:235–238
29. Wagner JG (1974) A safe method for rapidly achieving plasma concentration plateaus. Clin Pharmacol Ther 16:691–700
30. Wood M (1989) Variability of human drug response. Anesthesiology 71:631–634
31. Wood M (1991) Pharmacokinetic drug interactions in anesthetic practice. Clin Pharmacokinet 21:285–307

Feedback Control of Intravenous Anesthetics by Quantitative EEG

J. Schüttler and H. Schwilden

Introduction

The use of a feedback system to control intravenous anesthetic drug delivery based on the spontaneous EEG requires at first mapping the anesthesia-induced EEG changes onto a figure which can be easily calculated and used for control. The power spectrum of the EEG signal has been widely investigated as a basis for the derivation of EEG parameters. The power spectrum is nothing but a distribution; thus, the derivation of spectral EEG parameters is equivalent to the derivation of descriptors of a distribution. It should, however, be mentioned here that the estimation of the power spectrum is not a unique procedure. The transformation from the time domain into the frequency domain requires a signal extending from $-\infty$ to $+\infty$ in time. Because an EEG epoch is finite in time, methods for extrapolating the signal to the future and into the past are required. Fourier transformation assumes that the epoch under consideration is repeated indefinitely to $\pm\infty$, while other methods of power spectrum estimation, such as maximum entropy analysis [28], assume other methods of extrapolation. For the purpose of EEG monitoring during anesthesia, these differences in estimating the power spectrum are of minor importance if the EEG epoch is long enough. Figure 1 gives the scheme of an EEG power spectrum and the three monoparametric descriptors of distribution which were used. The simplest one is mean EEG frequency, defined as the mean of the power spectrum regarded as a distribution. As is known from ordinary statistics, the mean can give inappropriate measures of the center in the case of skew symmetric distributions and is, in addition, rather sensitive to outliers. Another descriptor which has been used is edge frequency [9], defined as that frequency below which 95% of total power (95% quantile) is located. The 50% quantile, i.e., median EEG frequency [15], is generally recommended as the most stable quantile with respect to outliers for the description of the center of a distribution.

Median EEG Frequency

Median EEG frequency has been studied in various groups of surgical patients and volunteers [13, 17, 18–22, 25, 26] treated with different agents and drug combinations. In a group of 60 patients who were treated with a variety of drugs and drug combinations, the dosing of which was left to the discretion of the anesthetist, we

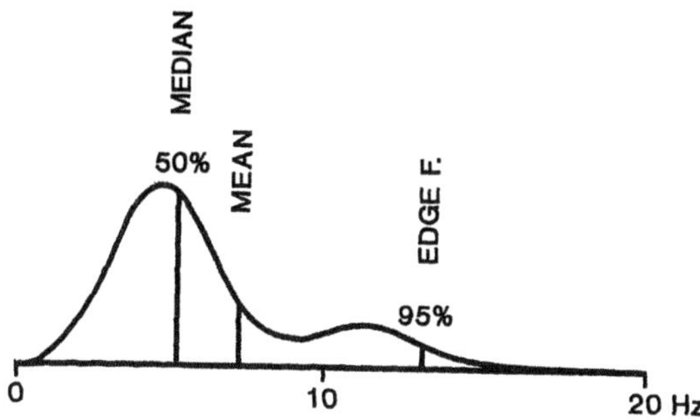

Fig. 1. Electroencephalogram (EEG) power spectrum regarded as a distribution, and three parameters which have been used to describe EEG frequency shifts during anesthesia

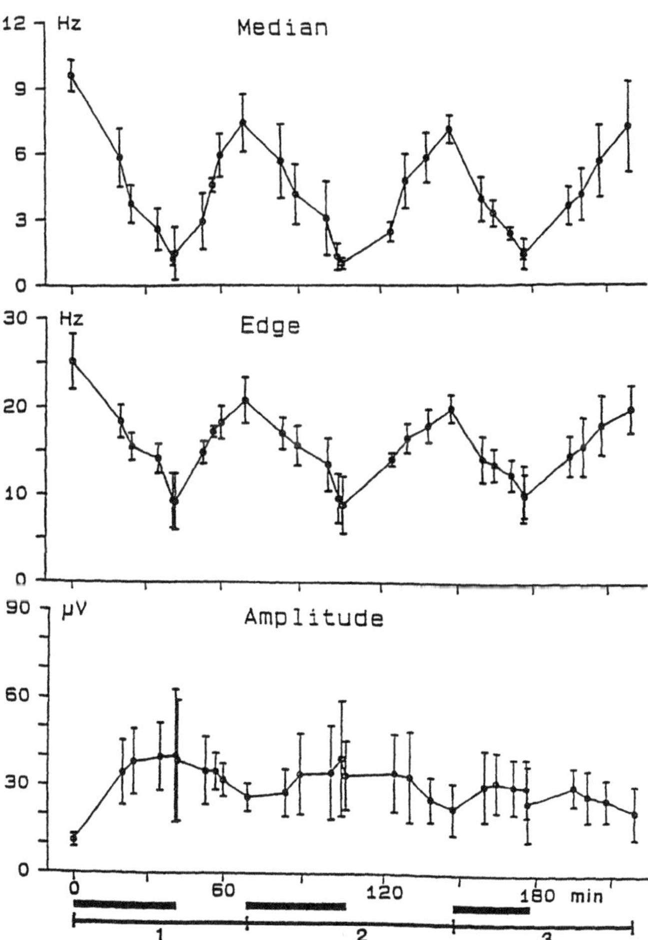

Fig. 2. Mean ± SD of median EEG frequency, edge frequency, and mean amplitudes at defined clinical end points (see text) in a group of five volunteers during a triple-slope infusion of methohexitone

observed a distribution of median EEG frequency which peaked at 2.5 Hz [26]. The 75% quantile of all observed values was below 5 Hz.

The relationship between median EEG frequency and clinical signs has been studied in volunteers treated with intravenous hypnotics such as etomidate [12, 21], methohexitone, and propofol [13]. The methodological approach was to generate linearly increasing drug concentration, the slope of which was chosen such that the onset of drug action and diverse clinical effects could be followed with reasonable precision. Such a method, which has already been described elsewhere [11, 12, 16, 17], requires a computer-controlled infusion for the calculation of the infusion scheme, as well as transmission of the steadily changing infusion rates to the pump. The linear increase of blood concentrations was maintained as long as burst suppression pattern occurred in the EEG trace. At this point, the infusion was stopped and the recovery phase observed. After the patient had regained consciousness with respect to time and location, the infusion was restarted. This cycle was performed three times for each volunteer. Figure 2 depicts a typical time course of median EEG frequency, edge frequency, and mean amplitude for a volunteer treated with propofol. During onset and offset of drug action, the following clinical events and associated values of spectral EEG derivations were recorded: baseline (A), falling asleep (ES), loss of eyelash reflex (0L), loss of corneal reflex (0C) and occurrence of burst suppression (BS). During recovery, the following signs were documented: disappearance of burst suppression (0BS), recurrence of corneal reflex (+C), recurrence of eyelash reflex (+L) reaction to verbal commands (+R), early orientation (FO), and full orientation (VO).

Figure 3 depicts two cumulative distributions as a function of median EEG frequency. The right curve gives the empirical probability derived from the above-mentioned volunteer studies for the occurrence of signs of undue light planes of anesthesia as a function of median EEG frequency. Around a value of 6 Hz, the probability is approximately 50%. The curve on the left gives the empirical prob-

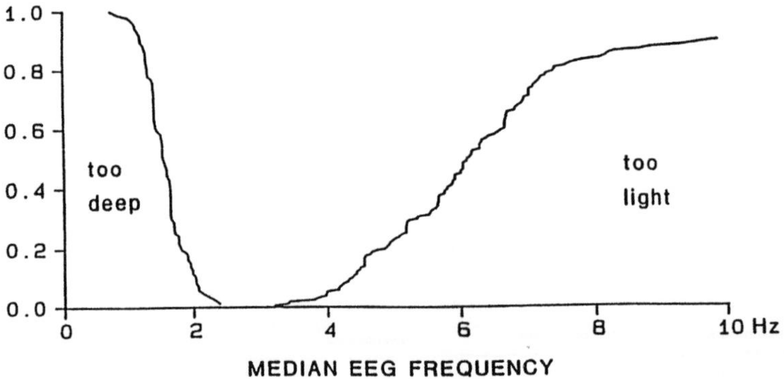

Fig. 3. Empirical probability of the occurrence of clinical signs which were considered an indication of too light an anesthesia (*right*) and too deep an anesthesia (*left*) as a function of median EEG frequency

ability of occurrence or disappearance of burst suppression pattern as a function of median EEG frequency. If one allows the optimal range of median EEG frequency to be defined as having probabilities of 5% or less for the occurrence of signs of undue anesthesia, Fig. 3 defines the interval between 2 and 4 Hz as the optimal range.

Model-based Adaptive Feedback Control of Anesthesia

If the pharmacodynamic effect of drug administration can be measured online, e.g., median EEG frequency or neuromuscular blockade, one can take into consideration the possibility of automatically delivering the drug such as to induce and maintain a given value of pharmacodynamic response.

Control theory distinguishes between open-loop control and closed-loop control. In open-loop control, the input (e.g., drug dosage) is independent of the output (e.g., depth of anesthesia). In closed-loop control systems, the input at any particular time depends on the previous output. Both control systems require a controller to determine the optimum dosage strategy. This might be the anesthesiologist and/or a model of the process to be controlled. When the input to the system is controlled by a model, this control is commonly referred to as being model based. Model-based closed-loop control systems may use the measured output of the system not only to determine the next input, but also to update the model describing the relationship between input and output. This method is referred to as model based and adaptive. Among the models used, one can distinguish between heuristic and deterministic models. PID (proportional-integral-differential) control is a very often used heuristic model for feedback control. In this case, it is assumed that the input to the system needed to correct for a difference between measured output set point is related to the difference between the set point and the output itself, the integral of the output as well as the derivative. Pharmacokinetic-dynamic models are examples of deterministic models used to control drug dosage.

For methohexitone and propofol [19, 20] we used median EEG frequency as pharmacodynamic signal and the interval of 2–3 Hz as desired range of control. Figure 4 depicts the results in 11 volunteers who were submitted to feedback control of methohexital anesthesia [19]. As target range of control, the interval of 2–3 Hz was chosen. Figure 4 depicts the time course of median EEG frequency (mean ± SD) for the 120-min procedure and the subsequent recovery. To achieve this result, a steady random stimulation of the volunteers by acoustic sensations, verbal commands, cold stimuli, pin picks, and testing of eyelid and corneal reflex was necessary. Though this figure demonstrates the functioning of feedback-controlled methohexitone administration in stimulated volunteers, it does not add anything beyond our expectations. The true added value of feedback-control systems is the dose which was required to maintain median EEG frequency at the set point. The cumulative amount (mean ± SD) of methohexitone required is depicted in Fig. 5. In this context, a special feature of feedback systems has to be

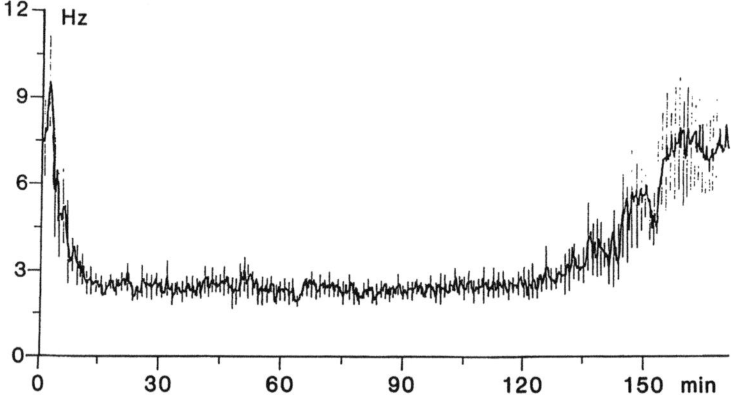

Fig. 4. Mean ± SD of median EEG frequency in 11 volunteers receiving methohexitone to maintain a median EEG frequency between 2 and 3 Hz for 2 h

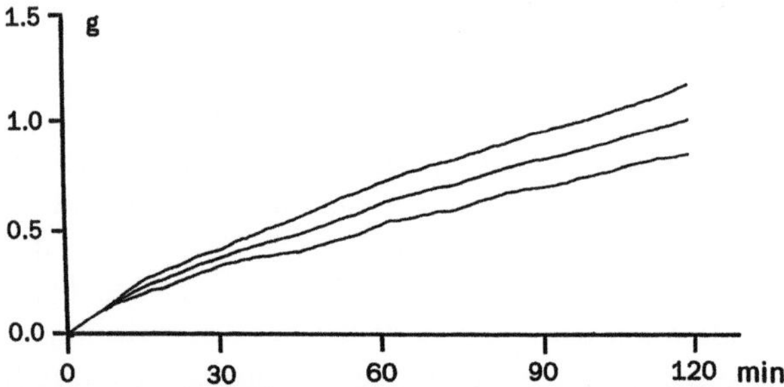

Fig. 5. The cumulative dose requirement (*y axis*) of methohexitone (mean ± SD) for 120 min (*x axis*) in the 11 volunteers for whom median EEG frequency was maintained between 2 and 3 Hz (see Fig. 4)

noted: In conventional therapeutic studies, a specified dose is given and the time course of effect emerges. Feedback-control systems invert this handling of the dose-effect relationship. Instead of giving a dose and observing the emerging effect, a feedback system allows us to preset an effect and to observe the dose necessary to achieve and maintain this effect. This feature could, for instance, be of high value in dose-finding studies. Using such a feedback system for propofol administration, we were able to identify dose-requirement curves similar to those with methohexitone. Comparing the dose requirement of both, one is now able to exactly define the relative potency of propofol with respect to methohexitone by determining the ratios of the cumulative dose-requirement curves. This ratio as a function of time is depicted in Fig. 6. It can be seen from Fig. 6 that the relative potency of propofol with respect to methohexitone is relatively stable with time and lies in the order of 0.72.

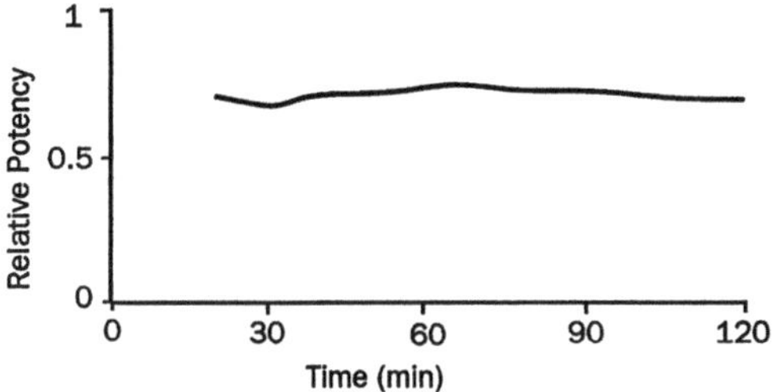

Fig. 6. The relative potency of propofol with respect to methohexitone as determined from the ratio of cumulative dose requirement during feedback-controlled drug administration to maintain median EEG frequency between 2 and 3 Hz

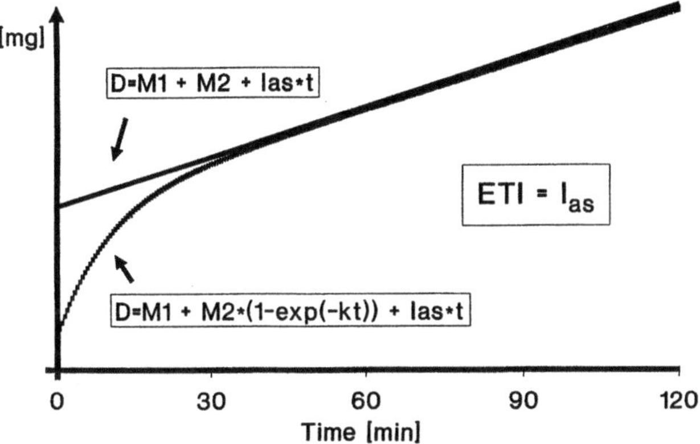

Fig. 7. Idealized dose-requirement curve during feedback-controlled drug delivery. The asymptote to the curve is defined by its intercept and its slope. The intercept is the total amount of drug in the body at steady state; the slope I_{as} gives the rate of infusion to maintain the set point at steady state. In maintaining a given effect, I_{as} is thus an effective rate of infusion. If the effect is chosen such that it lies within the therapeutic range, it obviously defines an effective therapeutic infusion (ETI)

The Concept of Effective Therapeutic Infusions

Figure 7 depicts an idealized cumulative dose-requirement curve together with its asymptote. The asymptote is defined by its intercept and slope, and both may be readily interpreted. The intercept gives the amount of drug in the body at steady state (so-called body load), and the slope gives the rate of infusion to maintain the desired effect. As this rate of infusion is determined by the feedback system as the infusion maintaining a given effect, it is an effective infusion. Where the effect was chosen such that it is within the therapeutic range, we named it effective therapeutic infusion (ETI) [22, 23]. Figure 8 depicts the cumulative distribution of the ETI of methohexitone in 11 surgical patients during a steady-state fentanyl infusion of 0.22 mg/h for a median EEG frequency between 2 and 3 Hz [23]. From Fig. 8, one

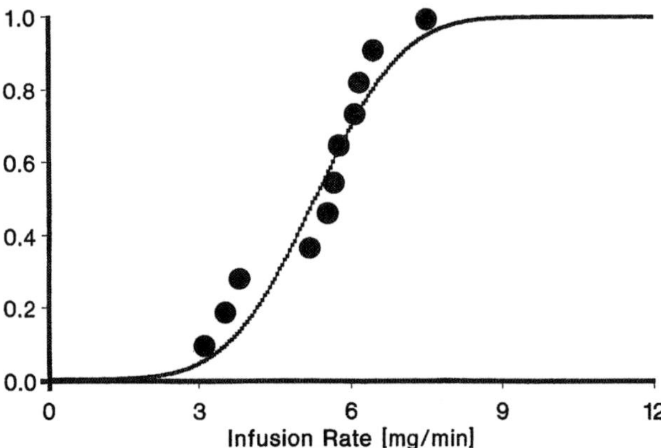

Fig. 8. Cumulative distribution of the effective therapeutic infusion of methohexitone in 11 surgical patients who were co-adminisitered fentanyl at a steady-state infusion of 0.22 mg/h

may easily derive the ETI_{50} (by analogy to ED_{50}) or any other quantile. Unlike the determinations of MAC [6, 8] or the minimum infusion rate [7], which by definition require that 50% of the investigated patients are not treated in the therapeutic range (movement in response to skin incision), this approach allows similar and even more conclusions, but each individual is treated within his or her therapeutic optimum. The ETI concept, together with the feedback-control method, is also a suitable tool for studying drug-drug interactions. The characterization and quantitation of drug-drug interaction in terms of additivity or nonadditivity requires the identification of pairs of doses dA-dB of drug A and drug B, leading to the specified effect E, at which the drug-drug interaction is studied. The common approach used today is a search among numerous doses dA with numerous doses dB until eventually enough dose pairs are identified yielding the effect E. Using a feedback system, such a trial and error approach may be streamlined to a few straightforward studies. The first drug A is given at various doses and the second drug B is administered by the feedback system maintaining effect E; i.e., the feedback system identifies immediately those dose pairs leading to the effect E, and superfluous studies of dose pairs not leading to effect E are avoided. Figure 9 depicts the interaction of methohexitone with fentanyl. Methohexitone given alone to volunteers required an ETI_{50} of 7.5 mg/min (right curve), and co-administration of fentanyl at a steady-state infusion rate of 0.22 mg/h yielded an ETI_{50} of 5.3 mg/min. Hence, the fentanyl administration reduced the methohexitone requirement by approximately 30%. These are not enough data to decide whether this interaction is additive or supra- or infra-additive. Gross estimations, however, lead to the conclusion that an infusion of 0.8 mg/h fentanyl at steady state will yield a median EEG frequency between 2 and 3 Hz. Given this estimation, the index of additivity is computed to 0.22 mg per h/0.8 mg per h + 5.3 mg per min/7.5 mg per min = 0.98~1. As the sum of both fractional doses of methohexitone and fentanyl

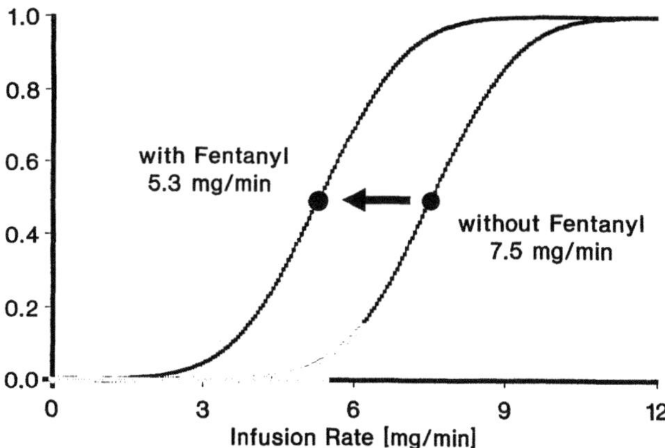

Fig. 9. Comparison of the distribution of the effective therapeutic infusion of methohexitone for the 11 surgical patients (see Fig. 8) and the distribution in 11 volunteers receiving no fentanyl. From this data it can be estimated that the co-administration of fentanyl (0.22 mg/h) reduces the methohexitone requirement by 2.2 mg/min at steady state

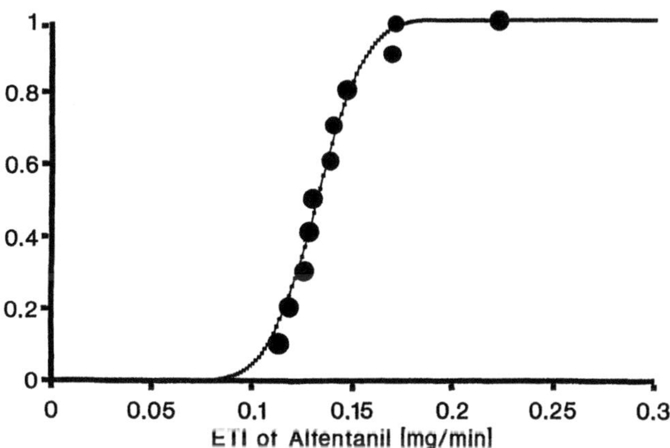

Fig. 10. Cumulative distribution of the effective therapeutic infusion of alfentanil in a patient undergoing major abdominal surgery during anesthesia with 60% nitrous oxide and alfentanil. The mean ETI is about 0.140 mg/min, being in reasonable agreement with other estimations of alfentanil requirement for surgical patients (see "Discussion")

add up to 1, it is concluded that, given the available information, there are no indications for a nonadditive interaction between both agents. So far, only hypnotic compounds have been considered for administration by EEG-based feedback systems. In a recent study we investigated feedback-controlled delivery of alfentanil during anesthesia with alfentanil-nitrous oxide [24]. Table 1 gives the data for the individual ETI of alfentanil, duration of surgery, and recovery times for the 11 surgical patients studied. We found a mean ETI of alfentanil of 0.140 ± 0.032 mg/min. Figure 10 depicts the cumulative distribution of the ETI in the group of 11 patients.

Table 1. Effective therapeutic infusion (ETI), duration of surgery, and recovery time in a study of feedback-controlled delivery of alfentanil

Patient	ETI (mg/min)	Duration of surgery (min)	Recovery time (min)
1	0.139	200	19
2	0.217	75	7
3	0.135	105	17
4	0.108	255	6
5	0.113	125	14
6	0.121	120	13
7	0.122	125	20
8	0.165	190	20
9	0.163	130	31
10	0.134	155	22
11	0.121	170	35
Mean	0.140	150.0	18.5
SD	0.032	50.7	8.9

SD, Standard deviation.

Feedback Control of Intravenous Agents in the ICU

Another application of closed-loop feedback control is in sedation. Critically ill and mechanically ventilated patients in ICU therapy often require prolonged sedation. At present, an opiate-benzodiazepine combination is most commonly employed, but propofol has also been utilized successfully. To date, there are no clear objective clinical signs to ensure an adequate and not excessively deep state of sedation. Thereby, drug accumulation might occur with undesired side effects and/or unnecessarily long recovery periods. In this study the median frequency of the patient's EEG power spectrum was obtained and used as a correlate of depth of sedation. This biosignal was then used as input function for a computer-based, closed-loop feedback system for the administration of propofol. Two representative cases (Fig. 11, post-op patient; Fig. 12, multitrauma patient) are shown in the figures (upper panel: median EEG frequency, lower panel: propofol blood levels). All patients were sedated successfully with the EEG median feedback closed-loop system, on average for 18.7 ± 7.1h (mean $\pm$ SD). In trauma patients the duration of closed-loop therapy was 22.8 ± 3.5h; we then continued with open-loop control of propofol and alfentanil. Different dosing requirements became apparent for surgical vs. trauma patients. Surgical patients ($n = 11$) tolerated a lighter sedation regimen (sedation score: 3.2 ± 0.8. EEG median: 2.5–3.5Hz), whereas trauma patients ($n = 5$) were maintained on 1.4 ± 0.3 of our clinical sedation scale ($p < 0.05$) and an average EEG median between 1 and 2Hz to ensure ICU therapy tolerance. This corresponded with the cumulative propofol/alfentanil doses

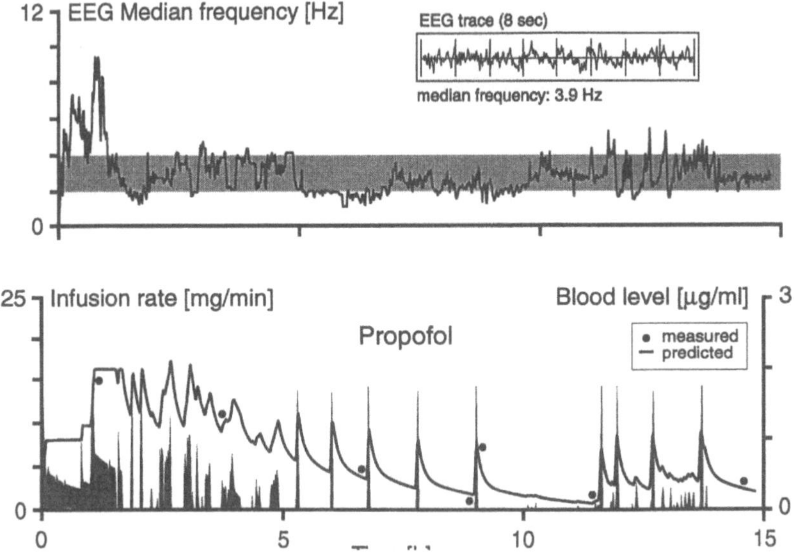

Fig. 11. Median EEG frequency and propofol blood concentrations in a postoperative patient during sedation in the ICU

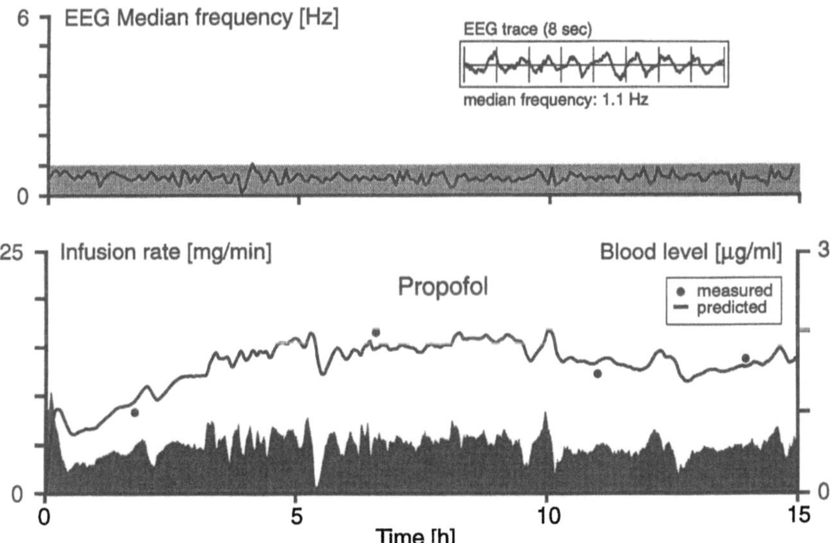

Fig. 12. Median EEG frequency and propofol blood concentrations in a multitrauma patient during sedation in the ICU

needed (surgical: propofol = 1.8 ± 0.9 mg/kg/h, alfentanil = 0.024 ± 0.009 mg/kg/ h; trauma: propofol = 3.6 ± 1.2 mg/kg/h, alfentanil = 0.04 ± 0.023 mg/kg/h). Statistical tests showed significant differences between the two groups for EEG median frequencies, sedation scores, and cumulative doses (all $p < 0.05$).

Discussion

In considering the use and usefulness of EEG-controlled feedback systems, two major points have to be addressed: first, does the EEG, and especially the derived-quantity median EEG, frequency reflect therapeutic drug action, and second, does feedback-controlled drug administration lead to "better" anesthesia? It has been argued that different anesthetic agents produce different EEG patterns, and thus it might not be possible to use the EEG for the control of anesthetic drug administration. Indeed, approaches such as the pharmaco-EEG try to identify differences in drug action on the EEG with the aim of anticipating the pattern of behavioral effects a drug and especially a new compound will exhibit. The use of the EEG for monitoring anesthesia and anesthetic drug action takes an opposite approach: Obviously, there is a plethora of anesthetic drugs and their combinations, all used with the same goal of inducing and maintaining anesthesia. Given this fact, the natural question is whether this common aim and achievement is reflected in some (not all) characteristics of the EEG. In trying to answer this question, a parametrization of EEG is necessary which is gross enough not to be influenced by the differences of different anesthetics on the EEG, but specific enough to reflect the induced mental state of reduced or lacking perception of stimuli. We believe that median frequency is at least a candidate for such parametrization. As shown in this review, many drugs used for anesthesia such as methohexitone, etomidate, thiopental, propofol, alfentanil-nitrous oxide [24], fentanyl, and fentanyl-methohexitone are able to slow EEG frequency. In addition, we have shown that a median EEG frequency between 2 and 4 Hz could be a reasonable set point for clinical uses. Especially for studies using alfentanil-nitrous oxide, there is enough worldwide experience to compare the feedback approach with other approaches to handling this drug combination for the maintenance of anesthesia. Several years ago, on the basis of pharmacokinetic investigations and clinical experience [10, 14, 27], our group proposed a target concentration for alfentanil of 400–500 ng/ml during anesthesia with 60% nitrous oxide for major surgery. Given the pharmacokinetic data of Schüttler et al. [10], this concentration corresponds to a maintenance infusion rate of approximately 0.14 mg/min for adult patients. Meanwhile, several authors have performed studies to identify appropriate dose requirements for alfentanil, mostly in addition to 66% nitrous oxide. They usually used blood pressure and heart rate to define additional alfentanil requirements. Ausems et al. [1] reported an average rate of infusion of 1.72 ± 0.15 μg/kg per min during intra-abdominal surgery, corresponding to 0.123 ± 0.011 mg/min for a patient with 72 kg body wt. This group used 66% nitrous oxide. Lemmens et al. [4] reported for a group of elderly patients ($n = 18$, 65–86 years) with an average body weight of 67 kg a total requirement of 23.5 ± 10.7 mg alfentanil for an average duration of anesthesia of 162 ± 42 min with the addition of 66% nitrous oxide. For patients with Crohn's disease with an average weight of 58.8 kg, Gesink-van der Veer et al. [3] found a mean rate of infusion of 2.1 μg/kg per min and for a control group with an average weight of 64.4 kg a mean rate of 1.05 μg/kg per min, corresponding to 0.151 mg/min and 0.076 mg/min, respectively, for a 72-kg patient. A later study by

Ausems et al. [2] found an average rate of infusion of $1.43 \pm 0.55\,\mu g/kg$ per min for lower abdominal surgery and $1.99 \pm 0.55\,\mu g/kg$ per min for upper abdominal surgery, with 66% nitrous oxide necessary to avoid "response", as defined by a set of criteria with respect to hemodynamics and autonomic signs. These data correspond to $0.1 \pm 0.04\,mg/min$ and $0.14 \pm 0.04\,mg/min$, respectively, for a 72-kg patient. In the study by Ausems et al., again 66% nitrous oxide was administered. The comparison of these data with the data presented in this review indicates that median EEG frequency may alternatively serve as a guide in defining appropriate doses of alfentanil during alfentanil-nitrous oxide anesthesia. In answering the second question, as to whether feedback-controlled drug delivery leads to better anesthesia, the key point is "better". It has many aspects, including outcome in terms of morbidity/mortality, patients' and doctors' comfort and convenience, as well as economic and ecological aspects. With respect to none of these aspects has it been proven or disproven that feedback-controlled drug delivery is superior to other techniques. There are, however, arguments why this might be so. One may consider feedback-controlled drug administration as a very careful computer-controlled titration of drug dosing within the very narrow limits of the set point. As such, it mimics the anesthetist, but on the grounds of sound pharmacokinetic-pharmacodynamic models and their handling. On the other hand, the feedback system as used in the presented studies has very limited information (the EEG only) compared with the anesthetist. Given this limited information, it is not surprising that these feedback systems have one major disability, and that is in terms of anticipating action. While the anesthetist can take measures and action before, for example, a skin incision or celiotomy, the feedback system in its present state lacks the ability to foresee such events and therefore does not have the advantage of anticipatory action. We therefore conclude that supervisory feedback control might be a reasonable compromise at this moment in time for the use of feedback-controlled drug delivery in the clinical setting. Another evaluation of the use and usefulness of EEG feedback-controlled anesthetic drug delivery is achieved if one considers it as a research tool in the clinical pharmacology of anesthesia. In this field, it appears to be useful in objectively determining drug requirements at constant and therapeutic effects. It helps in studying drug-drug interactions or the interaction of drugs with other circumstances, it eliminates the otherwise existing need to under- or overdose a certain portion of patients or volunteers, it reduces the number of individuals to be studied, and allows a more straightforward study design for a number of questions. Thus, it is a more effective and economic tool compared with trial-and-error or other research methods.

References

1. Ausems EM, Hug CC, de Lange S (1983) Variable rate infusion of alfentanil to nitrous oxide anesthesia for general surgery. Anesth Analg 62:982–986
2. Ausems EM, Hug CC, Stanski DR, Burm AGL (1986) Plasma concentrations of alfentanil required to supplement nitrous oxide anesthesia for general surgery. Anesthesiology 65:362–373

3. Gesink-van der Veer BJ, Burm AGL, Hennis PJ, Bovill JG (1989) Alfentanil requirement in Crohn's disease. Anaesthesia 44:209–211
4. Lemmens HJM, Burm AGL, Bovill JG, Hennis PJ (1988) Pharmacodynamics of alfentanil as a supplement to nitrous oxide anaesthesia in the elderly. Br J Anaesth 61:173–179
5. Levy WJ, Shapiro HM, Maruchak G (1980) Automated EEG processing for intraoperative monitoring – a comparison of techniques. Anesthesiology 53:223–236
6. Merkel G, Eger El 11 (1963) A comparative study of halothane and halopropane anesthesia including a method for determining equipotency. Anesthesiology 24:346–352
7. Prys-Roberts C, Davis JR, Calverley RK, Goodman NW (1983) Haemodynamic effects on infusions of diisopropyl phenol (ICI 35868) during nitrous oxide anaesthesia in man. Br J Anaesth 55:105–111
8. Quasha AL, Eger EI 11, Tinker JH (1980) Determination and applications of MAC. Anesthesiology 53:315–334
9. Rampil IJ, Sasse FJ, Smith NT (1980) Spectral edge frequency – a new correlate of anesthetic depth. Anesthesiology 53:S12
10. Schüttler J, Stoeckel H (1982) Alfentanil (R 39209). Ein neues kurzwirkendes Opioid. Pharmakokinetik and erste klinische Erfahrungen. Anaesthesist 31:10–14
11. Schüttler J, Schwilden H, Stoeckel H (1983) Pharmacokinetics as applied to total intravenous anaesthesia. Practical implications. Anaesthesia [Suppl] 38:53–56
12. Schüttler J, Schwilden H, Stoeckel H (1985) Infusion strategies to investigate the pharmacokinetics and pharmacodynamics of hypnotic drugs: etomidate as an example. Eur J Anaesthesiol 2:133–142
13. Schüttler J, Schwilden H, Stoeckel H (1985) Pharmacokinetic and pharmacodynamic modelling of propofol ("diprivan") in volunteers and surgical patients. Postgrad Med J 61[Suppl 3]:53–54
14. Schüttler J, Stoeckel H, Schwilden H, Lauven PM (1986) Pharmakokinetisch begründete Infusionsmodelle für die Narkoseführung mit Alfentanil. In: Doenicke A (ed) Alfentanil. Springer, Berlin Heidelberg New York, pp 42–51
15. Schwilden H, Stoeckel H (1980) Untersuchunger über verschiedene EEG-Parameter als Indikatoren des Narkosezustandes, Der Median als quantitative Maß der Narkosetiefe. Anaesth Intensivther Notfallmed 15:279–286
16. Schwilden H, Schüttler J, Stoeckel H (1983) Pharmacokinetics as applied to total intravenous anaesthesia. Theoretical considerations. Anaesthesia [Suppl] 38:51–52
17. Schwilden H, Schüttler J, Stoeckel H (1985) Quantitation of the EEG and pharmacodynamic modelling of hypnotic drugs: etomidate as an example. Eur J Anaesthesiol 2:121–131
18. Schwilden H. Stoechel H (1987) Quantitative EEG analysis during anaesthesia with isoflurane in nitrous oxide at 1.3 and 1.5 MAC. Br J Anaesth 59:738–745
19. Schwilden H, Schüttler J, Stoeckel H (1987) Closed-loop feedback control of methohexitone anesthesia by quantitative EEG-analysis in humans. Anesthesiology 67:53–59
20. Schwilden H, Stoeckel H, Schüttler J (1989) Closed-loop feedback control of propofol anaesthesia by quantitative EEG analysis in humans. Br J Anaesth 62:290–296
21. Schwilden H (1989) Use of the median EEG frequency and pharmacokinetics in determining depth of anaesthesia. In: Jones JG (ed) Bailliere's clinical anaesthesiology. Baillieres, London, pp 603–622
22. Schwilden H, Stoeckel H (1990) Effective therapeutic infusions produced by closed-loop feedback control of methohexital administration during total intravenous anesthesia with fentanyl. Anesthesiology 74:225–229
23. Schwilden H, Schüttler J (1990) Bestimmung effektive therapeutischer Infusionsraten (ETI) für intravenöse Anaesthetika durch feedback-geregelte Dosierung. Anaesthesist 39:603–606

24. Schwilden H, Stoeckel H (1993) Closed-loop feedback controlled administration of alfentanil during alfentanil-nitrous oxide anaesthesia. Br J Anaesth 70:389–393
25. Stoeckel H, Schwilden H, Lauven PM, Schüttler J (1981) EEG parameters for evaluation of depth of anaesthesia. The median of frequency distribution. In: Vickers MD, Crul J (eds) Proceedings of the European Academy of Anaesthesiology 1980. Springer, Berlin Heidelberg New York, pp 73–78
26. Stoeckel H, Schwilden H (1984) Quantitative EEG-analysis and monitoring depth of anaesthesia. In: Gomez QJ, Egay LM, de la Cruz-Odi MF (eds) Anesthesia safety for all. Elsevier, Amsterdam, p 151
27. Stoeckel H, Schüttler J, Schwilden H (1985) Grundlagen der Infusionsnarkose mit Alfentanil. In: Zindler M, Hartung E (eds) Alfentanil. Ein neues, ultrakurzwirkendes Opioid. Urban and Schwarzenberg, Munich, pp 141–150
28. Ulrych TJ, Bishop TN (1975) Maximum entropy spectral analysis and autoregressive decomposition. Rev Geophys Space Phys 13:183

Adaptive Control of Intravenous Anaesthesia by Evoked Potentials

G.N.C. Kenny and D.A.A. Ray

Awareness Under Anaesthesia

The state of anaesthesia has proved to be difficult to define, but certain features would be agreed on widely. For example, the principal concern of the surgeon will be to ensure no movement of the patient during the procedure. In contrast, the major concern of the patient is to remain oblivious of any events during surgery and to recover with minimum pain or emesis after the procedure. Considerable distress may be caused to patients who are completely aware and who experience pain during surgery. Reports from patients who suffered this experience provide a dramatic insight into the trauma involved [1, 2].

Incidence

The incidence of awareness during anaesthesia is difficult to quantify but has probably decreased in real terms over the past 20 years (Table 1). However, recent reports of the incidence range from 0.8 to 8 cases per 1000 anaesthetics [3, 4]. In spite of the reduction, awareness during anaesthesia represents a significant proportion of the claims of negligence made against anaesthetists.

Definition of Awareness

Awareness during anaesthesia may not be identifiable from the observation of cardiovascular data but may cause major psychological trauma during surgery and lead to longer term effects such as mental depression, personality transformation and sleep disturbances, including dreams, nightmares and insomnia [5]. In addition, it may not be simple to detect that patients were aware during general anaesthesia from postoperative questioning of the patient. Five states of awareness can be defined, ranging from complete awareness with recall to total lack of responsiveness and recall (Table 2).

Russell reported the results of a study conducted in patients undergoing hysterectomy where anaesthesia was provided with midazolam and alfentanil [6]. The isolated forearm technique was used to detect patient awareness following the administration of muscle relaxants [7]. Of the 32 patients studied, 72% responded

Table 1. Incidence of awareness during anaesthesia. (From [45])

Reference	Year	Awareness (%)	Dreams (%)	Sample size (n)
Hutchison et al. [41]	1960	1.2	3.0	656
Harris et al. [42]	1971	1.6	26.0	120
McKenna and Wilton [43]	1973	1.5	–	200
Wilson et al. [44]	1975	0.8	7.7	490
Liu et al. [3]	1991	0.2	0.9	1000

Table 2. Classification of awareness during anaesthesia

1. Conscious awareness with spontaneous or prompted recall (explicit recall)
2. Conscious awareness with amnesia
3. Dreaming
4. Unconscious awareness with amnesia (implicit recall)
5. No evidence of awareness

correctly to commands spoken to them during surgery, with 63% indicating that they were experiencing pain. None of these patients had spontaneous and un-prompted recall and only 10% had evidence of recall on prompting. The majority of these patients would therefore be classified in category 2, as having experienced conscious awareness with amnesia. Lack of explicit recall does not, therefore, always indicate lack of awareness during anaesthesia.

Monitoring Anaesthetic Depth

There are several techniques proposed for assessing the adequacy of anaesthetic depth (Table 3), but one of the main problems of evaluating the different methods is that there is no agreed standard available. Any monitor of anaesthetic depth must be able to provide sufficient information to enable satisfactory general anaesthesia to be produced during surgery. When muscle relaxants are employed, the most valuable sign of inadequate anaesthesia, which is movement, is lost. Another extremely valuable sign of light or deep anaesthesia is respiration in a patient breathing spontaneously. However, when the ventilation is controlled, depression of respiration is not available as a sign of excessively deep level of anaesthesia.

The closest control of anaesthesia is required when the patient is breathing spontaneously during surgery, since excessively light anaesthesia leads to the patient moving, while excessively deep anaesthesia results in depression of respiration. Therefore, any monitor of anaesthetic depth should provide information to allow the anaesthetist to deliver satisfactory anaesthesia to a patient breathing

Table 3. Criteria for monitoring depth of anaesthesia

- Movement of the patient
- Autonomic effects such as changes in blood pressure and heart rate
- Lower oesophageal contractility
- Analysis of the EEG
  Median frequency
  Spectral edge
  Bispectral analysis
- Evoked responses

Table 4. Required features of a monitor of anaesthetic depth

- Similar values for different types of anaesthetic agents
- Values at recovery from anaesthesia similar to those obtained before induction
- Appropriate change during surgical stimulation
- Unaffected by alterations in the cardiovascular system or by cardioactive drugs
- Marked difference in the signal between consciousness and unconsciousness

spontaneously while undergoing a surgical procedure. Satisfactory anaesthesia requires:

- Adequate cardiovascular and respiratory stability
- Ideally no, or at least only minimal, patient movement
- No awareness or recall of events during the procedure

These conditions are one part of a standard against which any monitor of the depth of anaesthesia can be judged. Table 4 indicates other features which should be present. For example, there is little value in a monitor which provides adequate information when only some types of anaesthetic agents are used but is of no value with different anaesthetics. It is important that the monitor should result in a similar signal when the patient has recovered from anaesthesia to that recorded before induction of anaesthesia, and surgical stimulation should cause an appropriate change in the signal. There should be no effect caused by alterations in the cardiovascular system, such as haemorrhage, or by cardioactive drugs. Ideally, there should be an obvious, marked change in the signal from awake to asleep and vice versa, since it is the inadvertent transition from the anaesthetised to the awake state which must be avoided or at least detected rapidly.

Clinical Signs

The vast majority of anaesthetists will control the administration of anaesthetic agents by clinical signs. Where muscle relaxants have not been administered, patient movement is probably the most important clinical sign and can be taken to indicate an inadequate level of anesthesia. However, it should be remembered that the MAC of a volatile anaesthetic is the concentration at which 50% of patients make a gross, purposeful move in response to surgical stimulation but do not generally have recall of the event. When relaxants have been administered, movement is lost as a sign of inadequate anaesthesia and reliance must be placed on indirect signs of the patient's arousal.

Autonomic effects such as changes in blood pressure and heart rate are the most frequently used measures for the adequacy of anaesthesia, but they do not always provide an accurate assessment [8], even when quantified [9].

Lower Oesophageal Contractility

The lower oesophageal sphincter is not affected by neuromuscular blocking drugs, and changes in oesophageal contractility correlate well with the MAC of volatile agents. However, there is not such a good correlation with intravenous agents [10], and even with volatile agents some patients will have no oesophageal activity when inadequately anaesthetised [11].

Analysis of the EEG

The EEG changes considerably both with level of anaesthesia and with degree of stimulation, but obtaining a reliable index of depth of anaesthesia has not proved easy. Analysis of the raw EEG data is too complex for use in this field (although the use of neural networks may make this possible in the future), and it has proved necessary to process the raw signal in order to obtain useful data. The compressed spectral array (CSA) involves multiple Fourier analyses of the raw EEG, producing a display of the power level of each component frequency; this has shown that under anaesthesia, the power spectrum shifts towards the lower frequencies. Use of this shift to produce a single figure of depth of anaesthesia has been investigated: The spectral edge frequency and the median frequency are two such derivations, these being the frequencies representing 95% (sometimes 90% or even 80%) and 50% respectively of the total power in the CSA. Again, these analyses produce useful values with one particular agent [12], but there is considerable variability between the different types of anaesthetic agent [13] and between maintenance and recovery from anaesthesia with intravenous and volatile agents [14,15]. This has limited the usefulness of this (and similar) methods in producing a reliable depth-of-anaesthesia monitor. Bispectral analysis is a more recent system of EEG analysis which provides a measure of depth of anaesthesia based on the interfrequency phase relationships of the EEG [16, 17]. While this has proved a more reliable system than those based on the CSA [18], it still suffers from some degree of interagent variability [19].

Auditory Evoked Response

The auditory evoked response (AER) has been investigated as an alternative measure of the depth of anaesthesia and is obtained by delivering auditory stimuli in the form of clicks to earphones at a frequency of 6–12 Hz. The EEG activity is recorded after each click from three electrodes placed on the scalp, and a total of between several hundred and several thousand EEG sweeps are filtered and averaged to produce the AER. The consistent stimulus and the resulting consistent waveform mean that analysis can be targeted at a particular part of the EEG signal.

The AER has been reported to provide a reproducible guide to the level of anaesthesia produced with different volatile anaesthetics [20, 21] and intravenous agents [22–24]. In addition, it appears to respond appropriately to different levels of surgical stimulation [25, 26].

Transition Between Consciousness and Unconsciousness

The value of AERs to discriminate between patients who were conscious and those who were unconscious has been reported for 11 patients who underwent orthopaedic surgery [27]. AERs were obtained by recording the EEG from electrodes attached to the mastoid and forehead for 144 ms after applying clicks at a rate of 6.9 Hz. The EEG signal was amplified and connected to a microcomputer via a 12-bit analogue-to-digital converter. A level of arousal score (LAS) was derived from analysis of a 3-s moving time average of the AER. Baseline LAS was measured before inducing anaesthesia with a target-controlled infusion which used a pharmacokinetic model [28] to deliver a target blood propofol concentration. This infusion system was used to increase and decrease blood propofol concentrations and so to alternate between periods of unconsciousness and consciousness. Patient response to a verbal command to squeeze the investigator's hand and the presence or absence of an eyelash reflex were determined every 30 s. The presence of a response to command and a positive eyelash reflex were taken as indicating awareness, and their absence was taken to indicate loss of consciousness.

The initial LAS was normalised to 100%, and in all patients the value decreased with the transition from consciousness to unconsciousness and increased with the transition from unconsciousness to consciousness (Table 5). Only two of

Table 5. Changes in the level of arousal score (LAS) between consciousness and unconsciousness (mean and 95% CI)

	Cons	Uncon	Con	Uncon	Con	Uncon
LAS (%)	100	56	92	56	94	57
		(50–62)	(83–100)	(49–64)	(83–105)	(49–65)

the 11 patients had any recollection of events after the onset of the propofol infusion. This consistent reduction in the AER derivative found with the transition from awareness to unconsciousness and the consistent increase from unconsciousness to consciousness confirm that analysis of the AER may provide a guide to awareness occurring during anaesthesia.

Closed-Loop Control of Anaesthesia

The ultimate proof for the accuracy of a measurement for depth of anaesthesia is that the signal should be capable of controlling automatically the delivery of an anaesthetic agent so as to produce satisfactory anaesthesia as defined previously in a patient breathing spontaneously during surgery.

Requirements for a Closed-Loop System

Any closed-loop control system must be reliable, robust and rapid in response. There is no point in having a system which is capable of intermittent satisfactory performance. It must be able to withstand the rigours of the operating environment and to deal with the high-voltage surges during diathermy. It is absolutely essential that the system be able to respond with sufficient speed to a change in the input signal, since there is little point in detecting that the patient was aware some minutes before. A response time of about 30 s would seem to be adequate to maintain satisfactory control, but a response time of several minutes would probably be unacceptable.

Closed-loop anaesthesia (CLAN) using the systolic arterial blood pressure as the input signal has been described by Robb and his colleagues [29]. This system altered the administration of a volatile agent during surgery and advised on the need for supplementary morphine, but the system was used only when satisfactory anaesthesia had already been established and in patients who were paralysed during surgery. The median frequency of the CSA has also been used to control the administration of intravenous anaesthetics, but not in patients breathing spontaneously during surgery [30–32].

Closed-Loop Control with AER

We have developed a closed-loop control system based on the AER which has been used to control the delivery of propofol in patients breathing spontaneously during surgery [33]. The system uses a 386-based microcomputer to deliver clicks to standard earphones. EEG activity is recorded using a purpose-built, high-quality amplifier after each click delivered at a frequency of 6.9 Hz. The AER is analysed on line to produce the level of arousal score (LAS) described previously [27].

The LAS is transferred into the control algorithm which attempts to minimise the error between the measured LAS value and the value selected by the anaesthetist. The controller calculates a target blood concentration of propofol and transmits the required value to the infusion system [28]. The infusion system incorporates a three-compartment pharmacokinetic model which controls the target blood concentration of propofol by delivering to the patient a rapid infusion to achieve the desired blood concentration, and then calculates and delivers the necessary infusion rates to maintain this value. When a lower target blood concentration is required, the infusion system stops delivery of the drug until the predicted concentration has declined to the new value and then restarts drug delivery at the appropriate rates. Thus, the infusion system handles the attainment and maintenance of the predicted propofol concentration determined by the control algorithm.

A baseline value of LAS is measured before induction of anaesthesia and subsequent measurements are calculated as a percentage of the baseline value. The target LAS is entered into the computer, and gradually increasing blood concentrations of propofol are achieved until the target LAS is achieved. Thereafter, a proportional-integral control algorithm is used to maintain the measured LAS close to the target value.

The CLAN system was used to control the induction and maintenance of anaesthesia in 27 spontaneously breathing patients who underwent body surface surgery. Alfentanil was infused to achieve a predicted plasma concentration of 15 ng/ml before induction of anaesthesia, and this value was maintained during surgery. Patients also breathed a mixture of 66% nitrous oxide in oxygen. The median LAS value required during surgery was 40 (range 35–44) which compares with the mean value of 56 recorded in patients who had just lost consciousness [27]. The median value at recovery of consciousness was 101 (range 87–111).

There was no occurrence of awareness during the surgical procedures in any patient, and the last memory all patients had before loss of consciousness was of the clicks being played through the earphones. All patients were prepared to have the same anaesthetic in the future. This is the first reported CLAN system operating from induction, during surgery, to recovery in patients breathing spontaneously. The quality of anaesthesia was controlled within acceptable limits, as assessed by satisfactory PRST scores and the occurrence of only minimal movement during surgery. Most patients had satisfactory values of end-tidal carbon dioxide during the entire procedure, although five did require assisted ventilation for a short time.

This system is the first enabling closed-loop control of anaesthesia from induction, during surgery, to recovery in nonparalysed patients. The principal requirement of a closed-loop system is a reliable input signal. The use of LAS as the input for closed-loop control of propofol anaesthesia validates it as a reliable index of anaesthetic depth with this technique. However, it is essential that other anaesthetic agents and types of patients be assessed to determine whether this index of anaesthetic depth can be applied more widely.

Use of CLAN as a Research Tool

Closed-loop control systems have a major advantage for research in providing completely unbiased drug administration and have been used to compare a variety of therapeutic procedures for the control of blood pressure [34, 35], sedation [36, 37] and analgesia [38, 39]. In a similar manner, CLAN using the LAS as the input signal provided a measure of the propofol requirements in 12 patients who underwent body surface surgery [40]. The quality of anaesthesia provided by the CLAN system was judged to be satisfactory, in that slight movement occurred in one patient during insertion of the final sutures but did not disturb the operation. Respiration was assisted after induction in two patients for less than 5 min, but otherwise, all patients breathed spontaneously during surgery and no patient experienced dreams or recalled any events during the procedure.

The median, maximum and minimum predicted and measured blood propofol concentrations required during surgery are shown in Table 6 (medians and ranges). The maximum blood propofol concentration required to control anaesthesia automatically for each patient was divided by the minimum value to calculate the percentage variation during surgery. The median variation in the predicted propofol concentrations was 225% (range 132–422%) and 273% (range 122–539%) for the measured values.

The relationship between the predicted and measured blood values in this study had a precision of 34.5%. This is a measure of the degree of scatter of the data about the line of perfect prediction and reflects the variability between the pharmacokinetics of different patients. CLAN provides an objective assessment of this variation in propofol requirements within patients and has demonstrated that the pharmacodynamic difference within each patient during surgery was six to seven times greater than the median pharmacokinetic variability between patients. It is obvious that any improvement in the relationship between the predicted and the measured concentrations of pharmacokinetic-based infusion systems would not result in marked improvement in the ability to provide satisfactory anaesthesia. The need to titrate target blood concentration against the patient's response to surgery is clearly shown by this study, and the pharmacodynamic variation is considerably greater than that caused by the difference between an individual's pharmacokinetic parameters and those of the general population.

Table 6. Predicted and measured blood propofol concentrations during closed-loop anaesthesia

	Median	Maximum	Minimum
Predicted (μg ml^{-1})	3.5 (0.9–10.9)	4.0 (2.9–10.9)	2.4 (0.9–6.1)
Measured (μg ml^{-1})	4.2 (1.0–11.4)	6.2 (4.0–11.4)	3.1 (1.0–4.3)

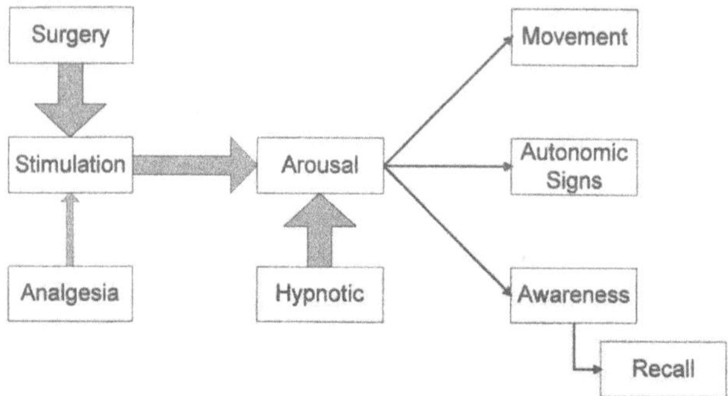

Fig. 1. Surgical stimulation leads to an increased level of arousal. A higher dose of hypnotic will be required to maintain satisfactory anaesthesia if the patient receives a small amount of drug

Balance Between Stimulation, Hypnosis and Analgesia

Use of the closed-loop control system has clarified the contribution of the different components which make up anaesthesia. Satisfactory anaesthesia involves a balance between the stimulating effects of events such as surgery or intubation and the effects of hypnosis and analgesia. Where a low dose of analgesic is administered to a patient, for example, when spontaneous respiration is desired, alterations in the degree of surgical stimulation must be controlled by alterations in the concentration of the hypnotic delivered to the patient, and moderately high blood concentrations of propofol may be required to produce satisfactory anaesthesia (Fig. 1).

If larger doses of analgesia can be given to the patient, as would be the case for patients undergoing cardiac surgery, then relatively small amounts of hypnotic will be required to maintain satisfactory anaesthesia. When general anaesthesia is supplemented with a local block, the amount of hypnotic required to produce satisfactory anaesthesia is greatly decreased since almost no surgical stimulation will reach the central nervous system. With careful psychological preparation of the patient or small amounts of sedation, no general anaesthesia may be required at all and the patient will remain quiet during surgery with no disturbing movements or evidence of increased sympathetic activity (Fig. 2).

Gross movement of patients in response to surgical incision will provide only a limited estimate of the depth of anaesthesia. Clearly, when a local block has been placed and is functioning effectively, there should be no patient movement following the start of surgery, even though the patient is completely awake. In contrast, studies to measure the MAC of volatile anaesthetics are designed to have 50% of patients moving purposefully in response to incision, but these patients show no evidence of conscious awareness and have no recall of events.

Satisfactory levels of anaesthesia can be obtained using a combination of different techniques, which will be selected based on the different requirements of individual patients. By developing techniques to monitor the effect of the

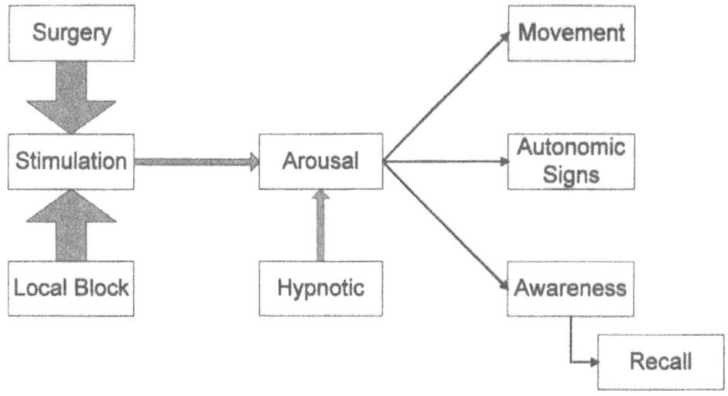

Fig. 2. When a local block has been placed successfully, the amount of surgical stimulation which has reached the central nervous system will be decreased. This will result in a marked reduction in the amount of hypnotic required to maintain satisfactory anaesthesia

anaesthetic agents administered to patients, we can better understand the methods used to provide anaesthesia and ideally improve our control of this relatively intangible state.

References

1. Tracy J (1993) Awareness in the operating room: a patient's view. In: Sebel PS, Bonke B, Winograd E (eds) Memory and awareness in anesthesia. Prentice Hall, Englewood Cliffs, NJ, pp 349–353
2. Moerman N, Bonke B, Oosting J (1993) Awareness and recall during general anesthesia. Facts and feelings. Anesthesiology 79:454–464
3. Liu WH, Thorp TA, Graham SG, Aitkenhead AR (1991) Incidence of awareness with recall during general anaesthesia. Anaesthesia 46:435–437
4. Osborne GA, Webb RK, Runciman WB (1993) The Australian Incident Monitoring Study. Patient awareness during anaesthesia: an analysis of 2000 incident reports. Anaesth Intensive Care 21:653–654
5. Cobcroft MD, Forsdick C (1993) Awareness under anaesthesia: the patients' point of view. Anaesth Intensive Care 21:837–843
6. Russell IF (1993) Midazolam-alfentanil: an anaesthetic? An investigation using the isolated forearm technique. Br J Anaesth 70:42–46
7. Tunstall ME (1979) The reduction of amnesic wakefulness during caesarean section. Anaesthesia 34:316–319
8. Breckenridge JL, Aitkenhead AR (1983) Awareness during anaesthesia: a review. Ann R Coll Surg Engl 65:93–96
9. Evans JM, Davies WL (1984) Monitoring anesthesia. In: Sear JW (ed) Clinics in anesthesiology. Saunders, Philidelphia, pp 242–262
10. Sessler DI, Stoen R, Olofsson CI, Chow F (1989) Lower esophageal contractility predicts movement during skin incision in patients anesthetised with halothane but not with nitrous oxide and alfentanil. Anesthesiology 70:42–46
11. Cox PN, White DC (1986) Do oesophageal contractions measure the depth of anaesthesia? Br J Anaesth 58:131–132
12. Scott JC, Ponganis KV, Stanski DR (1985) EEG quantitation of narcotic effect: the comparative pharmacodynamics of fentanyl and alfentanil. Anesthesiology 62:234–241

13. Burhrer M, Maitre PO, Ebling WF, Stanski DR (1987) Pharmacological quantitation of midazolam's CNS drug effect in hypnotic doses. Anesthesiology 67:A501
14. Arden JR, Holley FO, Stanski DR (1986) Increased sensitivity to etomidate in the elderly: initial distribution versus altered brain response. Anesthesiology 65:19–27
15. Drummond JC, Brann CA, Perkins DE, Wolfe DE (1991) A comparison of median frequency, spectral edge frequency, a frequency band power ratio, total power, and dominance shift in the determination of depth of anaesthesia. Acta Anaesth Scand 35:693–699
16. Sebel PS, Rampil I, Cork RC et al (1993) Bispectral analysis for monitoring anesthesia. Anesthesiology 79:A178
17. Sebel PS, Rampil IJ, Cork RC et al (1994) Bispectral analysis (BIS) for monitoring depth of anesthesia: comparison of anesthetic techniques. Anesthesiology 81:A1488
18. Kearse LA jr, Manberg P, DeBros F, Chamoun N, Sinai V (1994) Bispectral analysis of the electroencephalogram during induction of anesthesia may predict hemodynamic responses to laryngoscopy and intubation. Electroencephalogr Clin Neurophysiol 90:194–200
19. Vernon JM, Bowles S, Sebel PS, Chamoun N (1992) EEG bispectrum predicts movement at incision during isoflurane or propofol anesthesia. Anesthesiology 77:A502
20. Heneghan CP, Thornton C, Navaratnarajah M, Jones JG (1987) Effect of isoflurane on the auditory evoked response in man. Br J Anaesth 59:277–282
21. Thornton C, Heneghan CP, James MF, Jones JG (1984) Effects of halothane or enflurane with controlled ventilation on auditory evoked potentials. Br J Anaesth 56:315–323
22. Thornton C, Konieczko KM, Knight AB et al (1989) Effect of propofol on the auditory evoked response and oesophageal contractility. Br J Anaesth 63:411–417
23. Thornton C, Heneghan CP, Navaratnarajah M, Jones JG (1986) Selective effect of althesin on the auditory evoked response in man. Br J Anaesth 58:422–427
24. Thornton C, Heneghan CP, Navaratnarajah M, Bateman PE, Jones JG (1985) Effect of etomidate on the auditory evoked response in man. Br J Anaesth 57:554–561
25. Schwender D, Golling W, Klasing S et al (1994) Effects of surgical stimulation on midlatency auditory evoked potentials during general anaesthesia with pro-pofol/fentanyl, isoflurane/fentanyl and flunitrazepam/fentanyl. Anaesthesia 49:572–578
26. Thornton C, Konieczko K, Jones JG et al (1988) Effect of surgical stimulation on the auditory evoked response. Br J Anaesth 60:372–378
27. Kenny GN, Davies FW, Mantzaridis H (1993) Transition between consciousness and unconsciousness during anesthesia. Anesthesiology 79:A330
28. Kenny GN, White M (1992) A portable target controlled propofol infusion system. Int J Clin Monit Comput 9:179–182
29. Robb HM, Asbury AJ, Gray WM, Linkens DA (1991) Towards a standardized anaesthetic state using enflurane and morphine. Br J Anaesth 66:358–364
30. Schwilden H, Stoeckel H, Schüttler J (1989) Closed-loop feedback control of propofol anaesthesia by quantitative EEG analysis in humans. Br J Anaesth 62:290–296
31. Schwilden H, Stoeckel H (1990) Effective therapeutic infusions produced by closed-loop feedback control of methohexital administration during total intravenous anesthesia with fentanyl. Anesthesiology 73:225–229
32. Schwilden H, Schüttler J, Stoeckel H (1987) Closed-loop feedback control of methohexital anesthesia by quantitative EEG analysis in humans. Anesthesiology 67:341–347
33. Kenny GN, McFadzean WA, Mantzaridis H, Fisher AC (1992) Closed-loop control of anesthesia. Anesthesiology 77:A328
34. Mackenzie AF, Colvin JR, Kenny GN, Bisset WI (1993) Closed-loop control of arterial hypertension following intracranial surgery using sodium nitroprusside. A comparison of intra-operative halothane or isoflurane. Anaesthesia 48:202–204

35. Colvin JR, Kenny GN (1989) Automatic control of arterial pressure after cardiac surgery. Evaluation of a microcomputer-based control system using glyceryl trinitrate and sodium nitroprusside. Anaesthesia 44:37–41
36. Chaudhri S, Kenny GN (1992) Sedation after cardiac bypass surgery: comparison of propofol and midazolam in the presence of a computerized closed-loop arterial pressure controller. Br J Anaesth 68:98–99
37. McMenemin IM, Church JA, Kenny GN (1988) Sedation following cardiac surgery: evaluation of alfentanil and morphine in the presence of a computerized closed–loop arterial pressure controller. Br J Anaesth 61:669–674
38. Burns JW, Aitken HA, Bullingham RE, McArdle CS, Kenny GN (1991) Double-blind comparison of the morphine-sparing effect of continuous and intermittent i.m. administration of ketorolac. Br J Anaesth 67:235–238
39. McLintock TTC, Aitken HA, Downie C, Kenny GN (1989) Intraoperative suggestions and postoperative analgesia. Br J Anaesth 63:629–630P
40. Kenny GN, McFadzean WA, Mantzaridis H (1993) Propofol requirements during closed-loop anesthesia. Anesthesiology 79:A329
41. Hutchinson R (1960) Awareness during surgery: a study of its incidence. Br J Anaesth 33:463–469
42. Harris TJB, Brice DD, Hetherington RR, Utting JE (1971) Dreaming associated with anaesthesia: the influence of morphine premedication and two volatile adjuvants. Br J Anaesth 43:172–178
43. McKenna T, Wilton TN (1973) Awareness during endotracheal intubation. Anaesthesia 28:599–602
44. Wilson SL, Vaughan RW, Stephen CR (1975) Awareness, dreams, and halluncinations associated with general anesthesia. Anesth Analgesia 54:609–617
45. Aitkenhead AR (1993) Conscious awareness. In: Sebel PS, Bonke B, Winograd E (eds) Memory and awareness in anesthesia. Prentice Hall, Englewood Cliffs, pp 386–399

IV Control and Automation of Drug Delivery

c) Neuromuscular Blocking Agents and Vasoactive Drugs New Drug-Delivery Devices

Model-Based Adaptive Control
of Neuromuscular Blocking Agents

K.T. OLKKOLA

Introduction

Given a certain therapeutic aim, preprogrammed drug delivery can achieve the desired effect only within a certain range of interindividual variation. A reduction of this variation can be obtained by observing the patient's response and the individual titration of the dose. If the effect can be measured continuously, one may consider the approach of an automatic drug-rate control. The effects of neuromuscular blocking agents during anesthetic treatment can nowadays be measured rather precisely and nearly continuously. Several systems have been described for the automatic feedback control of drug administration [3, 22], and especially for the control of neuromuscular blocking agents [1, 2, 5, 12, 24, 27]. A widely used control algorithm is PID control, which assumes that drug input to correct measured effect to the set point is proportional to the effect itself, to its integral, and to its derivative. Such a control, which is widely used in engineering sciences, integrates no information about the dosing-effect relationship. It is therefore suitable rather for the control of stochastic processes. Given a pharmaco-kinetic-dynamic model of the dose-effect relationship, one may consider an approach to integrating this model into the feedback control system. This review aims to examine the characteristics of a model-based adaptive closed-loop feedback control system which can be used to achieve and maintain neuromuscular block at a relatively constant level.

Theory

Figure 1 depicts the schematics of the model-based adaptive feedback loop. Drug input to the patient produces a certain measured effect E, which is compared with the set point and the predictions of the model. The model assumes average pharmacokinetic-dynamic parameters as starting values. Based on these data, an administration scheme is calculated to achieve and maintain the desired effect (set point). Subsequently, the difference between the measured effect and the set point can be used to update the model parameters so that the initial values are adapted to the individual patient under consideration. This updated model may then be used to calculate the drug administration to minimize the error signal.

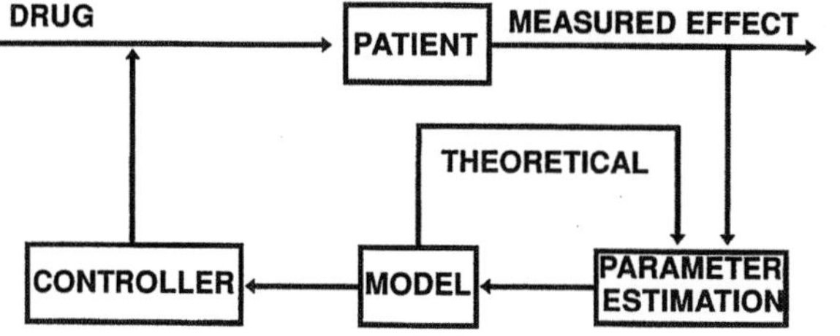

Fig. 1. Structure of a model-based adaptive feedback loop

Control Algorithm

A two-compartment, open mammillary model having a hypothetical effect compartment linked to the central compartment is assumed to represent a valid model of the pharmacokinetics of muscle relaxants [8, 21]. The integrated pharmacokinetic and pharmacodynamic model consists of two formulas (both given as a function of time, (t), one representing the relationship between the function for drug input, I(t), and the concentration of the drug in the effect compartment, $c_e(t)$, i.e.,

$$c_e(t) = \int_0^t dt'\, G(t - t') I(t') \tag{1}$$

and one representing the relationship between concentration $c_e(t)$ and effect E(t) [23]

$$E(t) = \frac{E_{max}[c_e(t)]^{\gamma}}{c_0^{\gamma} + [c_e(t)]^{\gamma}} \tag{2}$$

The function G(t) is given by the effect compartment concentration after bolus administration of a unit dose [7]:

$$G(t) = k_{e0}\left[\frac{C_1}{k_{e0} - \lambda_1}e^{-\lambda_1 t} + \frac{C_z}{k_{e0} - \lambda_z}e^{-\lambda_z t} \right.$$
$$\left. + \frac{C_1(\lambda_z - k_{e0}) + C_z(\lambda_1 - k_{e0})}{(\lambda_1 - k_{e0})(\lambda_z - k_{e0})}e^{-k_{e0}t}\right] \tag{3}$$

C_1 and C_z are the zero-time intercepts, and λ_1 and λ_z are the exponential disposition rate constants describing the decay of plasma concentrations $c_p(t)$ after bolus administration of a unit dose [$c_p(t) = C_1 e^{-\lambda_1 t} + C_z e^{-\lambda_z t}$]. K_{e0} is the elimination rate constant for the effect compartment, E_{max} is the maximum effect, and c_0 is the concentration at half-maximal effect. γ is a value describing the steepness of the concentration-response curve. The initial values used for the parameters are based on previously reported pharmacokinetic and pharmacodynamic data and previous computer simulations.

By applying the superposition principle, it is possible to calculate the concentration of muscle relaxant in effect compartment at any moment and during any drug administration scheme. Equations 1–3 give a full description of the drug input-effect relationship. Given a set point, Eq. 2 may be solved for the necessary concentration in effect compartment. The pharmacokinetic model, Eq. 1, may be subsequently used for the calculation of the drug input function [19].

If the measured neuromuscular block is within 2% of the desired neuromuscular block, an infusion scheme is used to keep the effect at its current level, as predicted by the pharmacokinetic-dynamic model (that is, Eqs. 1 and 2). Otherwise, the difference between the measured and predicted neuromuscular block is used to correct the model parameters. The updated values are then used to calculate the new infusion scheme for achieving and maintaining the desired level of neuromuscular block. This cycle is performed every 20 s. Adjustment of the parameters of the pharmacokinetic-dynamic model begins 2 min after activation of the closed-loop system.

Adaptation Algorithm

One observes that Eq. 2 is scale invariant with respect to the transformation $(c_e, c_0) \rightarrow (\lambda c_e, \lambda c_0)$ for any number $\lambda \neq 0$. Consequently, the insertion of equation 1 to equation 2 does not depend on C_1, C_z and c_0, but only on the ratios C_1/c_0 and C_z/c_0, thus not allowing to estimate clearance or volume of distributions but only microconstants k_{el}, k_{12}, k_{21} and the amount of drugs in diverse compartments. This is, however, sufficient for determining the drug input function. A complete adaptation would require the estimation of C_1/c_0, C_z/c_0, λ_1, λ_z and k_{e0}. We have chosen to update during the feedback control only the parameters C_1/c_0 and C_z/c_0. This allows the adaptation of the initial bolus to achieve a certain effect (short-term control) and of the steady-state infusion rate to maintain the given effect (long-term control).

The effect E may be regarded as a function of C_1 and C_z and the drug input $I(t)$:

$$E(t) = E(C_1, C_z, I(t))$$

Denoting by $C_1 + \delta C_1$ and $C_z + \delta C_z$ the true hybrid constants for an individual subject, the difference between measured and predicted effect (ΔE) can be expanded in a Taylor series, as follows:

$$\Delta E = E(C_1 + \delta C_1, C_z + \delta C_z, I(t)) - E(C_1, C_z, I(t))$$
$$= (\partial E/\partial C_1)\delta C_1 + (\partial E/\partial C_z)\delta C_z + \ldots \tag{4}$$

In conjunction with the condition to minimize the expression $\delta C_1^2 + \delta C_z^2$, Eq. 4 can be used to solve for δC_1 and δC_z. A change in the range of $\pm 10\%$ of the previous values is allowed in each update. From the updated values, new microconstants are calculated that serve to correct the drug input function.

Controller Performance

Controller performance can be measured by calculating the mean offset from set point and mean standard deviation from set point during feedback infusion.

Feedback infusion is said to begin when block returns from overshoot to set point after the initial bolus. Mean offset is calculated by

$$\text{Mean offset} = \sum_{i=1}^{n} \frac{s - b_i}{n}$$

where s = set point,
b_i = neuromuscular block measured every 20 s during feedback infusion,
n = number of measurements.

Mean standard deviation from set point is standard deviation for mean offset defined above.

Use of Model-Based Adaptive Control of Neuromuscular Blocking Agents in Clinical Practice

So far, the developed model-based adaptive controller has been used for the administration of atracurium [14, 16, 20], mivacurium [13, M. Kansanaho and K. Olkkola, unpublished results], rocuronium [15], and vecuronium (K. Olkkola and M. Kansanaho, unpublished results). These studies have been aimed at either optimizing the controller or studying interactions of neuromuscular blocking agents with other drugs used during anesthesia. With approval of the local medical ethics committee, and after obtaining informed consent from the patient or from the parents (of patients younger than 18 years of age), altogether 201 patients have been studied. The age of the patients has varied from 1 to 75 years. Patients with muscular dystrophies, myopathy or cerebral palsy, significant renal, hepatic, or cardiac dysfunction, marked ventilatory impairment due to underlying respiratory disease, and raised intracranial pressure, and patients on concomitant medication known to affect neuromuscular transmission were excluded from the studies.

After induction of anesthesia with intravenous anesthetics according to the study protocols in the different studies, but before administration of the muscle relaxant for neuromuscular block, a Relaxograph neuromuscular transmission monitor (Datex, Helsinki, Finland) was used to obtain control electromyographic values. Specifically, the train-of-four sequence was assessed (frequency of stimuli, 2 Hz; pulse width, $100\,\mu s$) by means of stimulating surface electrodes placed adjacent to the ulnar nerve at the wrist. Recording electrodes were placed on the first dorsal interosseus muscle and second finger [9]. The stimulus output is a rectangular wave with a current range of 0–70 mA, and the machine calibrates automatically by searching for the optimum signal levels before setting the supramaximal level. A stable baseline calibration signal was awaited before muscle relaxants were administered. The degree of neuromuscular block, assessed every 20 s with the Relaxograph, was defined as the ratio of the measurement of first response in the train-of-four sequence (T1) to the corresponding control value. Cardiorespiratory parameters were measured according to our routine, which included noninvasive measurement of blood pressure, heart rate, continuous ECG, minute ventilation, respiration rate, end-tidal CO_2, inspiratory O_2, airway pressure and pulse oximeter. Palmar skin temperature was measured and kept above 32°C. End-tidal CO_2 tension was maintained at 4–5 kPa.

The patients were intubated after bolus administration of either atracurium, mivacurium, rocuronium, or vecuronium, according to the protocols in the different studies. Bolus administration of muscle relaxant was followed by model-driven closed-loop feedback-controlled infusion. An infusion pump (Fresenius Infusomat CP-IS, Fresenius AG, Bad Homburg, Germany) and the Relaxograph were attached to an IBM-compatible computer by means of a serial RS232 interface. The solution was administered through an indwelling catheter in a forearm vein.

Figure 2 gives as an example the time course of neuromuscular block, the rate of the infusion of rocuronium, the cumulative dose, and the fitted cumulative dose for an individual patient [15]. Table 1 shows the controller performance in 201 patients given either atracurium, mivacurium, rocuronium or vecuronium by model-based adaptive controller. There appear to be no major differences in controller performance between the drugs. However, if we look at the values for the mean standard deviation from set point of those drugs where two levels of neuromuscular blocks have been studied, we see that it was greater at lower levels of neuromuscular block ($p < 0.05$). This is not surprising, because the concentration-response curve has a sigmoid shape. The concentration-response curve is steeper when the effect is 20–80% of the maximum. When the effect is around 50% of the maximum, even a small change in muscle-relaxant concentration at the site

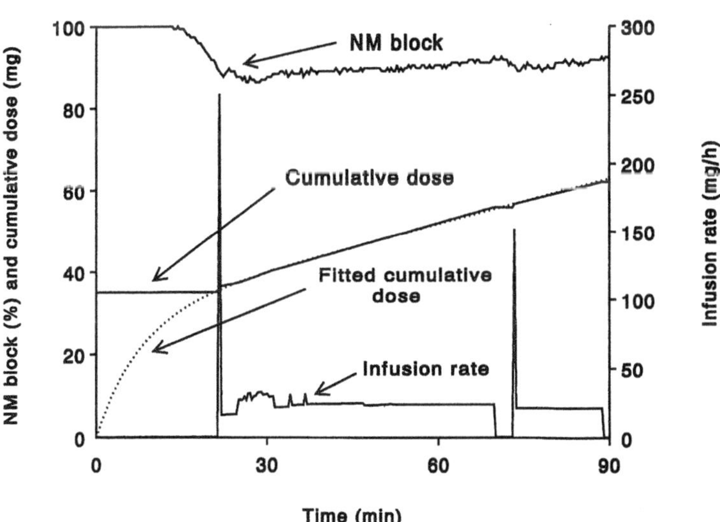

Fig. 2. Neuromuscular (*NM*) block, the infusion rate, cumulative dose, and fitted cumulative dose of rocuronium in a representative patient during closed-loop administration of rocuronium for 90% neuromuscular block

Table 1. Controller performance in patients given atracurium, mivacurium, rocuronium, or vecuronium with model-based computerized infusion (mean ± SD)

Drug	Neuromuscular block (%)	Number of patients	Mean offset from set point (%)	Mean standard deviation from set point (%)
Atracurium	90	22	−0.2 ± 0.8	1.9 ± 0.9
	50	20	−0.3 ± 0.7	3.0 ± 1.0
Mivacurium	95	38	0.3 ± 0.5	2.2 ± 1.2
	50	21	−0.5 ± 1.3	8.1 ± 2.7
Rocuronium	90	60	0.5 ± 0.7	1.7 ± 0.6
Vecuronium	90	40	1.0 ± 0.7	2.5 ± 0.9

of action causes a relatively large change in effect. Near the ceiling effect, even large changes in concentration change the effect only a little. This phenomenon is further illustrated in Fig. 3, which shows the time course of targeted 95% and 50% neuromuscular blocks and the cumulative infusion requirements of mivacurium [13]. The targeted neuromuscular block was maintained relatively stable within a

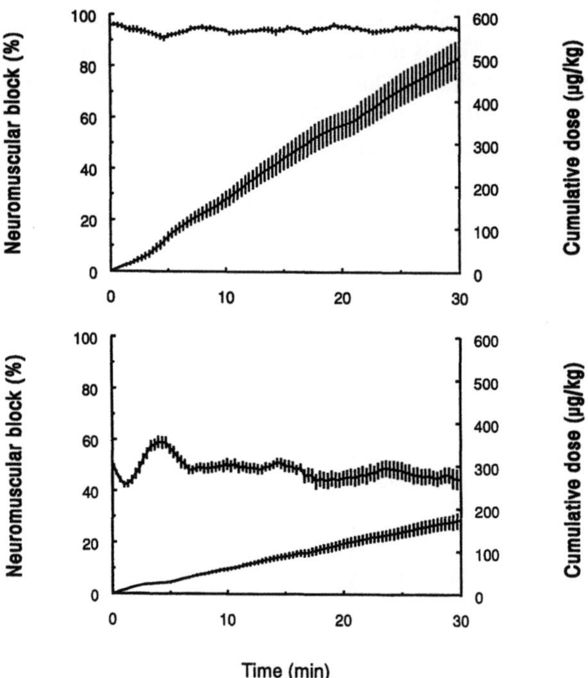

Fig. 3. Time course of targeted 95% (*upper graph*) and 50% (*lower graph*) neuromuscular blocks (*upper curves*) and the cumulative infusion requirement of mivacurium (*lower curve*); mean ± SEM. The targeted neuromuscular block was maintained relatively stable within a few minutes of the block first passing the target value. However, the initial oscillations were greater at 50% than at 95% neuromuscular block

few minutes of the block first passing the target value. However, the initial oscillations are greater at 50% than at 95% neuromuscular block.

Use of Model-Based Adaptive Control of Infusion of Muscle Relaxants as Research Tool for Clinical Pharmacological Investigations

Besides being useful for the administration of intermediate-acting and short-acting neuromuscular blocking agents during long anesthesias, model-based adaptive controllers can be applied as a clinical pharmacological tool. Studies report that prior administration of succinylcholine augments the neuromuscular blocking effects of competitive neuromuscular blocking drugs, i.e., vecuronium, pancuronium, and d-tubocurarine [4, 6, 10, 18]. Some reports have questioned this effect for the latter two agents [25, 26]. To investigate the possible interaction between succinylcholine and atracurium, our study group used a closed-loop feedback control method of administering atracurium to produce and maintain a relatively constant neuromuscular block of 90% or 50%. Interaction between atracurium and succinylcholine was quantified by determining the asymptotic steady-state rate of infusion necessary to produce 90% or 50% neuromuscular block with atracurium [14, 16].

After induction of anesthesia patients were randomly assigned to one of two sequences: (a) bolus administration of succinylcholine (1 mg/kg), intubation, complete recovery from the depolarizing block, and intravenous bolus administration of atracurium (0.5 mg/kg); or (b) bolus administration of atracurium (0.5 mg/kg) and intubation, with no prior administration of succinylcholine. Bolus administration of atracurium was followed by infusion of atracurium controlled by a model-driven closed-loop feedback system. For both groups, the desired level of neuromuscular block (i.e., the set point) was set at 90% or 50%. To estimate the asymptotic steady-state rate of infusion (I_{ss}), we used nonlinear curve fitting (see Fig. 2) to fit the following formula to the curve representing the cumulative dose requirement of atracurium [11]:

$$\text{Cumulative dose of atracurium} = D \cdot (1 - e^{k \cdot t}) + I_{ss} \cdot t,$$

where D = amount of atracurium contained in its apparent distribution volume,

k = relative rate of distribution of atracurium,

I_{ss} = asymptotic steady-state rate of infusion of atracurium,

t = duration of atracurium administration.

Figures 4 and 5 show the mean ($\pm$ SEM) cumulative dose requirements for atracurium for the two groups at 90% and 50% neuromuscular block. In both studies, the model-driven computerized infusion of atracurium kept the desired degree of neuromuscular block at a reasonably constant level, and the controller performance was similar in the groups with and without prior administration of

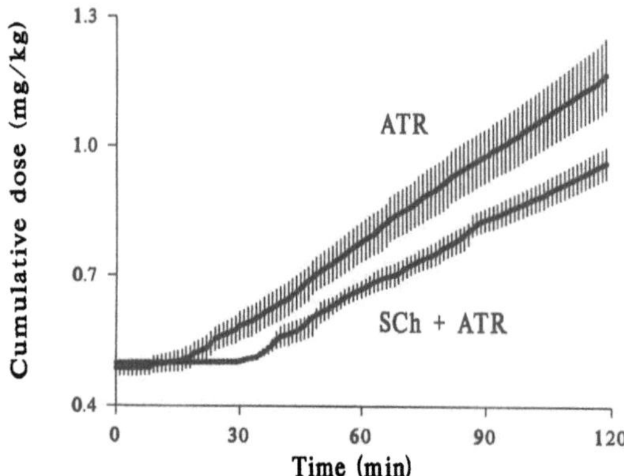

Fig. 4. Cumulative dose ($\pm$ SEM) calculated as milligrams of atracurium per body weight in the two groups given atracurium with (*SCh + ATR*) and without (*ATR*) prior administration of succinylcholine to produce a constant 90% neuromuscular block by closed-loop administration of atracurium

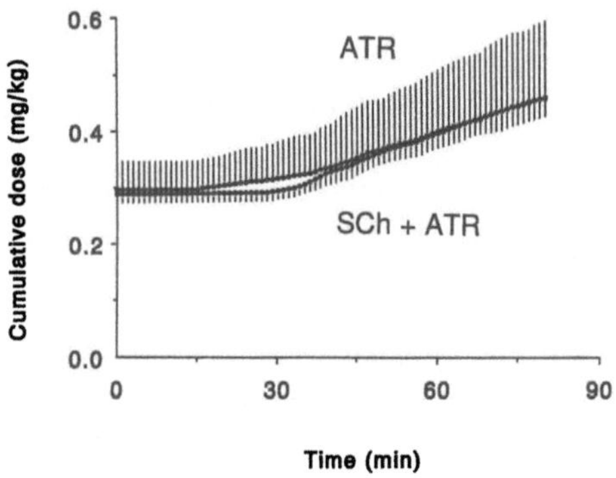

Fig. 5. Cumulative dose ($\pm$ SEM) calculated as milligrams of atracurium per body weight in the two groups given atracurium with (*SCh + ATR*) and without (*ATR*) prior administration of succinylcholine to produce a constant 50% neuromuscular block by closed-loop administration of atracurium

succinylcholine. This allowed the assessment of the possible interaction between atracurium and succinylcholine. At 90% neuromuscular block the mean average rate of infusion of atracurium was 1.4 times higher for patients with no prior administration of succinylcholine than for patients given succinylcholine for intubation ($p < 0.05$). At 50% neuromuscular block the infusion requirements were similar in both groups.

The described model-based adaptive controller has been also used to investigate the possible interactions of rocuronium with etomidate, fentanyl, midazolam, propofol, thiopental, and isoflurane [15]. Sixty patients were randomly assigned to one of six sequences where anesthesia was maintained with etomidate, fentanyl, midazolam, propofol, or thiopental and nitrous oxide, or with isoflurane and

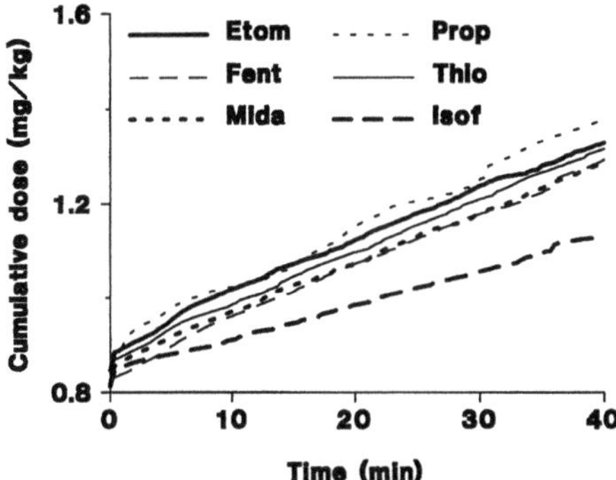

Fig. 6. The cumulative dose of rocuronium given by model-driven computerized infusion to produce a constant 90% neuromuscular block in the six groups anesthetized with etomidate (*Etom*), fentanyl (*Fent*), midazolam (*Mida*), propofol (*Prop*), thiopental (*Thio*), or isoflurane (*Isof*). The cumulative dose is expressed as mg per lean body mass. Time 0 refers to the moment when the model-driven computerized infusion started for the first time, i.e., at T1 it had recovered to 10% of control after an initial bolus of rocuronium. For clarity, error bars are not shown

nitrous oxide. The possible interaction of rocuronium with the anesthetics was quantified by determining the asymptotic steady-state rate of infusion (I_{ss}) of rocuronium necessary to produce a constant 90% neuromuscular block. Patient characteristics and controller performance did not differ significantly between the groups. I_{ss} values calculated per lean body mass were 0.64 $\pm$ 0.22, 0.60 $\pm$ 0.15, 0.61 $\pm$ 0.21, 0.67 $\pm$ 0.31, 0.63 $\pm$ 0.15, and 0.39 $\pm$ 0.17 mg·kg^{-1}·h^{-1} in the etomidate, fentanyl, midazolam, propofol, thiopental, and isoflurane groups, respectively (Fig. 6). The isoflurane group had a lower steady-state rate of infusion of rocuronium than the other five groups ($p < 0.05$). Compared with the intravenous anesthetics, etomidate, fentanyl, midazolam, propofol, or thiopental, isoflurane reduced the infusion requirement of rocuronium by 35–40%.

Discussion

In common anesthesia practice neuromuscular blocking agents are administered by repetitive bolus doses. Such a method necessarily implies over- and under-shooting of effect. Furthermore, it requires drugs with durations of action that are not too short. On the other hand, there is a strong need to enhance the controllability of neuromuscular block by using shorter-acting agents, which is especially of value during the recovery from anesthesia. The ongoing development of shorter-acting neuromuscular blocking agents with increased controllability thus requires dosing strategies alternative to repetitive bolus dosing. Continuous infusion techniques, however, easily result in systematic deviations from desired degree of block unless the effect is measured. If the effect is measured, it is a logical development to use this information for an automatic closed-loop feedback control. The data presented here prove the clinical applicability of model-based feedback control for the administration of muscle relaxants.

The performance of the developed model-based adaptive controller appears to be at least as good as those of previously described controllers [1, 2, 5, 12, 24, 27]. Model-based adaptive controllers have, however, two major advantages over PID- and "on-off" controllers [2, 5, 12, 24, 27]. PID controllers are not universally applicable to nonlinear concentration-response curves. They use, in general, the approach of linear approximation of the concentration-response curve around the set point. By using the entire pharmacokinetic-dynamic model, this limitation can be overcome and the algorithm can be used in principal, for any degree of effect, allowing variation of the degree of neuromuscular block intraoperatively according to the needs of the surgeon.

Another major aspect is the stability of the controller with respect to artifacts. In case of sensor failure, PID control methods have no means of predicting the future dose requirements for maintaining the effect within reasonable margins. The model-based controller, however, can be used to calculate the drug requirement during such failure periods where no feedback is possible on the basis of the adapted pharmacokinetic-dynamic model.

Besides the possible usefulness of such a method for drug treatment during anesthesia, it can be used as a research tool for clinical pharmacological investigations. The establishment of cumulative dose requirement can be used to quantify the drug-drug interactions of concomitantly administered anesthetic drugs and neuromuscular blocking agents at identical clinical effects. By fitting a straight line as asymptote to the data on the cumulative dose requirement of atracurium, it has been shown, for instance, that prior administration of succinylcholine augments the neuromuscular block induced by atracurium at 90%, but not at 50% block. Furthermore, the described model-based adaptive controller has been of great value during the study of possible interactions between rocuronium and intravenous anesthetics.

References

1. Bradlow HS, Uys PC, Rametti LB (1986) On-line control of atracurium-induced muscle relaxation. J Biomed Eng 8:72–75
2. Brown BH, Asbury J, Linkens DA, Perks R, Anthony M (1980) Closed-loop control of muscle relaxation during surgery. Clin Phys Physiol Meas 1:203–210
3. Cosgrove RJ (1985) Automatic, feedback controlled drug delivery devices. In: Smolen F, Bull LA (eds) Controlled drug bioavailability. John Wiley, New York, pp 109–183
4. d'Hollander A, Agoston S, Barvais L, Massaut, Baurain M (1985) Evolution of vecuronium requirements for stable mechanical effect: comparison with or without previous succinylcholine administration. Anesth Analg 64:319–322
5. De Vries JW, Ros HH, Booij LHDJ (1986) Infusion of vecuronium controlled by a closed-loop system. Br J Anaesth 58:1100–1103
6. Foldes FF, Wnuk AL, Hammer Hodges RH, DeBeer EJ (1957) The interaction of depolarizing and non-depolarizing neuromuscular blocking agents in dog and cat. J Pharmacol Exp Ther 119:145

7. Holford NHG, Sheiner LB (1981) Understanding the dose-effect relationship: clinical application of pharmacokinetic-pharmacodynamic models. Clin Pharmacokinet 6:429–453
8. Hull CJ, Van Beem HBH, McLeod K, Sibbald A, Watson MJ (1978) A Pharmacodynamic model for pancuronium. Br J Anaesth 50:1113–1123
9. Kalli I (1990) Effect of surface electrode positioning on the compound action potential evoked by ulnar nerve stimulation during isoflurane anaesthesia. Br J Anaesth 65:494–499
10. Katz EL (1971) Modification of the action of pancuronium by succinylcholine and halothane. Anesthesiology 35:602–606
11. Keéri-Szanto M (1960) Drug consumption during thiopentone-nitrous oxide-relaxant anaesthesia: the preparation and interpretation of time/dose curves. Br J Anaesth 32:415–423
12. MacLeod AD, Asbury AJ, Gray WM, Linkens DA (1989) Automatic control of neuromuscular block with atracurium. Br J Anaesth 63:31–35
13. Meretoja O, Olkkola KT (1993) Pharmacodynamics of mivacurium in children by using a computer-controlled infusion. Br J Anaesth 71:232–237
14. Olkkola KT, Schwilden H (1990) Quantitation of the interaction between atracurium and succinylcholine using closed-loop feedback control of infusion of atracurium. Anesthesiology 73:614–618
15. Olkkola KT, Tammisto T (1994) Quantifying the interaction of rocuronium (ORG 9426) with etomidate, fentanyl, midazolam, propofol, thiopental, and isoflurane using closed-loop feedback control of rocuronium infusion. Anesth Analg 78:691–696
16. Olkkola KT, Tammisto T (1994b) Assessment of the interaction between atracurium and suxamethonium at 50% neuromuscular block using closed-loop feedback control of infusion of atracurium. Br J Anaesth 73:199–203
17. Olkkola KT, Kansanaho M (1995) Quantifying the interaction of vecuronium with enflurane using closed-loop feedback control of vecuronium infusion Acta Anaesthesiol Scard (in press)
18. Ono K, Manabe N, Ohta Y, Morita K, Kosaka F (1989) Influence of suxamethonium on the action of subsequently administered vecuronium or pancuronium. Br J Anaesth 62:324–326
19. Schwilden H (1981) A general method for calculating the dosage scheme in linear pharmacokinetics. Eur J Clin Pharmacol 20:379–386
20. Schwilden H, Olkkola KT (1991) Use of a pharmacokinetic-dynamic model for the automatic feedback control of atracurium. Eur J Clin Pharmacol 40:293–296
21. Sheiner LB, Stanski DR, Vozeh S, Miller RD, Ham J (1979) Simultaneous modeling of pharmacokinetics and pharmacodynamics: application to d-tubocurarine. Clin Pharmacol Ther 25:358–371
22. Vozeh S, Steimer J-L (1985) Feedback control methods for drug dosage optimisation. Concepts, classification and clinical application. Clin Pharmacokinet 10:457–476
23. Wagner JG (1968) Kinetics of pharmacological response. I. Proposed relationships between response and drug concentration in the intact animal and man. J Theor Biol 20:173–201
24. Wait CM, Goat VA, Blogg CE (1987) Feedback control of neuromuscular block: a simple system for atracurium. Anaesthesia 42:1212–1217
25. Walts LF, Dillon JB (1969) Clinical studies of the interaction between d-tubocurarine and succinylcholine. Anesthesiology 31:39–44
26. Walts LF, Rusin DW (1977) The influence of succinylcholine on the duration of pancuronium neuromuscular block. Anesth Analg 56:22–25
27. Webster NR, Cohen AT (1987) Closed-loop administration of atracurium: steady-state neuromuscular block during surgery using a computer-controlled closed-loop atracurium infusion. Anaesthesia 42:1085–1091

Supervisory Adaptive Control
of Arterial Blood Pressure by Vasoactive Agents

N. Ty Smith, J.F. Martin, J. Mandel, A.M. Schneider, and M.L. Quinn

This workshop dwelt at length on the many potential and implemented uses of control systems in anesthesia. We can briefly summarize some of these uses here: the control of the administration of inhaled and injected anesthetic agents, as well as of ancillary agents; the control of ventilation, in all of its aspects; the control of oxygen concentration; and the control of a closed-circuit volume. The advantages of a control system have also been dealt with at length and include the following. (a) Continuous monitoring of the patient and continuous adjustment for the appropriate input or inputs. (b) As a corollary, implementation of a more rapid response to an emergency. (c) Elimination of the factors that can lead to an accident or error: boredom, fatigue, irritation, or distraction. (d) Relief of the anesthetist from simple or boring tasks in complex cases.

However, we should emphasize the disadvantages of a clinical control system, partly because they have not been addressed in this workshop and partly because discussing them openly helps all of us construct better control systems. In essence, control systems are potentially dangerous. (a) They can use the wrong data. For example, if an arterial line is flushed, the numerical value of the blood pressure increases dramatically. If a sodium nitroprusside infusor believes these high values, it could infuse an enormous amount of drug and possibly kill the patient. (b) They can interpret the correct data incorrectly. For example, historically, many blood pressure control systems have interpreted a decrease in MAP as being due to the agent, when it might have been due to one or more of the many causes described below. An adaptive control system, for example, may then adapt itself incorrectly. (c) They can break down, either through mechanical problems, through the software, or through the monitors supplying the information. (d) If they work properly, they can essentially eliminate one or more vital signs as a monitor.

This last disadvantage has been one of the least expected. For example, if a system maintains tight control over blood pressure with nitroprusside, or heart rate with esmolol, blood pressure or heart rate, respectively, are lost as monitors. With our nitroprusside controller, our residents learned to use the infusion rate, which was displayed as a trend graph, as a substitute. As a matter of fact, perhaps because of the novelty, they appeared to learn to use infusion rate even better than arterial pressure, although we did not evaluate that impression. One must ask, however, if an anesthesiologist would be able to adapt so facilely to a multi-drug and/or multivariate controller, where infusion rates may be a function of complex and nonintuitive algorithms.

The early story of control systems in anesthesia – our current stage – could be compared with that of mechanical ventilation. Mechanical ventilation has been a great boon to anesthesiologists, freeing their hands to accomplish other tasks. One could argue that mechanical ventilation has been partly responsible for the development of modern anesthesia. There has been a price to pay for this convenience, however. The accidental airway disconnect was with manual ventilation a quickly discoverable nuisance and with spontaneous ventilation a somewhat greater nuisance that could result in an awake patient. With mechanical ventilation, the disconnect became a fatal mishap, vaulting its way to the most common of critical incidents. These disconnects were frequently responsible for deaths or permanently comatose patients. An entire special group of monitors had to be developed to deal with this serious situation, and it was over a decade before all of the problems were worked out of these monitors. We must not let the history of mechanical ventilation repeat for control systems.

One of many approaches to preventing a repeat of the history of mechanical ventilation is the use of a supervisor, which essentially controls the controller. The rest of this essay describes the control system that we used, the supervisor, and a trial of the system during cardiac surgery. We should first also describe briefly the types of drugs used for control in anesthesia, since understanding these drugs helps us understand the need for supervisory control. The description that follows actually fits most anesthetic drugs, almost by definition. Anesthetists love the type of drugs that have survived the test of time in their field. They act rapidly, they have a short half-life, and they are used extensively and frequently, so that the anesthetist feels comfortable with them. They elicit measurable effects, such as a change in blood pressure or a change in the EEG. These very features also make these drugs dangerous, so that they often also elicit undesirable side effects, such as hypotension or death. These side effects can occur rather rapidly, not surprisingly. Thus, they require continuous, close supervision. The epitome of these drugs is sodium nitroprusside (SNP), a useful drug that can be rapidly lethal. Nitroprusside is a deceptive drug. On the surface, it is very easy to control; pharmacologically, it is dangerous. The potential for death is always there. We have felt, therefore, that any lessons learned from the control of nitroprusside could be useful for the control of other drugs where the potential for disaster is not so immediate.

Our approach to the control of nitroprusside has been two-pronged: the development of a robust controller and of supervisory control. A robust controller is one that does not break down under adverse conditions. This term is best explained by giving some examples. If the anesthetist mixes or enters the wrong concentration of the controlled drug, the controller must realize that fact quickly and adapt to the situation. Similarly, a robust controller must be able to quickly adapt to changes in patient gain. In anesthesia, changes in gain can be caused by several factors, including changes in position, especially Trendelenburg and reverse Trendelenburg, injection of an anesthetic agent, injection of a cardiovascular agent, the initiation of various reflexes, or sudden hemorrhage.

A second example of a situation that controllers find very difficult to handle is a delay, in this case between a change in infusion rate and the achievement of the resulting effect. A good analogy for the reader not acquainted with control systems is to think about what would happen if you were driving an automobile that didn't respond for 30 s to your turning the steering wheel.

Still another difficult situation for the clinical controller occurs when an infusion line becomes disconnected, the disconnection is discovered, and the line is simply reconnected. If the disconnection lasts for several minutes, the mean pressure may be considerably higher than the set point, and the nitroprusside may be infusing at a very rapid rate by the time the line is reconnected. Worse yet, if the controller uses integral control, a phenomenon known as "integral windup" can delay the decrease in infusion rate that should result when MAP starts plummeting. We call this sequence a "double whammy." In addition, it should be intuitive that a combination of delay and a disconnect can create a particularly difficult situation for a controller. The following is a summary of our controller and supervisor, a description of which has appeared in other publications [1–5]. These publications contain many figures, and the interested reader who wishes to explore these controllers in more detail should refer to these papers.

To implement a robust controller, we used a multiple-model adaptive controller (MMAC). Our MMAC contained nine simple models, similar to those described by Slate [7]. Multiple-model adaptive control is based upon the assumption that the patient can be simply represented by one of a finite number of models. For each such model there exists a separate controller. An adaptive mechanism, based on the relative residuals between the models' responses and the patient's response, determines the a posteriori probabilities that the models represent the "patient." These a posteriori probabilities are referred to as the "weights" of the models, and the MMAC controller output is a weighted sum of the outputs from the individual controllers associated with each model. Our MMAC had nine models, which were graded by their sensitivity to SNP, with 1 being very sensitive and 9 being very insensitive.

For each new patient we had to identify the model that was the closest to that patient. To accomplish this task, we chose one of two paths. The conservative approach started with a very slow infusion rate and increased the rate slightly once. If there was little or no response of blood pressure after an appropriate time period, the controller became more aggressive, that it, went to a higher model. It required about 6 min to learn about the patient with this method. Alternatively, an impulse response to a brief bolus of SNP could be used to identify the model.

For each model in the adaptive scheme there has to be a unique regulator. We chose to use a regulator that was a combination of a Pl (proportional-integral) and a series compensator. The Pl was chosen to ensure zero steady-state error for a constant value of the desired pressure ("set point"). The series compensator was designed using pole placement, to achieve our specified step-response characteristics. To achieve greater design flexibility, the state of the Pl was fed back into the series compensator. To minimize the effects of the SNP infusion delay, a Smith predictor was added to the feedback loop. A single Pl was common to all models.

A unique series compensator and Smith predictor were designed specifically for each of the different models.

The need for supervisory control in the clinical situation, especially cardiac surgery, can be stated simply. An aggressive controller is needed to respond to the many and rapid crises that occur. An aggressive controller is dangerous. Something, then, is needed to "control the controller." Thus, although our MMAC controller exceeded the specified design goals, as determined by model and animal studies, it was not ready for the clinical environment. The aggressiveness designed into it to meet the step-response criteria caused it to overreact to large disturbances. Therefore, we designed around the MMAC regulator a supervisor [3, 5, 6] that was able to modify controller gains, to limit infusion rates and rates-of-change of infusion, to stop or start adaptation, to hold infusion rates constant, and to use predicted model response to determine the next infusion rate when MAP measurements were deemed in error.

To provide a comprehensive safety net, the supervisor had three interlocking levels. Each level by itself was designed to add a measure of safety to the controller. The first level set limits on infusion rate and limits on the rate-of-change of infusion rate. The second level was concerned with detecting and reacting to artifactual changes in MAP, such as the changes occurring during a flush of the arterial line. The third level was designed to respond appropriately to potentially dangerous physiological changes in MAP, such as severe hypertensive or hypotensive episodes. Since in a hemodynamically unstable patient a 30-s delay in response to a disturbance can be dangerous, the supervisor was invoked every 2 s, which was also the MMAC control interval.

In all, 30 safety features were incorporated into our supervisor. Why all this fuss about increasing safety in an already robust controller? We felt it necessary because we were testing the system in one of the worst possible situations, cardiac surgery. Cardiac surgery provides a unique testing ground for a control system. The stakes are very high, and a malfunctioning controller could quickly be disastrous. In addition, a large variety of perturbations occur during cardiac surgery. There are about 50 different perturbations, and we have categorized them into five classes. Not only are there a large number of perturbations that can seriously affect a control system, there is also considerable overlap in time, so that several perturbations can occur at once. It is difficult to duplicate this sort of situation with simple models and with animal studies, and the controller can be fine-tuned to only a certain extent prior to clinical studies.

The first level of the supervisor is an extension of a safety feature common to most SNP controllers. SNP is metabolized by the body into cyanide; hence, excess SNP can be toxic to the patient. Therefore, a maximum allowable infusion rate (based on patient weight and drug concentration) is a feature that most SNP controllers have. This maximum infusion rate may protect the patient from cyanide toxicity, but it does not protect the very sensitive patient from experiencing severe hypotensive episodes as a result of an overly aggressive controller chasing a disturbance. To address this problem, we base the infusion rate limit (and limit infusion rate changes) on the models of the model bank. The maximum allowable infusion rate is based on the model with the highest weight. Model 1, the lowest gain model, has the highest maximum allowable infusion rate. All other, higher gain, models have decreasing maximum infusion rates. The maximum infusion rates for each model were determined by the amount of SNP needed to drop the model's MAP by 100 mmHg. When the maximum infusion rate is reached, the supervisor will notify the operator.

This model-based maximum infusion rate is not sufficient to eliminate controller overreaction. As soon as the pressure starts increasing, the model with the highest weight changes from 5 to 1. Thus, the highest maximum allowable infusion rate (model 1) is the only limiting factor. To avoid this shifting of weights impacting on safety of control during a disturbance, we defined the "best" model as the model with the highest weight during the last successful control period (i.e., MAP within ±5 mmHg of the desired pressure). This "best" model is then the model on which the infusion rate limits are based. Therefore, when a disturbance occurs that suddenly changes the weights erroneously (by changing MAP suddenly), the safety of the controller is not impacted. The cyanide toxicity limit on SNP infusion is also present, and if this level is more restrictive than the "best" model-based limit, it becomes the limiting factor on SNP infusion rate.

This first level of the supervisor has an additional feature that rapidly changes (increases) the "best" model and resets the controller if an error is detected during initial identification of patient sensitivity. These identification errors can be caused by an incorrectly filled SNP infusion line or a significant increase in the patient's baseline (no SNP) MAP. Either of these will result in an initial underestimation of patient sensitivity, resulting in poor initial control. Therefore, if such a problem is encountered, the "best" model is increased (e.g., from model 3 to model 4) and the control variable is reset to match that model.

The second level of the supervisor detects unphysiological changes in MAP (artifact). Such changes are a product of arterial blood sampling and flushing or manipulation of the arterial line. In these cases there is an extremely rapid change in MAP (often rising to 300 mm Hg). To prevent the controller from overreacting to such a disturbance, a routine was developed to detect bad MAP measurements and discard them. Rather than simply basing control on the last good MAP measurement throughout the artifact, which could lead to problems if the patients's MAP were changing, the controller predicts the MAP response of the patient based on the "best" model. This predicted MAP is then used for control calculations. Control continues using the predicted MAP until either the end of the disturbance is detected, or the disturbance has continued for more than 2.5 min, in which case the controller will notify the operator of a problem and stop the infusion.

In addition to detecting arterial line flushes and blood drawings, this level of the supervisor can also detect a clogged arterial line. If this occurs, as with the previous situation, control is based on the "best" model's predicted MAP until the problem is fixed, or until a specified period of time has elapsed.

The third level of the supervisor responds to potentially dangerous physiological changes in MAP. If the patient suddenly hemorrhages or is given a bolus of a vasodilating drug, his MAP can decrease dramatically. With SNP still being infused this could result in a severe hypotensive episode or even death. Therefore, this supervisor level looks for rapidly, but still physiologically, decreasing MAP and/or very low MAP and responds by immediately turning off the SNP infusion. In both cases, SNP infusion is maintained at zero until MAP rises above a threshold, at which time the controller is reset to a conservative steady-state infusion rate, based on the "best" model, to try to reduce the amount of hypertensive rebound and avoid repeating the drop in MAP.

Hypotensive episodes can also occur as a result of controller action, for example, as an overreaction to a bolus of a vasoconstricting drug. The first level of the supervisor reduces this problem, although there still can be a significant hypotensive rebound. Therefore, in addition to looking for and responding to rapid drops in MAP, the third level of the supervisor also responds to rapid increases in MAP. A rapid rise in MAP may not be simply caused by a vasoconstricting drug injection; it may be a true physiological change. If MAP rises too high, a weak artery could rupture, stitches might leak, or a stroke could occur. It would appear then that the controller should respond to such increases by aggressively increasing the infusion rate (within limits of the first level of the supervisor). However, this can result in a hypotensive rebound if the increase is only transient. Therefore, this part of the supervisor allows the controller to respond quickly to an increasing MAP, but when it determines (by peak MAP followed by a sharply decreasing MAP) that it was only a transient rise, the supervisor takes over and uses a form of expert control to bring MAP back to the set point without severe overshoot. The expert control algorithm includes such features as not allowing the SNP infusion rate to increase once MAP has passed a peak (but only for a specific amount of time), and making large-step decreases in SNP according to the slope of the MAP decrease. The controller (PID with pole placement) is reset and restarted when MAP nears the set point or after a specified period of time.

As a backup to the rapid-drop feature, the third level of the supervisor also modifies the controller, and control signal, in response to a MAP that is decreasing sharply as it passes through the set point, but not at a rate sufficient to trigger the automatic rapid-drop shut off. SNP infusion rate is decreased, outside of the PI/pole-placement controller, as a function of the slope of MAP as it crosses the set point. This feature attempts to minimize the amount the MAP drops below the set point.

The system described above was studied in 19 patients undergoing cardiac surgery, after Institutional Review Board Approval and individual written consent were obtained. In the 19 patients analyzed, control was maintained for a total of 61 h.

The cardiac surgery environment was even more hostile to a control system than we had anticipated. There was a greater variety of disturbances and a much greater frequency of disturbance than we had previously thought. Table 1 contains a list of events that were judged by the anesthesia team to have significantly altered MAP and, therefore, to have challenged the controller. In most instances, the controller, through the action of the supervisor, was able to respond to the disturbance in an acceptable manner and continue control. For example, there were 103 flushes of the arterial line. The controller, through the supervisor, correctly identified 97 flushes (94.2%) and simply ignored the erroneous pressure measurements. In four of the six remaining flushes, the supervisor recognized the return of the signal and adjusted the rate itself. Two of the episodes required manual intervention. These were the only two occurrences of intervention in the entire 61 h, about one intervention every 30 h.

We defined a hypotensive episode as one where MAP fell more than 10 mm Hg below the set point and lasting more than ten seconds. There were 178 episodes during the 61 h of control. In response to these episodes, the controller turned off the SNP 100 times, decreased the infusion rate 65 times, and maintained a constant infusion rate the remaining 13 times. The infusion rate was never maintained constant for more than 90 s, and no intervention was required during the hypotensive episodes. We do not have data on the comparable response of the human controller to such hypotensive episodes.

These studies were begun more than 10 years ago, and the results were perhaps more successful than we deserved. The clinical system was implemented on a Macintosh Plus, with the only Macintosh A-D board available at the time. An upgraded system was implemented on a Macintosh II and used an internal board. The lessons that we learned can be implemented on the better computers that are available today. For example, by examining the waveform of the arterial pressure, it will be much easier to do on-line signal analysis and determine more reliably when a true pressure is not available.

The supervisor was tested on simulations and animal studies with artificially induced disturbances. During these preliminary studies the controller was given sufficient time (20–30 min) to respond to each disturbance, to fully judge its performance, before another disturbance was initiated. During cardiac surgery, the supervisor did not have this luxury. We estimated 600 disturbances during the 61 h of control, or about one disturbance every 5–6 min. Of course the disturbances did not occur at regular 5-min intervals. Rather, they often occurred in groups, severely testing the supervisor.

The controller responded appropriately to the majority of disturbances, including the rapidly occurring ones. One of the events we were interested in was the controller's response to hypotensive episodes. We defined a hypotensive episode as any period of 10 s or more in which the MAP started within or above a ± 5 mmHg bound around the set point and then fell to 10 mmHg or more below the set point. There were 178 such episodes, many of which occurred in rapid succession, that matched these criteria. The controller responded appropriately, by rapidly dropping the SNP infusion rate, to 165 (93%) of them. We have not evaluated the potential benefit of the controller's appropriate response to hypotensive episodes in the 165 instances in which a distracted anesthesiologist might have failed to lower the SNP infusion rate.

In summary, we hope that others may benefit from our experiences, especially those factors that need improvement. We are optimistic about the future of control systems in the fields of anesthesia and critical care but suggest that great caution and care are advisable.

References

1. Martin JF, Schneider AM, Smith NT (1987) Multiple-model adaptive control of blood pressure using sodium nitroprusside. IEEE Trans Biomed Eng 34(8):603–611
2. Martin J, Smith N Ty, Quinn M, Schneider A (1991) Supervisory adaptive control of arterial pressure during cardiac surgery. IEEE Trans Biomed Eng 39:389–393
3. Martin J, Schneider A, Quinn M, Smith N Ty (1991) Improved safety and efficacy in adaptive control of arterial blood pressure through the use of a supervisor. IEEE Trans Biomed Eng 39:381–388
4. Smith N Ty, Quinn ML, Scanlon TS, Martin JF, Voss GI (1992) Performance evaluation of a closed-loop sodium nitroprusside delivery device during hypotensive anesthesia in mongrol dogs. In: Ikeda et al (eds) Computing and monitoring in anesthesia and intensive care. Springer, Berlin Heidelberg New York, pp 147–149
5. Martin JF, Smith N Ty, Quinn MB, Masuzawa T, Mandel J (1992) Adaptive control of arterial pressure: a supervisor can improve safety and efficacy. In: Ikeda et al (eds) Computing and Monitoring in anesthesia and Intensive Care, K. Springer, Berlin Heidelberg New York, pp 150–152
6. Martin JF (1987) Multiple-model adaptive control of blood pressure using sodium nitroprusside. PhD dissertation, Department of Applied Mechanics and Engineering Sciences, University of California, San Diego
7. Slate JB (1980) Model-based design of a controller for infusing sodium nitroprusside during post surgical hypertension. PhD dissertation, Department of Electrical Engineering, U. Wisconsin-Madison

New Drug-Delivery Devices for Volatile Anesthetics

E.-G. Scharmer

Introduction

Modern inhalational anesthesia is strongly connected with the administration of volatile anesthetic agents. Most of these agents exist at ambient temperature and pressure as a mixture of liquid and saturated vapor. Only nitrous oxide is in the gaseous phase under these conditions.

The vapor component of the volatile anesthetic has to be separated from the liquid component by technical means and has to be transported together with a carrier-gas flow via the breathing system to the patient. The amount of vapor which reaches the patient must be controlled very carefully during this process.

Most devices used today for enriching the carrier gas with the vapor of an anesthetic agent are so-called plenum vaporizers. New plenum vaporizer devices are under development for dosing the new agent sevoflurane.

Whereas vaporization of volatile anesthetics in the fresh gas flow is the most common method of adding these agents to the breathing system, direct liquid injection is a very old technique. A revival of direct injection has been described by Weingarten and Lowe [1]. The only device available on the market which uses direct liquid injection is the Physioflex anesthesia machine.

Other principles for administration of halogenated anesthetic agents have been discussed in the literature, for example the Boston Anesthesia System by Cooper and co-workers in 1978 [2] and the Penlon microprocessor controlled Vaporizer by Hahn and co-workers in 1986 [3]. These devices are not commercially available to date.

The purpose of this paper is to describe new devices for the dosing of volatile anesthetics which are available on the market or will be available in the near future.

These devices can be classified according to three different physical principles:

1. Evaporation without the utilization of external energy
   The well-known plenum vaporizers are developed according to this principle, which was recently applied to the new Dräger 19.3 sevoflurane vaporizer.
2. Evaporation by heating and pressurizing
   Electrical energy can be used to support and control evaporation of anesthetic agents. Gambro Engström applied this principle to the Elsa and to the new EAS

9010 Anesthesia System and Ohmeda designed the Tec 6 desflurane vaporizer using this technology.
3. Dosing of liquids
   Direct liquid injection into the breathing system is used in the Physioflex anesthesia machine.
   Dosing of liquids into the fresh gas will be the technological basis of the Dräger electronic anesthetic agent dosing device.

Despite all the different technical possibilities for administering volatile anesthetics, new devices have to meet certain design criteria there must be:

High standards in quality and reliability
High accuracy of the delivered vapor concentration
Independence of the delivered vapor concentration from
- fresh-gas flow
- carrier-gas composition
- ambient temperature and temperature variation due to evaporation
- ambient pressure and back pressure variation due to artificial ventilation

Plenum Vaporizers

Most of the modern calibrated vaporizers for volatile anesthetics are plenum vaporizers. They are available for the most common agents and from many manufacturers.

The functional principle is mainly gas-flow partitioning (see Fig. 1); i.e., the incoming gas flow is divided into two parts: F_1 and F_2. F_1 bypasses the vaporization chamber and is led directly to the output. It has no contact with the liquid anesthetic agent. F_2, the smaller part, can be adjusted and is fed through the vaporizing chamber where it becomes saturated with the vapor of the anesthetic agent. The final concentration of the anesthetic gas leaving the vaporizer at the fresh-gas outlet depends on the splitting ratio F_1/F_2.

Plenum vaporizers have very sophisticated designs in respect of temperature compensation, independence of anesthetic concentration of the total flow, and alternating back-pressure compensation due to artifical ventilation. These general specifications are defined in national and international standards.

Although these vaporizers fill most demands of standard anesthesia with respect to safety and reliability, they have limited accuracy at the edges of the specified operation, as was described by Gilly [4]. In addition, they have no electronic interface for communication with data-management systems, and there is no possibility for external control. Thus they can normally not be a part of an anesthetic agent control device.

The Dräger 19.3 sevoflurane vaporizer is a new plenum vaporizer. The new volatile agent sevoflurane requires a redesigning of the plenum vaporizer for halothane, enflurane, and isoflurane to achieve the same technical performance. Because of the higher MAC value of sevoflurane compared with the other volatile

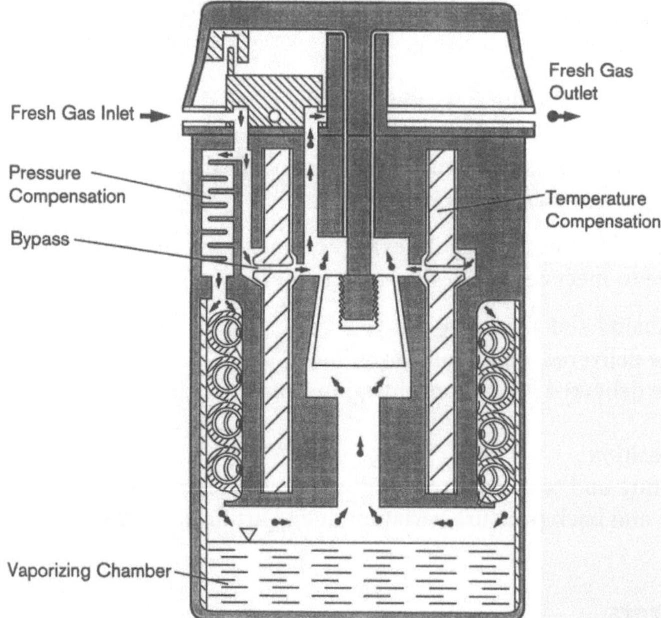

Fig. 1. Dräger plenum vaporizer vapor 19

anesthetics, the dosing range of the sevoflurane vaporizer has been increased to 8% V/V. The very high evaporative cooling at 8% V/V makes it necessary to redesign the temperature-compensating mechanism.

The Tec 6 Desflurane Vaporizer

Desflurane is a new anesthetic agent which has unusual pharmacological and physical properties in comparison to other agents commonly in use. Desflurane reveals a moderate potency with a MAC value of 6–7% V/V [5]. The vapor pressure of desflurane is three to four times higher than that of the other inhaled anesthetics [6]. Its boiling point is 23.5°C [7], which is very near to room temperature.

For these reasons, conventional vaporizer technology is unsuitable for desflurane. To solve these problems, Ohmeda has introduced the Tec 6 vaporizer, with electric heating and pressurizing to achieve controlled vaporization of desflurane.

The Ohmeda Tec 6 vaporizer is designed to dose desflurane up to 18% V/V in the fresh gas. It is equipped with a "Selectatec" mechanical interface, needs electrical power for heating, but has no electronic interface for external communication.

External heating is necessary, because the absolute amount of desflurane vaporized during a given time period is considerably higher than that of other

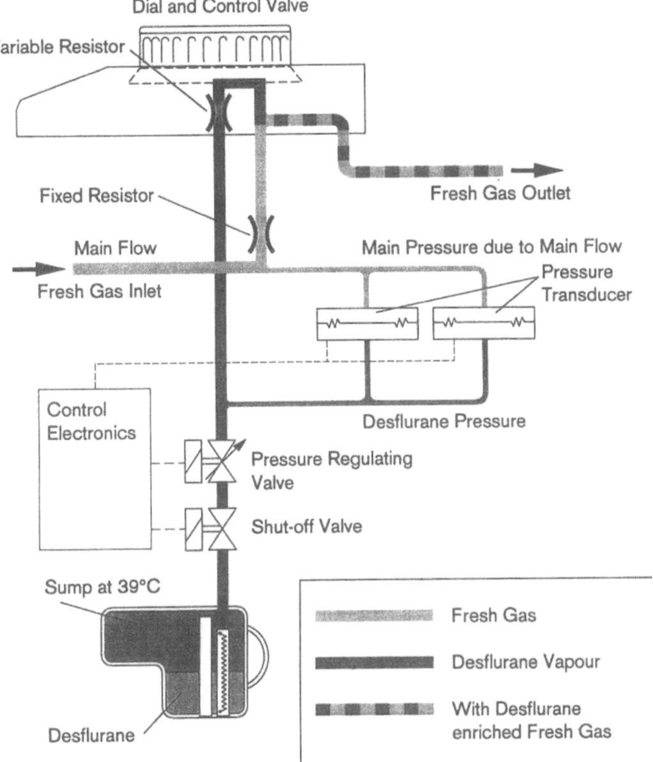

Fig. 2. Tec 6 desflurane vaporizer. (From [9])

anesthetics. Because of the excessive cooling, traditional methods of mechanical temperature compensation will fail.

The functional principle is shown in a simplified diagram (Fig. 2). Andrews and Johnston [9]. There are two independent gas circuits, the fresh-gas (light gray) and the vapor circuit (dark gray). The incoming fresh gas passes through a fixed resistor and exits at the fresh-gas outlet.

Desflurane is evaporated at the sump, which is electrically heated to 39°C; this is well above the boiling point of desflurane. The vapor passes through a pressure-regulating valve and a manually controlled variable restrictor which determines the desflurane output concentration.

Internal electronic control regulates the vapor pressure to equal the main pressure due to the fresh-gas flow. This working pressure is constant at a fixed fresh-gas flow rate. If the operator increases the fresh-gas flow, more back pressure is exerted upon the transducer and the working pressure of the vaporizer increases. There is a linear relationship between fresh-gas flow rate and working pressure.

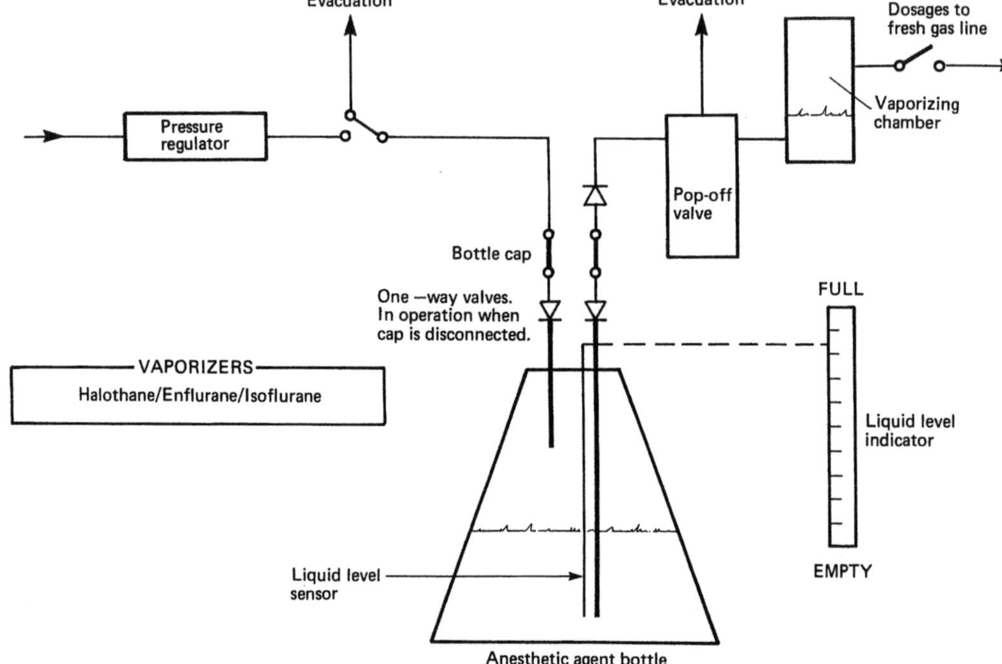

Fig. 3. Engström Elsa vaporizer. (Courtesy of Gambro Engström, Sweden)

The Engström Elsa Vaporizer

The Engström vaporizer is an integral part of the Elsa anesthesia system. There are three independent vaporizing systems for halothane, enflurane, and isoflurane. The vaporizing principle is based on pressurizing and heating, as shown in Fig. 3.

Normally, three separate volatile anesthetic agents are connected in their original bottles at the rear of the machine. The required agent is selected by pressing a key on the front panel. As a result, the corresponding vaporizing chamber is heated to a constant temperature, which is specific for each agent.

The active vaporizer system is charged with oxygen at a constant pressure of about 0.4 bar. This pressure forces the liquid anesthetic to flow from the original bottle to the vaporizing pressure chamber. The evaporation generates a counterpressure which is controlled by the temperature of the heating element. At the pressure equilibrium there is 100% anesthetic agent vapor at a pressure of 0.4 bar.

Opening of the digital magnetic valve adds known quanta of anesthetic vapor to the fresh-gas flow. The stroke frequency is controlled according to the desired concentration of the anesthetic agent, which can be set up to 8% V/V in the fresh gas.

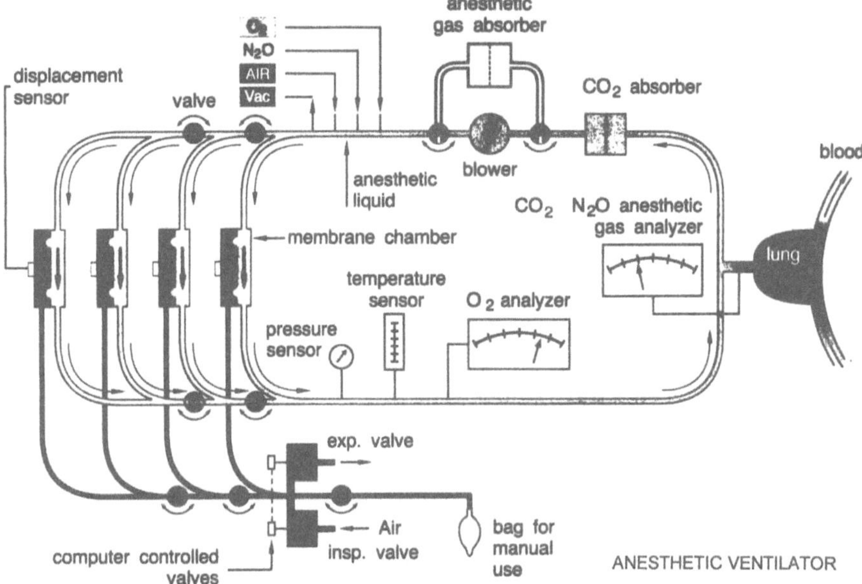

Fig. 4. Physioflex vaporizing system

The Physioflex Vaporizer

The anesthetic vaporizer integrated in the Physioflex anesthesia system is based on the principle of liquid anesthetic injection from a syringe directly into the breathing system (see Fig. 4). The amount of liquid anesthetic is immediately evaporated by a high constant gas flow of 70 l/min, which is generated by a blower. Quick transport of the agent and equilibration of concentration are therefore guaranteed.

A gas analyzer, which is an integral part of the system, measures the inspired and expired anesthetic gas concentration. According to this measurement, the motor of the syringe pump is controlled via a PID algorithm to keep the end-tidal anesthetic gas concentration constant. This end-tidal concentration can be adjusted up to 2.5% V/V.

Thus the electronic control of the anesthetic vapor-dosing unit is used to create an automated anesthesia feedback system. In a recent development, Physio changed the control to keep the inspiratory gas concentration constant.

Similar to the Engström machine, the Physioflex accepts the original bottles as the liquid agent supply for halothane, enflurane, and isoflurane. The syringe is automatically filled with the selected agent at the beginning of the anesthesia and in the meantime, if necessary.

Digital Volumetric Dosing

A digitally controlled volumetric metering system for volatile agents consists mainly of a liquid pump mechanism. A fixed volume V of a known quantum is filled with liquid agent at a frequency f. The total liquid flow rate $\dot{V}_A$ is the product of volume V times frequency f:

$$\dot{V}_A = V * f$$

This volume is added to the fresh-gas flow, where the evaporation is supported by adding the necessary amount of heat.

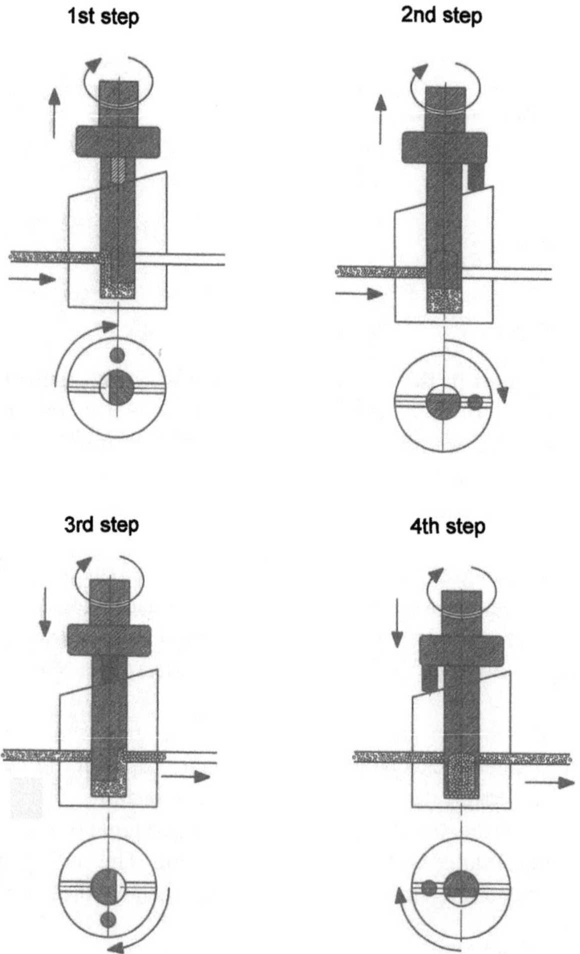

Fig. 5. Micropump for liquid anesthetic agent. First step, loading of the volume with liquid agent; second step, closing the liquid inlet; third step, dumping the liquid agent to the liquid outlet; forth step, closing the liquid outlet and return to the first position

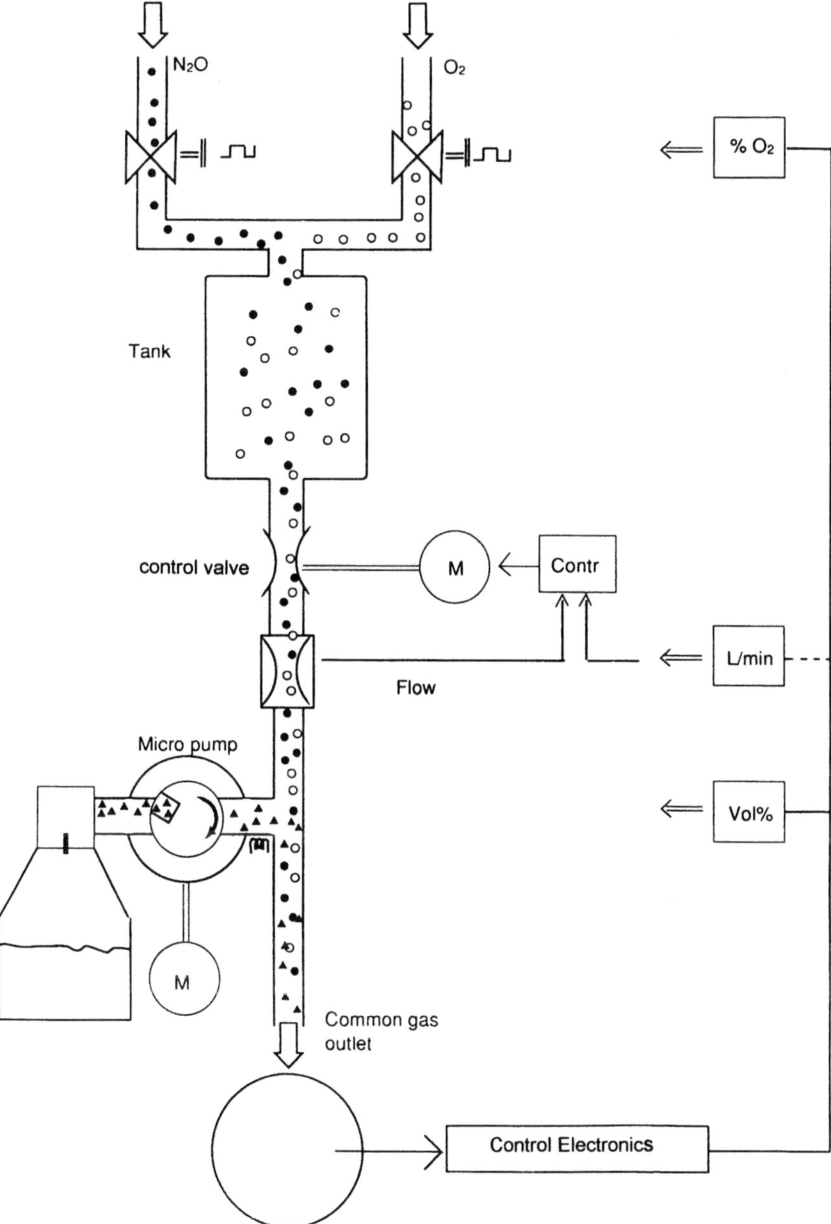

Fig. 6. Digitally controlled anesthetic gas and agent delivery system

This dosing mechanism possesses an inherently high accuracy, because the volume and the frequency can be determined very precisely. On the other hand, there is a linear relationship between the delivered liquid flow rate and the product of frequency and volume; therefore a corrective algorithm is not necessary for this dosing process. In addition, temperature effects are very small compared with conventional plenum vaporizers. Back pressure, gas type, and total flow effects are negligible [8].

In designing a suitable micropump for this application, one has to ensure sufficient lifetime and deal with the sticking effects of thymol (a stabilizing chemical additive in halothane). Based on their experience in this field, Dräger developed a micropump which has no valves and no seals and is inherently safe from unintentional liquid agent flow in case of a failure.

The micropump consists of a cylinder with liquid inlet and outlet and a piston. The cylinder has a tilted surface, so that the movement of the piston has an additional oscillatory component besides rotation. The pump operates in four steps, as shown in Fig. 5.

During one revolution $5.3\,\mu l$ of liquid agent is transported. The whole device is designed to deliver up to 18% V/V anesthetic vapor in the fresh gas, which has a maximum total flow of 12 l/min. This means that the liquid rate has to have an extremely high dynamic range, from about $10\,\mu l$/min to 8.9 ml/min.

The described micropump is embedded in an digitally controlled anesthetic gas-delivery device, as shown in Fig. 6. The tank is filled with the desired gas mixture (air is not shown in the picture) until a defined pressure is reached. This pressure is held constant during the time of operation. The desired oxygen concentration is defined by the stroke freqencies of the digital magnetic valves.

A magnetic valve with a proportional control defines the amount of fresh gas which is led to the common gas outlet. This valve is set according to the pressure drop across the laminar flow resistance. The pressure drop is proportional to the total fresh-gas flow.

Similar to the Engström and the Physioflex systems, the liquid is taken out of the original bottle, but in contrast to them, the described device is suitable for administering all anesthetics which are now used or which will be in use in the future: halothane, enflurane, isoflurane, sevoflurane, and desflurane. The dosing of liquids is carried out without overpressure; therefore, the total leakage of the device is minimized to 0.5 ml/24 h. Modular and compact design allows dosing in the fresh-gas as well as closed-loop application with control of inspiratory or expiratory concentration.

Conclusion

Besides the well-known plenum vaporizers, there are some new devices for dosing liquid anesthetics on the market which are based on electronic technology and control. These electronic devices are suitable as integral parts of modern anesthesia work stations with internal data communication and control. Although not yet routinely used, new electronic devices for volatile anesthetics will be the basis of the future anesthesia work station, which will include:

- Closed-loop control for volatile agents and oxygen
- Ergonomic control, making low-flow anesthesia easy to use
- Precise evaluation of drug consumption
- Communication to data-management systems
- Minimal pollution of the environment

References

1. Weingarten M, Lowe HJ (1973) A new circuit injection technic for syringe-measured administration of methoxyflurane: a new dimension in anaesthesia. Anesth Analg 52:634
2. Cooper JB, Newbower RS, Moore JW, Trautman ED (1978) A new anesthesia delivery system. Anaesthesiology 49:310
3. Hahn CEW, Palayiwa E, Sugg BR, Lindsay-Scott D (1986) A microprocessor controlled anaesthetic vaporizer. Br J Anaesth 58:1161
4. Gilly H (1989) Limitations of present dosing systems for gases and volatile anaesthetics. In: van Ackern K, Frankenberger H, Konecny E, Steinbereithner K (eds) Quantitative anaesthesia. Springer, Berlin Heidelberg New York (Anaesthesiology and intensive case medicine, vol 204)
5. Rampil IJ, Lockhart SH, Zwass MS et al (1991) Clinical characteristics of desflurane in surgical patients: minimum alveolar concentration. Anestesiology 74:429
6. Andrews JJ, Johnston RV, Kramer GC (1993) Consequences of misfilling contemporary vaporizers with desflurane. Can J Anesth 40:71
7. Jones RM (1990) Desflurane and sevoflurane: inhalation anaesthetics for this decade? Br J Anesth 65:527
8. Wallroth CF, Jaklitsch R, Wied HA (1989) Technical realisation of quantitative metering and ventilation. In: van Ackern K, Frankenberger H, Konecny E, Steinbereithner K (eds) Quantitative anaesthesia. Springer, Berlin Heidelberg New York (Anaesthesiology and intensive case medicine, vol 204)
9. Andrews JJ, Johnston RV (1993) The new tec 6 desflurane vaporizer. Anesth Analg 76:1338

New Drug-Delivery Systems for Intravenous Anesthetics

P.S.A. GLASS, J.R. JACOBS, and T. QUILL

Introduction

The development of intravenous drug administration was initiated by Wren when he utilized a quill and bladder to administer substances intravenously following the description by Harvey of the circulatory system in 1628 [1]. The next major advance in drug-delivery systems was the development of the hollow needle and syringe by Alexander Wood [1]. Today, the needle and syringe remains the most commonly used drug delivery system for the administration of intravenous anesthetics. The introduction of several newer drugs and a greater appreciation of pharmacokinetics and pharmacodynamics, combined with technological advances, have resulted in several new developments in intravenous drug-delivery systems.

An important concept (beginning to enjoy general acceptance) is that it is more rational to give intravenous anesthetic drugs continuously, rather than intermittently or by high dose at the initiation of anesthesia. Furthermore, while there is a significant degree of interindividual variability in the response of the patient to a particular drug plasma level attained, the application of pharmacokinetic principles to administer a drug on the basis of *plasma level* rather than *dose* moves the clinician one step closer to better control of the drug at its effect site. The application of pharmacokinetics to the dosing scheme may be achieved manually or it may be incorporated directly into the drug-delivery system. On this basis, there are either manual or automated intravenous drug-delivery systems.

Automated drug delivery implies that some form of electronic and/or mechanical instrumentation performs dose *rate* adjustments independent of human intervention. This is in contrast to a manual drug delivery system, for which the human operator makes all dose rate adjustments.

Manual Intravenous Drug-Delivery Systems

As described above, it is desirable to manipulate the plasma concentration of intravenously administered anesthetic drugs in a continuous and predictable manner analogous to the administration of the potent inhalation agents. Accordingly, an understanding of pharmacokinetics is likely to improve the clinician's ability to provide anesthesia with intravenous drugs when using a manual delivery system.

Mathematically rigorous approaches to the development of pharmacokinetically oriented manual infusion schemes for intravenous drugs have been described by many authors [2, 3]. Most notably, the two-step infusion technique developed by Wagner [4] is widely used. This and other schemes consist essentially of a loading bolus or infusion, followed by a maintenance infusion to achieve a relatively stable plasma drug concentration. The loading dose quickly raises the plasma concentration to the desired level, and the maintenance infusion replaces drug lost to metabolism or excretion. Simplistically, the loading dose could be a bolus of an amount adequate to fill the entire volume of distribution

$$\text{Bolus} = Cp_d \cdot V_d,$$

or just large enough to fill the central compartment

$$\text{Bolus} = Cp_d \cdot V_1,$$

either of which would be followed by an infusion to replace drug lost due to clearance. For a drug exhibiting one-compartment kinetics, the regimen

$$\text{Infusion Rate} = Cp_d \cdot k_{10} \cdot V_1 = Cp_d \cdot \text{Clearance},$$

would achieve Cp_d precisely. For drugs exhibiting multi- compartment kinetics, *as almost all do*, the loading dose based on the volume of distribution at steady state results in plasma concentrations that are much greater than Cp_d for an extended period of time, while the smaller loading does, based on the initial volume of distribution, results in plasma concentrations that fall below the desired level due to distribution until the infusion achieves its steady-state level. In neither case has drug distribution been appropriately considered.

In 1968, Kruger-Thiemer described the infusion regimen theoretically required to quickly achieve and maintain a constant plasma concentration of an intravenously administered drug whose kinetics are described by a two-compartment model [5]. This regimen was popularized as the "BET scheme" by Schwilden et al. [6–8]. A bolus ("B") to fill the central compartment to the desired concentration is followed by a constant infusion to replace drug being eliminated ("E") from the central compartment by excretion or metabolism. Superimposed on this is an exponentially declining infusion to replace drug being transferred ("T") into the peripheral compartment. The infusion scheme precisely obtains and maintains the desired concentration, as it appropriately accounts for redistribution. It is virtually impossible to manually compute and implement precisely a BET scheme. The clinical implication is that to maintain a desired concentration manually, a high infusion rate is initially implemented and then decreased with time.

The control of the infusion rate can be obtained by numerous mechanisms. The most simple is to control the rate of fluid flow produced by gravity. The CAIR clamp and Dial-a-Flo (Abbott Laboratories) are typical examples. They are not accurate devices, however, and infusion pumps that are capable of delivering very accurate infusion rates are therefore more suitable for the administration of the potent drugs given during anesthesia. These infusion pumps can be classified as either controller/gravimetric pumps or positive displacement pumps. Explicit in

Table 1. Essential features for infusion devices (from [9])

---

1. Electrical safety
2. Air detection
3. Occlusion alarm – time to alarm $<3\,$min
4. Maximum infusion pressure $<250\,$mmHg
5. Flow rate accuracy of $\pm2\%$
6. Prevention of free flow
7. Continuous flow (i.e., minimal intermittent flow)
8. Function unaffected by electromagnetic fields

---

their title, gravimetric pumps contain mechanisms that control the rate of flow produced by gravity, whereas positive displacement pumps contain active pumping mechanisms. Independent of the mechanism utilized to control flow rate, there are several features that are essential for all infusion devices used for the delivery of intravenous anesthetic drugs [9]. These features are listed in Table 1. Gravimetric pumps, though very accurate, are limited as to the maximal infusion rates they can deliver, and positive displacement pumps are therefore the primary infusion devices used for intravenous anesthetic drug delivery. Positive displacement pumps have either a peristaltic or a piston mechanism. Infusion pumps with a piston mechanism utilize either a to-and-fro or a screw motion to drive the piston. The screw mechanism utilizes the rotation of the screw to drive a plunger to displace fluid (e.g., a syringe pump). The thread of the screw and rate of rotation will determine the flow rate. Rack and pinion or belt-driven mechanisms provide a to-and-fro piston motion to pump fluid. There are many positive displacement pumps presently available; however, several have now been designed specifically for the administration of intravenous drugs during anesthesia. To aid in pharmacokinetic-based infusion schemes, the first requirement of an infusion pump used for intravenous anesthetics is that it can be programmed to administer both a rapid infusion (bolus) and a maintenance infusion.

There are also other features that make infusion pumps more suitable for the administration of intravenous anesthetics [9]. These are listed in Table 2. Several other new pumps have attempted to provide the features necessary for more optimal intravenous anesthetic drug delivery. The most significant advance in commercially available infusion pumps has been the incorporation of a calculator function within the pump. The calculator pump allows the user to enter the weight of the patient and the dose (i.e., mg/kg) or infusion rate (μg/kg/min) to be administered. The concentration of the drug is either preset or entered by the user. The pump automatically calculates the volume (ml) or infusion rate (ml/h) and administers this to the patient. This has markedly simplified the manual application of pharmacokinetically based infusion schemes of intravenous drugs during anesthesia.

Another area of pump development is in providing multiple channels in a single compact unit. Commercial pumps have successfully combined three or four channels into a unit similar in size to many presently available single-channel pumps.

Table 2. Desirable features for infusion pumps (from [9])

1. Versatility
    a) Choice of bolus or infusion mode
    b) Internal calculator for choice of dosing scheme
    c) Adaptable for use with all anesthetic drugs
    d) Choice of infusion rates from 0 to 1500 with 0.1-ml/h resolution in 0–100 ml/h and 1-ml/h resolution in the range 100–1500 ml/h
    e) Choice of up to four separate channels, with no opportunity for backflow or drug mixing proximal to the i.v. cannula
2. Light weight
3. Automatic priming of administration set
4. Clear display of drug administered and infusion rate
5. Simple protocols for initiation or change of infusion rates
6. Digital interface for record keeping or external automated control
7. Automated drug recognition
8. Alarm for tubing disconnect

Major advances have been made in pump technology and design, enabling intravenous anesthetics to be conveniently delivered by continuous infusion. However, no commercially available device for the delivery of intravenous anesthetics approaches the convenience of the present-day vaporizer. It is therefore desirable to take intravenous drug delivery systems one step further, beyond a "calculator" pump to a truly "smart" pump by utilizing automated drug delivery.

Automated Drug Delivery

As stated above, automated drug delivery implies that some form of electronic and/or mechanical instrumentation performs dose rate adjustments independent of human intervention (in contrast to the manual devices described above). The desired value (e.g., predicted drug plasma level or clinical response) is still chosen by the clinician. Preprogrammed dosing (either bolus or infusion) is the simplest form of automated drug delivery. An example of a preprogrammed automated infusion pump is that developed by Crankshaw, which enables the user to select a single target concentration [10]. This pump has been used succesfully in the administration of alfentanil, thiopental, and methohexital. The primary disadvantage of such systems is that the user cannot alter the set point; therefore, the intravenous anesthetic cannot be titrated to the desired effect.

More sophisticated automated drug delivery is either model-based (a form of open-loop control) or closed loop. Both model-based and closed-loop systems require a *set point* (Fig. 1). The set point is the quantifiable end point (e.g., plasma concentration or % T1 of the EMG) related to the clinical objective (level of anestheia, neuromuscular blockade, etc.) Thus, the set point is the value that the automated control system is attempting to control. The *feedback signal* is the actual measured (e.g., % T1 of the EMG) or simulated (e.g., predicted plasma

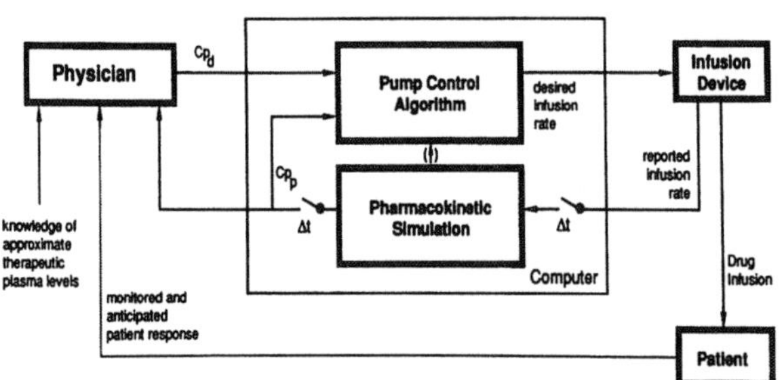

Fig. 1. Components of a typical automated drug delivery system. (With permission from [16])

concentration from pharmacokinetic simulation) value that results from the automated delivery process.

Closed-loop drug delivery is the ideal means of drug administration, but there is not always a measurable feedback signal. Model-based drug delivery is therefore an important alternative in circumstances where the feedback signal cannot be measured and an appropriate model is available. A mathematical equation that can simulate the process that produces the set point provides the model. Consequently, the efficacy of any model-based control system is dependent on how well the model represents the process under control. The *control signal* (which for automated drug delivery is the dosing scheme) is generated by a set of instructions known as an *algorithm*. An algorithm is ordinarily designed to keep the control variable as close as possible to the set point value. The set point and feedback values, in turn, act on the algorithm to generate the control signal. The control signal directs the *actuator* (i.e., instructs it to deliver the dosage regimen prescribed by the algorithm to the patient), thereby producing the intervention necessary to obtain the set point. This intervention results in a new feedback control signal, and the process repeats itself so as to maintain the patient at the set point. In an adaptive control system the algorithm is altered/ adapted to the individual's unique response to the intervention produced by the actuator. For example, in a closed-loop system to control T1 of the EMG the algorithm may prescribe an increase in the infusion of atracurium of 1 μg/kg/min when the T1 exceeds the set point (e.g., 10% of the control value). While this may generally be an appropriate prescription, a change in infusion rate of this magnitude may cause a much greater drop in T1 in a sensitive individual than desired. An adaptive controller will, after experience with the patient, learn the individual's sensitivity and utilizing this, will change the algorithm so that the control signal (dosing scheme) results in an intervention by the actuator that brings the feedback signal more closely to the set point.

Model-based Automated Drug Delivery

The complex dosage regimens, which require infusion rates that change continuously as a function of time until steady state is achieved, cannot be computed or implemented accurately manually but can be easily implemented using automated drug delivery. As personal computers began to become commonplace, Schwilden and his colleagues in Bonn [6–8] interfaced a microcomputer to an infusion pump and demonstrated the first clinical application of automated drug delivery utilizing the BET infusion scheme originally described by Kruger-Theimer 10 years earlier [5]. They wrote a software program using the theorem of superposition to compute and implement BET infusion regimens in real time to obtain plasma drug concentrations specified by the anesthesiologist.

Open-Loop Target-Control Drug Delivery

The BET infusion regimen is now just one of several algorithms that have been used to provide pharmacokinetic model-driven infusion of anesthetic drugs through *computer assisted continuous infusion* (CACI) devices [9]. All of these algorithms have been derived by manipulating a pharmacokinetic model. Each prototype CACI implementation has been somewhat different, but all are conceptually similar. Each consists of a microcomputer interfaced to a drug infusion pump, with a novel software program written by the investigators to implement the model-driven infusions. In using the device (Fig. 2), the anesthesiologist specifies (via the computer keyboard) a target (set point) plasma drug concentration, which is based on monitored and anticipated patient response, on the current

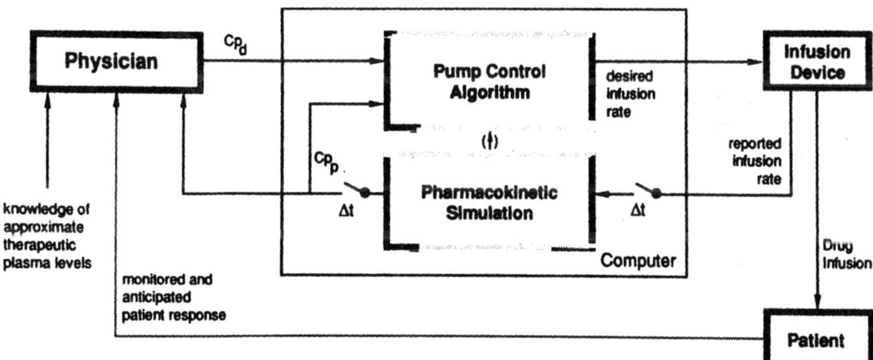

Fig. 2. Authors' approach to pharmacokinetic model-driven drug delivery. In this computer-assisted continuous infusion (CACI) device, the physician enters the desired plasma drug concentration (Cp_d). An infusion device-control algorithm uses a pharmacokinetic model for the drug being infused to determine what the infusion rate should be for the next infusion interval (e.g., 10 s). The infusion device delivers drug to the patient, and the infusion rate is fed into a simulation of the pharmacokinetic model to compute the current predicted plasma drug concentration (Cp_p). The state variables computed in the simulation are available to the algorithm. On the basis of monitored and anticipated patient response, knowledge of approximate therapeutic plasma drug concentrations (e.g., Cp50), and on Cp_p, the physician can titrate Cp_d as necessary. (From [17] with permission)

prediction of the plasma drug concentration, and on the pharmacological properties of the drug being administered. At frequent intervals (e.g., every 10–15 s), the software program compares the set point with the current prediction (feedback signal) of the plasma drug concentration, which is computed, implicitly or explicitly, by real-time simulation of a pharmacokinetic model of the drug being infused. A pump-control algorithm within the software program acts on any discrepancy between the predicted and desired concentrations to calculate a new infusion rate (control signal) to achieve or maintain the set point. The infusion rate is then transmitted electronically to the drug infusion pump (actuator), which delivers drug to the patient. The drug infusion rate is fed back into the pharmacokinetic simulation so that the next predicted plasma concentration can be computed.

The plasma is not the site of drug effect, and significant hysteresis may occur between the plasma concentration and the observed effect. Thus, the plasma concentration may not be the ideal target to provide the desired effect. The biophase (or effect compartment) may be considered the site of drug effect. Through the use of high-resolution pharmacokinetics and pharmacodynamic measurements it is possible to model the effect site concentration. Utilizing this, the pharmacokinetic parameters that incorporate the effect site can be calculated and employed in CACI devices to target the effect site concentration rather than a plasma concentration. (See chapter on Target of Control:Plasma or Effect.)

By communicating with the infusion device, the computer program can take into consideration, and help the user to be alerted to, error conditions, such as occlusion of the intravenous catheter. An adequate depth of anesthesia is dependent on the interaction of (a) drug concentration, (b) the individual's sensitivity to the drug, and (c) the surgical stimulus. It is therefore critical that the user be able to adjust the set point as frequently as he desires. CACI cannot remove drug from the blood, but it can continuously calculate the theoretical plasma concentration and predict the time required to reach a particular level after the infusion has been decreased or terminated; this may be helpful in guiding the titration as the surgical procedure nears completion.

As a result of the increasing popularity of intravenous anesthesia and continuous infusion techniques, the inherent reasonableness of pharmacokinetically based drug delivery, and the promising results achieved with CACI administration of a variety of drugs by research groups around the world, CACI is now undergoing commercial development. It is expected that CACI concepts and techniques will become increasingly prevalent and that CACI devices will become generally available in clinical practice. Standard infusion pumps, most of which already contain powerful microprocessors, will be equipped with the capability of performing pharmacokinetic model-driven infusions as a software-selectable option. Pharmacokinetic parameters for various drugs will be preprogrammed into the device to provide the model. The user will employ the pump's keypad or touch screen to select the drug to be infused and to enter some pharmacokinetically relevant information about the patient, such as weight, age, and sex, and will ensure that the infusion setup is primed with drug at a specified concentration. Then, the keypad or touch screen will be used to enter set points, in the same manner that the dial on a calibrated vaporizer is utilized in titrating the administration of an inhalation anesthetic.

Closed-Loop Automated Drug Delivery

Automatic mechanical feedback systems were first employed by James Watt in the eighteenth century for the control of steam engine speed. Electronic systems were developed in the 1930s and 1940s for control of aircraft and ships, giving birth to the subdivision of electrical engineering known as "control theory" – basically, the science of accurate indirect electronic control of a measured parameter. The basic building block of control theory is the "proportional controller", illustrated in generic terms in Fig. 3. Here a measured value of a parameter (the "output") is arithmetically subtracted from the desired value (the "set point"), producing a difference value (the "error"). This error signal is used to drive some device (the "prime mover") in such a way as to decrease the error (i.e., "negative feedback"). Thus, the system tends toward an equlibrium where the set point is equal to the output, and the error signal is zero. If the set point or output is subsequently changed, the system automatically corrects the situation. Proportional controllers are simple in concept but perform poorly where there is an appreciable delay in the response of the prime mover. Then they tend to overcorrect and oscillate. This limitation led to the development of the "Proportional-Derivative" (PD) controller, which generates an error signal based not only upon the difference between the set point and the output, but on the time rate of change of this difference as well. In principle, a PD controller will detect the condition where the error signal is rapidly approaching zero, and thus slow the corrective action of the prime mover. PD controllers perform well in mechanical servo applications, but a slight limitation exists whenever the output is biased by a constant factor such as a mechanical

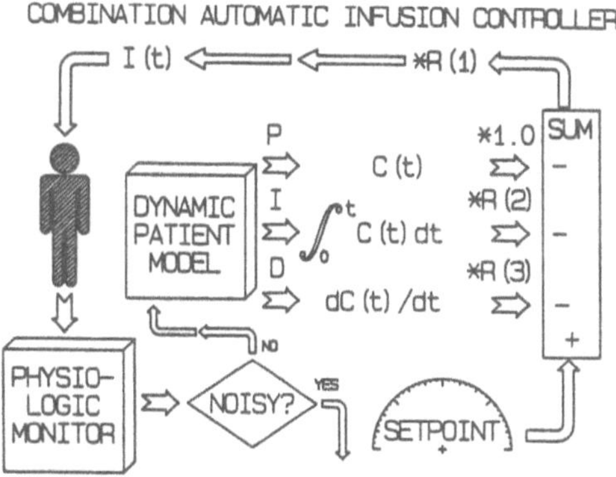

Fig. 3. PID controller incorporating an internal pharmacodynamic model and noise filter for reliable control of a physiologic variable. (From [16])

load. In this situation, the PD controller comes into equilibrium with a small constant error which exactly balances the effect of the load. Often the error is small enough to be negligable, but it can often be corrected by adding a third component consisting of the time integral of the error, forming a "Proportional-Integral-Derivative" (PID) controller. The integral component corrects for the constant error and forces the output to be exactly equal to the set point. Applied control theory in the form of the PID controller is essential to the operation of much modern electronic and mechanical equipment.

Since applied control theory works well in electronic applications, an obvious extension would be the automatic control of drug administration based upon objectively measured patient response. Closed-loop control is an example. Several formidable difficulties arise in practical situations, however, since physiologic drug response (a) is nonlinear and exhibits hysteresis, (b) varies with time, (c) varies from subject to subject, and (d) exhibits an absolute time delay which also varies with time and individual. These factors limit the performance of simple PID controllers in physiologic applications, since the differential equations resulting from a comprehensive system analysis are generally so complex as to be unsolvable, except by numerical approximation techniques. Although virtually every successful reported closed-loop drug-delivery scheme involves a PID controller, extensive empirical modifications and "tuning" are required before a practical device is developed which is capable of adequate performance of different subjects. Common empirical modifications include limitation or elimination of the integral component, variable proportional gain as the error increases, and continuous dynamic automatic optimization of parameters, so-called self-tuning or adaptive controllers. Other forms of controllers are also now being tested for complex biological systems. These types of controllers are discussed in detail in other chapters.

All closed-loop physiologic control systems incorporate several essential elements. A reliable monitor is critical for efficient and safe performance and is often the limiting component of the system. While monitoring is fairly routine for blood pressure or muscle relaxation, it can be very difficult to continuously measure, e.g., serum glucose or depth of anesthesia. The requirement to monitor possible adverse effects can likewise be a simple or complex problem, depending upon the drug. A logical filter for noise is generally required to eliminate improper operation from spurious input. Computer hardware developed impressively in the 1980s, with the advent of sophisticated, inexpensive microprocessors and memory. Presently available technology allows elegant and complex programming to be contained within an arbitrarily small package. Pumps themselves have likewise become smaller, as well as more sophisticated and reliable, and hardware itself is thus seldom a limiting factor in performance.

Systems for the automatic delivery of drugs based upon negative feedback from pharmacologic effects were developed and reported as early as 1950. A controller system administered anesthetic gases intraoperatively using blood pressure as the controlled parameter. Although forced to be large and awkward by the technology of the times, the system worked well. Other successful automatic drug administration systems were subsequently tested and described, but clinical applications were limited prior to the development of microprocessors. Thus, small and reliable devices without the numerous problems associated with analog controllers can be used.

Automatic muscle relaxant infusions using the electrically evoked response of skeletal muscle were described and tested in both animals and human beings by several authors [11–13]. Although there are sophisticated self-tuning controllers for this purpose, the most successful devices utilize fairly simple modifications of standard PID controllers. The shorter acting agents, vecuronium, atracurium, and succinylcholine, offer the best performance and the most practical applications.

The IVAC Titrator, a unit specifically designed to administer nitroprusside for blood pressure control in human beings, was the only commercially available automatic feedback drug-delivery system in the USA. Extensive clinical trials [14, 15] conclusively demonstrated outstanding and consistent performance in automatically maintaining desired blood pressure.

Almost without exception, automatic drug administration with a well-designed control algorithm and safety features outperforms, or at least equals, an average human operator accomplishing the same task.

Conclusion

Numerous intravenous anesthetic agents whose duration of action is relatively short have been released for use over the past few years. These agents lend themselves to administration via continuous infusion. Clinical studies have clearly demonstrated the advantages of continuous infusion over repeated bolus dosing. These two factors, combined with technological advances, have prompted manufacturers to produce pumps that simplify the administration of intravenous anesthetics by continuous infusion. It is concentration, rather than dose, that produces the desired effect. Utilizing pharmacokinetic principles, it is possible to provide automated drug-delivery systems that can provide, within the patient, a clinician-specified drug concentration. In addition, where there is an easily measurable effect closed-loop feedback control can be implemented to automatically control the desired parameter within a very narrow range. With this rapid development in intravenous drug delivery, it becomes imperative that clinicians familiarize themselves with these new drug-delivery devices so that they can, in the future, use these systems to optimally care for their patients.

References

1. Corssen G, Reves JG, Stanley TH (1988) Intravenous anesthesia and analgesia. Lea and Febiger, Philadelphia
2. Iliadis A, Bruno R, Cano JP (1988) Dynamical dosage regimen calculations in linear pharmacokinetics. Comp Biomed Res 21:203–220

3. Schwilden H, Stoeckel H, Schuttler J, Lauven PM (1986) Pharmacological models and their use in clinical anaesthesia. Eur J Anaesth 3:175–208
4. Wagner JG (1974) A safe method for rapidly achieving plasma concentration plateaus. Clin Pharmacol Ther 16:691–700
5. Kruger-Thiemer E (1968) Continuous intravenous infusion and multicompartment accumulation. Eur J Pharmacol 4:317–324
6. Schwilden H (1981) A general method for calculating the dosage scheme in linear pharmacokinetics. Eur J Clin Pharmacol 20:379–386
7. Schwilden H, Schuttler J, Stoekel H (1983) Pharmacokinetics as applied to total intravenous anaesthesia: theoretical considerations. Anaesthesia 38[Suppl]:51–52
8. Schuttler J, Schwilden H, Stoekel H (1983) Pharmacokinetics as applied to total intravenous anaesthesia: practical implications. Anaesthesia 38[Suppl]:53–56
9. Glass PSA, Jacobs JR, Reves JG (1990) Intravenous drug delivery systems. In: Miller RD (ed) Anesthesia, 3rd edn. Churchill Livingstone, New York
10. Crankshaw DP, Boyd MD, Bjorksten AR (1987) Plasma drug efflux – a new approach to optimization of drug infusion for constant blood concentration of thiopental and methohexital. Anesthesiology 67:32–41
11. Ritchie G, Ebert JP, Jannett TC, Kissan I, Sheppard LC (1985) A microcomputer-based controller for neuromuscular block during surgery. Ann Biomed Eng 13:3–15
12. DeVries JW, Ros HH, Booij LH (1986) Infusion of vecuronium controlled by a closed-loop system. Br J Anaesth 58:1100–1103
13. Jaklitsch RR, Westenskow DR (1987) A model-based self-adjusting two-phase controller for vecuronium-induced muscle relaxation during anesthesia. IEEE Trans Biomed Eng BME-34:583–594
14. Sheppard LC (1980) Computer control of the infusion of vasoactive drugs. Ann Biomed Eng 8:431–444
15. Cosgrove DM, Petre JH, Waller JL, Roth JV, Shepherd C, Cohn LH (1989) Automated control of postoperative hypertension: a prospective, randomized, multicenter study. Ann Thorac Surg 47:678–683
16. Jacobs JR, Glass PSA, Reves JG (1991) Automated drug delivery in anesthesia. ASA refresher course in anesthesiology, vol 19. ASA, Philadelphia
17. Jacobs JR, Glass PSA, Reves JG (1990) Opioid administration by continuous infusion. In: Estafamous FG (ed) Opioids in anesthesia, II. Butterworth, London
18. Glass PSA, Jacobs JR, Quill TJ (1991) Intravenous drug-delivery systems. In: Fragen RJ (ed) Drug infusions in anesthesiology. Raven, New York, pp 23–61

The Technical Point of View

U. Bovenkamp and H. Junker

There is no doubt that anaesthesia ventilators or infusion pumps should be safe during normal use. As every piece of technical equipment may become faulty, medical equipment may fail too, but even under a first-fault condition it should not create a danger to the patient, the operator or the environment. This means, technically, a well-defined safe state of the equipment, should it differ from normal operation (for example: stopping of an infusion pump, together with optical and acoustical alarms), but this does not mean redundancy, as is necessary for aeroplane engines.

Under such a first-fault condition, necessary or life-supporting functions must be guaranteed by the organisation of the medical treatment. For example, in case of an anaesthesia ventilator malfunction, it is sufficient if a hand-bag is available.

For "safe" equipment the following points are mandatory:

1. Under normal conditions the equipment operates as described by the manufacturer and according to generally accepted principles and standards.
2. Under a first-fault condition the equipment behaves in a clearly defined manner. This status shall be safe for the patient, even if this it valid only for a limited time. Additionally, the operator is informed of the malfunction by alarms, normally audible and visible.

In the following I will try to explain, using the example of a typical anaesthesia ventilator, how these requirements might be realised. Let us look at two safety functions: protection against excessive (positive) pressure, and protection against an unwanted increase of anaesthetic gas concentration.

It is assumed that the anaesthesia ventilator controls tidal volume and the inspiratory and expiratory timing. Depending on the patient's lung a changing lung pressure will result. By monitoring, this pressure can be compared with an independently set maximum(= safety) value, so that in case of overpressure – regardless of where it has originated – an alarm can be generated. As overpressure may damage the lung immediately, it is not sufficient to alarm the operator. The pressure monitor must also act as a protection device which stops the pressure build-up and releases the pressure. This implies that the monitor has direct access to the control system of the ventilator. Obviously, it must be guaranteed that the elements which control the flow can be switched off independently of the normal operation.

An analysis of this function (Fig. 1) shows two channels: one of them is for normal control and the other for the purpose of monitoring and protection. As both channels are independent and have their own user interface, the system is safe even under a first-fault condition.

If an anaesthesia ventilator works under pressure control the functional blocks will be equivalent, but the relations between them are slightly different. The output of the monitor now switches the flow generator from inspiration to expiration, which is now part of the normal function and not an alarm condition (Fig. 2). This means that the monitor has lost its alarm function and become a part of the normal control system – the ensurance against a first fault has been lost (concerning pressure).

Another example is that of classical anaesthesia ventilators, which use a vaporiser in line with the fresh gas. As long as the flow of the fresh gas is much higher than the patient uptake, the concentrations of volatile anaesthetics in the fresh-gas line and in the breathing circuit (circle system) are rather similar. A monitoring device looking for the inspiratory limb of the patient circuit or for the fresh-gas line may be used for surveillance of correct vaporiser function. As changes in gas concentration are not immediately critical, in contrast to pressure

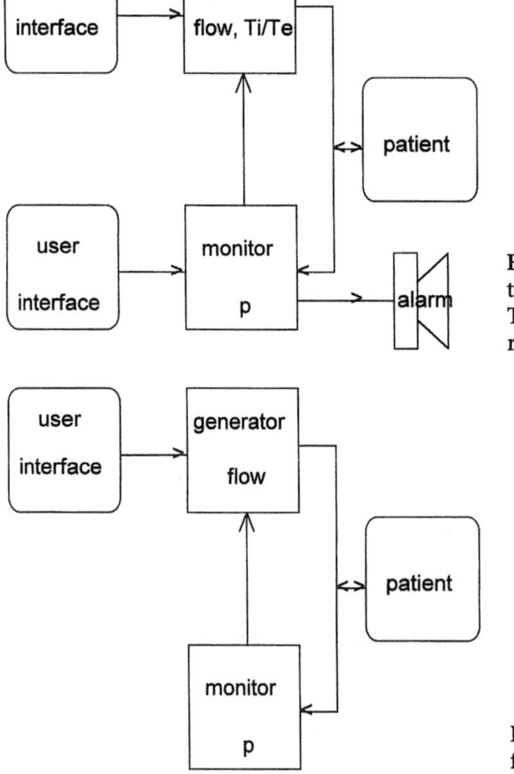

Fig. 1. Automatic systems must have two independent function channels; Ti/Te, inspiratory to exspiratory time ratio

Fig. 2. Monitoring without alarm function

V Nonmedical Aspects of Automated Control: Requirements and Liability for Automated Systems

build-up, it may be sufficient that a monitor only gives an alarm and that the operator is responsible for switching off a faulty or wrongly adjusted vaporiser.

If the same type of monitor is used for a low-flow or totally closed system, the monitor may check the vaporiser when it is in the fresh-gas line, but this concentration may be far away from that in the inspiratory branch, so that information about the patient's inspiratory gas concentration is missing. On the other hand, when the inspiratory gas is measured, the information about the correct functioning of the vaportiser is lost.

The general requirements for equipment which is safe even under first-fault conditions are shown in Fig. 3. The flow chart is valid for all types of equipment

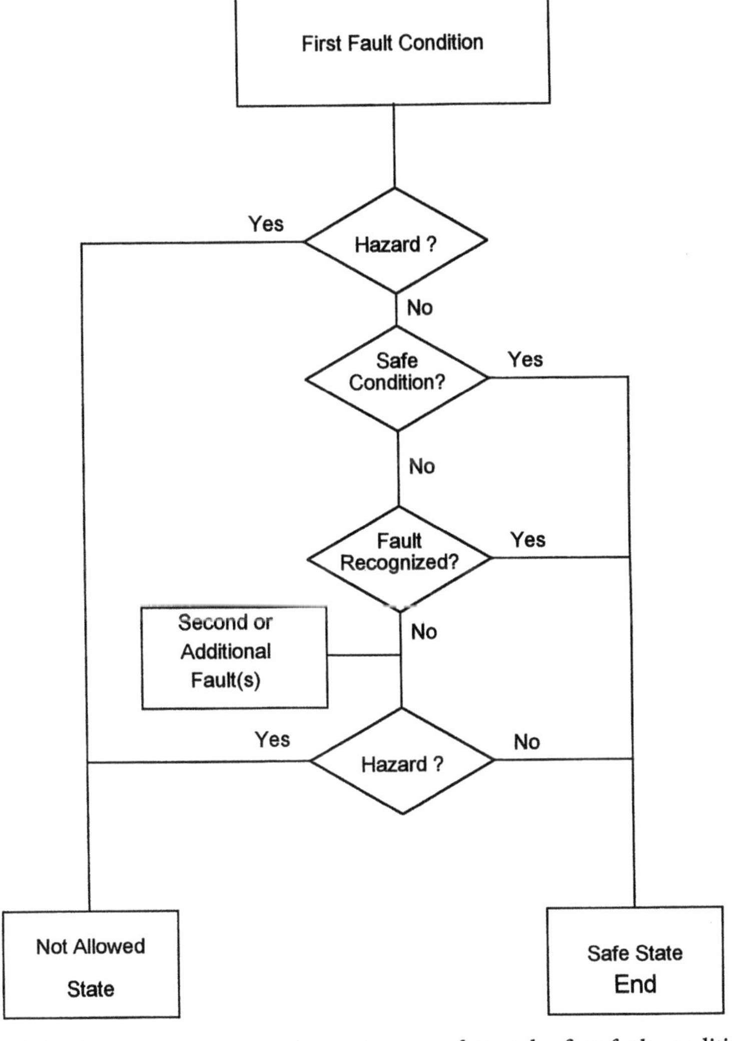

Fig. 3. General requirements for equipment safety under first-fault conditions

which should reach a safe state under first-fault conditions and where the safe state may be different from normal use.

If we look at newer developments, in which anaesthesia ventilation or intravenous drug delivery are dependent on monitoring devices, it becomes obvious that there is no longer protection against a first fault, even when the anaesthesia ventilator itself or an infusion pump is protected against a first fault. The reason is that measured values of EEG, blood pressure monitors, CO_2 monitors or others are now used instead of stable set values. As these monitors are normally not protected against internal first faults, the possible variations of control data must be limited to an acceptable range of tolerance (as one of several possibilities), or additional independent monitoring should be employed. In some cases the built-in monitoring of anaesthesia ventilators may be used for that purpose.

Normally, a monitor will not directly control a ventilator or an infusion pump; rather, a computer is used. Besides the monitors, the algorithms used must be sufficiently exact, and the computer itself must be safe under a first-fault condition. Standard PC designs do not fulfil these requirements, as everyone who uses PCs and software has experienced.

For control of ventilators, anaesthesia work stations and infusion pumps microcomputer-based control and monitoring systems are in use, which operate with more than one microcomputer. These concepts follow the first-fault philosophy and they can be considered safe. In many cases diversity of hardware and software further improves the safety.

A last point which should be addressed is Electromagnetic Compatibility (EMC). With more and more electronic components inside equipment, not only have the emissions but also the susceptibility of equipment to line voltage variations, transients, electrostatic discharges and electromagnetic fields has increased. Cases have been reported where the operation of cordless telephones has reprogrammed infusion pumps. The use of rf-surgery equipment may have similar effects. In the future, testing of noise immunity will be necessary, and not only this is addressed by the new Medical Device Directive (MDD). For every reasonably predictable hazard the MDD requires an appropiate risk reduction. This must be fulfilled by every medical device by 1998 at the latest!

Regulatory Aspects

E. Tschöpe

Present Regulations

The current situation concerning the regulation of automated systems in medicine, especially the automated control of drug delivery, is characterized by the laws and regulations applicable to this field. These are:

Drug law
Law on machine safety
Medical apparatus regulation
Calibration law
Radio protection regulation
Medical advertising law

These regulations partially cover the field of medical devices; none of them covers it totally and this is why the situation must be changed. Let me first explain some of the items of the order on the safety of medical devices:

Clarifications
General requirements
Introduction of medical devices
Type approval (test houses)
Provisions on setting up and operating
Training of the staff
Safety check
Inventory and equipment
Notification of accidents and damage

Regulations for Medical Devices (*Medizingeräteverordnung*)

The medical devices are divided into four groups. In the first two groups specified medical devices are explicitly enumerated. The anesthesia machine is, for instance, one of 25 devices belonging to group I. The definition of the groups is more than 10 years old. Thus it cannot cover all relevant points existing today. Group II includes implantable medical devices. Pacemakers, as far as they are implants, are subjected additionally to the German drug law. The third group deals with otherwise powered medical devices which are not implantable. Group IV covers all remaining medical devices.

Statute Covering Medical Products (*Medizinproduktegesetz*)

This is the situation to date. The European legislation has created two directives; directive 90/385, which is concerned with active implantable devices, and directive 93/42, applicable to all medical devices; a third directive on in vitro diagnostics is in preparation.

These three directives have to be transformed into national law, and this is the draft of the *Medizinproduktegesetz*, which may become effective in 1995. In order to help execute this law, 10–12 new orders have to be established. It is very hard to foresee at this moment in what period of time what will be elaborated in detail. For the establishment of the new orders we need the participation of the following bodies:

Federal government
Parliament
Federal council
Pressure groups

To return to the new *Medizinproduktegesetz*, what are the directives in the new law and what will be changed? The new law incorporates:

Definition of general safety requirements
The importance of standards
   It is assumed that the safety requirements are fulfilled if harmonized standards
   are applied.
Delegation of control functions from the national authorities to notified bodies
   The notified bodies may or may not be governmental. In Germany the notified
   bodies will be for example the test houses, for instance, TÜV or Dekra.

The general safety requirements establish protection against:

Lack of sterility
Adverse effects
Misuse caused by misleading information
   If, for instance, you have a good product which is sold in the USA, but only with
   information in German, it may be an unsafe product.
Damage caused by mechanical failure
Injury caused by mechanical failure
   The interface between medical devices and human beings is a critical one.
   Some years ago there was a publication by the paediatric clinic of the University
   of Bonn about the death of two newborns. The incubator had been connected
   to the oxygen supply by a certain tubing system which delivered the softener
   of the PVC, which may have caused the deaths. Another example is polyure-

thane as an insulator in pacemakers, which may degrade under the influence of body fluids.
Failure of energy supply
Other electrical risks
Hazards caused by deterioration due to aging
This is of relevance for orthopaedic implants.

Standardization

Standardization has got a new quality in regulation. We are aiming at the adoption of harmonized standards by the CEN on the basis, whenever possible, of international standards. Two types of standards, horizontal and vertical, are differentiated. Horizontal standards apply to all medical devices, vertical standards apply only to specific types of medical devices. The horizontal standards established include for example:

Quality assurance systems EN 29000
Sterile packaging
Labelling and symbols
Biocompatibility
Electromagnetic compatibility
Guides for clinical investigation

As an example, one may consider the standards for clinical investigations of medical devices as elaborated by the technical committee CEN TC258. For a properly designed clinical study, there must be a clinical investigation plan, and the functions of the clinical investigator, the promoter and the mentors are defined. The clinical performance of the medical device is defined and the ethics committee must give a positive vote before the clinical study commences. In addition, there are provisions regarding how to conduct multicenter clinical studies, and finally, at the end of the clinical trial, there must be a report about the clinical study, signed by the clinical investigator and the company sponsoring it.

Risk Assessment

Special attention is given in the new law to risk assessment, which is one of the tasks the federal health office will have to deal with. The law requires that the manufacturer evaluate information about incidents and notify the authorities. A member state has to ensure that information is available to the authorities in all other member states, if there is:

Deterioration of performance
Deterioration of characteristics
Inaccuracy in labouring
Any technical recall which might lead to death or to serious harm of a person

The threshold for notification and monitoring is much higher for medical devices than for the drug field, where even minor accidents have to be reported. The role of the national authorities is to control the application and to assess the risks as mentioned above. In addition, they have the final decision about classification, they have to register the persons responsible for placing medical devices on the market, and they have to supervise clinical investigations, and to notify other appropriate officials.

In summary, our office in Berlin is not responsible for marketing or for the central register; our main purpose is the evaluation of risk and information control within Germany and to head an expert committee.

Remaining Problems

The present *Medizinproduktegesetz* will not solve all problems, however. There will be three different bodies to manage and coordinate medical devices. Access to the market and a CE mark is controlled by the above-mentioned notified bodies, risk assessment is done by the BFArM (formerly BGA), and the collection of data is performed by the DIMDI. Another problem is that the CE mark is valid throughout Europe, which leads to difficulties with respect to labeling, product information, and translation. Last but not least, the manufacturer of the medical device is the only institution responsible for the product and its performance. This is much different from the situation in the field of drugs, where a mutual consensus must be reached by the manufacturer and the authority granting a license.

The Manufacturer's Point of View

B. Hermanrud

Goals and Questions

Automatic control systems are more complex than manual systems. Methods for automating anesthesia systems raise two sets of questions for the manufacturer. First, what is the cost of the introduced complexity? Second, what are the goals of automated control? The cost of complexity is not only a manufacturing cost but primarily a development cost. The goals of automated control are ultimately lower cost through increased quality of care and the use of new modalities. The cost of complexity must therefore be weighed against possible gains, and the manufacturer asks what complexity the hospitals can afford.

The cost of automated control systems in anesthesia is determined by the requirements and the validation and verification. Also, the legal and ethical implications are, to a large extent, determined by the definition and the testing of a product. Measured outcome of care will determine the appropriateness of technology used. Who bears the responsibility when automated control systems go wrong? This will be clarified by the method that is proposed below.

Performance

An automatic control system shows good performance when its behavior is completely predictable and intuitively understandable. This reflects, to a large extent, the manufacturer's point of view. The clinical user has the additional requirement that the equipment function well from a medical point of view in all clinical settings. It is, however, clear that whatever the level of improvement of the clinical performance, there will always be situations when the equipment performance is unacceptable. It might be with certain patients, due to improper initial settings, malfunction, or inadequate algorithms. These areas of unacceptable performance are artifacts in the system's behavior. It is important that these artifacts be detected and that the user be alerted to the situation. The only alternative to a well-performing system is human interaction. An "artifact detector" must therefore give a message to the user that "the machinery cannot process" (Fig. 1). This is also the standard start-up condition, when human interaction is always needed.

When an automatic control system does not perform well and, further, the artifact detector does not detect unacceptable performance, alerting the user to the

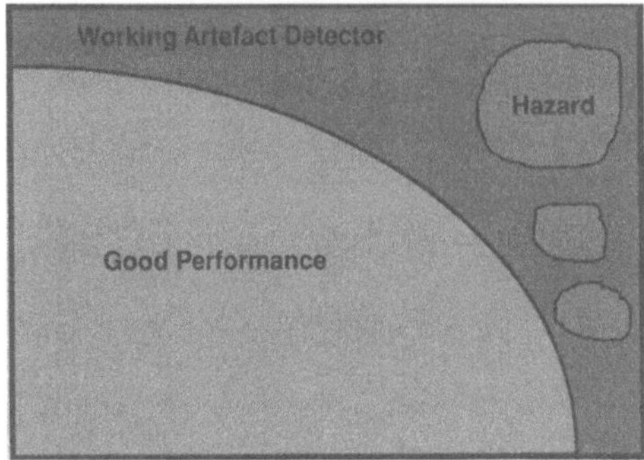

Fig. 1. Automatic systems with problems must have a working artifact detector

condition, a hazardous condition has developed. Hazardous conditions therefore exist when the system is not functioning properly, has not been able to detect the condition, and has therefore left both the user and the system unaware of the situation. The understanding and rigorous management of hazards in automatic systems is the key to the development and safe manufacturing of such control systems in anesthesia.

Human Interface

Human interaction with automatic control systems falls into three categories. First, the start-up conditions will be initiated by the human operator. Second, a phase of monitoring the status of the equipment and the patient occurs. With complex systems the necessary "cockpit" can become quite intimidating for the user. The third phase of human interaction is the "cannot process" information from the artifact detector. All three aspects of human interface must be clearly understood by both the operator and the manufacturer. The area that is poorly covered will very likely constitute the hazardous condition. The elimination of these hazards is the responsibility of the manufacturer.

Method

A medical product life cycle is inherently an iterative process. Six different steps in this process are isolated but might overlap with each other time-wise:

1. Requirements
2. Design
3. Implementation
4. Test
5. Installation and checkout
6. Operation and maintenance

A common way to describe a product life cycle is to view the different steps as parts of a waterfall. From the requirements, information flows into the design, from the design it flows into the implementation, and so on. If something goes wrong in the test, a change in the design might be necessary or even in the requirements.

A similar iterative process is necessary for the hazard analysis of the product. Each step in the product life cycle needs a mirror step in a "hazard analysis waterfall". Since the hazard analysis tries to uncover areas of unacceptable performance, it tends to be more iterative than the product life cycle process. In the manufacturing and development of an automatic anesthesia control system, the quality of each step in the hazard analysis waterfall determines the quality of the system itself.

Different methods of identifying and quantifying hazards are provided by different agencies. The MIL-1629A method divides patient hazards into categories 1–4, from catastrophic to minor. *Technischer Überwachungsverein* (TÜV) hazard analysis has been adopted by many medical-device manufacturers. The TÜV microprocessor safety requirement proposes both software diversification and the use of redundant hardware. Software diversification suggests the use of different algorithms, different program structures, different data access, different programming languages, and different compilers. The level of diversity is decided by analyzing what category of patient hazard might occur as seen in the hazard analysis waterfall.

A separate design tool for uncovering patient hazards, in the different steps, is the fault tree analysis. It provides an easy-to-understand overview of the safety architecture, and it can be applied late in the process in order to identify areas of required maintenance. An added advantage of medical fault tree analysis is the potential use of fuzzy logic. By estimating the failure rate for the different components in the system, the total criticality of the patient hazard can be assessed. It also helps in finding holes in the requirements and the need for simplification of the user interface. The sheer complexity of using an automatic system during critical conditions might render the device unsafe. Sometimes automatic systems are developed by experts who have an excellent understanding of the system's behavior during good performance but fail to analyze the hazards during artifacts or start-up conditions.

A Proposal

With the development and manufacturing of automatic systems in anesthesia, a new level of understanding between user and manufacturer is needed. When the user allows the machine to take over control and delivery of anesthetic agents and to adjust its own delivery according to measured parameters, the safety of the system is of prime importance. The clear understanding of the inherent hazards might decide if available technology should be used in a new product or not. The user of an automatic system in anesthesia should therefore demand all hazard analysis of the system to be made public. The advantage of this proposal is obvious. It makes it possible to choose the appropriate care technology with a better understanding of the potential outcome of care. It is the only reasonable way to assess the quality of a system before purchase. It forces the manufacturers to take on their part of the responsibility and to state where it ends.

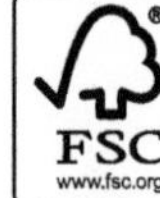

MIX
Papier aus verantwortungsvollen Quellen
Paper from responsible sources
FSC® C105338

If you have any concerns about our products,
you can contact us on
ProductSafety@springernature.com

In case Publisher is established outside the EU,
the EU authorized representative is:
**Springer Nature Customer Service Center GmbH
Europaplatz 3, 69115 Heidelberg, Germany**

Printed by Libri Plureos GmbH
in Hamburg, Germany